NEUROSCIENCE RESEARCH PR

AF682574

ADVANCES IN VISUAL PERCEPTION RESEARCH

NEUROSCIENCE RESEARCH PROGRESS

Additional books in this series can be found on Nova's website under the Series tab.

Additional e-books in this series can be found on Nova's website under the e-book tab.

NEUROSCIENCE RESEARCH PROGRESS

ADVANCES IN VISUAL PERCEPTION RESEARCH

THOMAS HEINEN
EDITOR

NOVA BIOMEDICAL

New York

Copyright © 2015 by Nova Science Publishers, Inc.

All rights reserved. No part of this book may be reproduced, stored in a retrieval system or transmitted in any form or by any means: electronic, electrostatic, magnetic, tape, mechanical photocopying, recording or otherwise without the written permission of the Publisher.

We have partnered with Copyright Clearance Center to make it easy for you to obtain permissions to reuse content from this publication. Simply navigate to this publication's page on Nova's website and locate the "Get Permission" button below the title description. This button is linked directly to the title's permission page on copyright.com. Alternatively, you can visit copyright.com and search by title, ISBN, or ISSN.

For further questions about using the service on copyright.com, please contact:
Copyright Clearance Center
Phone: +1-(978) 750-8400 Fax: +1-(978) 750-4470 E-mail: info@copyright.com.

NOTICE TO THE READER

The Publisher has taken reasonable care in the preparation of this book, but makes no expressed or implied warranty of any kind and assumes no responsibility for any errors or omissions. No liability is assumed for incidental or consequential damages in connection with or arising out of information contained in this book. The Publisher shall not be liable for any special, consequential, or exemplary damages resulting, in whole or in part, from the readers' use of, or reliance upon, this material. Any parts of this book based on government reports are so indicated and copyright is claimed for those parts to the extent applicable to compilations of such works.

Independent verification should be sought for any data, advice or recommendations contained in this book. In addition, no responsibility is assumed by the publisher for any injury and/or damage to persons or property arising from any methods, products, instructions, ideas or otherwise contained in this publication.

This publication is designed to provide accurate and authoritative information with regard to the subject matter covered herein. It is sold with the clear understanding that the Publisher is not engaged in rendering legal or any other professional services. If legal or any other expert assistance is required, the services of a competent person should be sought. FROM A DECLARATION OF PARTICIPANTS JOINTLY ADOPTED BY A COMMITTEE OF THE AMERICAN BAR ASSOCIATION AND A COMMITTEE OF PUBLISHERS.

Additional color graphics may be available in the e-book version of this book.

Library of Congress Cataloging-in-Publication Data

ISBN: 978-1-63482-455-2
Library of Congress Control Number: 2015934870

Published by Nova Science Publishers, Inc. † New York

Contents

Preface

The book "Advances in Visual Perception Research" provides a state-of-the-art discussion forum for topics that are of high interest in the field of visual perception research. Experts from different countries and different scientific disciplines, such as medicine, psychology, neuroscience, sport and movement science, provide a number of significant contributions covering recent theoretical developments, innovative methodical developments, current research evidence, as well as implications for practical applications in visual perception.

Ryan Hacklaender, David Eckert and Christina Bermeitinger (University of Hildesheim, Germany, and University of Louisville, Kentucky) focus on the visual processing of things that may be of particular importance. The authors utilize the response-priming paradigm while addressing the processing of motion stimuli. In a subsequent step, the authors consider the visual processing of threatening stimuli. Taken their theoretical and empirical evidence together, it can be argued that stimuli of higher importance (in terms of domain-specific and domain-general mechanisms), receive a preferential processing in the visual system.

William J. Brady and Emily Balcetis (New York University, USA) focus on the perception of facial expressions of emotions. The authors argue that peoples' ability to perceive or read the emotional expressions of other people may predict affective reactions to conflictive situations. The authors present empirical evidence on the impact of emotion perception accuracy on peoples' affective reactions. It is argued that variation in negative affect experienced during conflict can be predicted from the visual experiences people have when looking at others.

Ralf Kredel, André Klostermann and Ernst-Joachim Hossner (University of Bern, Switzerland, Germany) introduce an innovative automated vector-based system for analyzing gaze behavior in humans performing rather complex motor skills. A lot of currently available commercial systems suffer from technical and methodological limitations and thus experimentally gathered data needs to be interpreted with caution. The described system is strongly appealing for researchers (and potentially also practitioners) who are interested in assessing gaze behavior together with movement behavior in basic or applied scenarios.

Christoph von Laßberg, Karl A. Beykirch and Jennifer L. Campos (University of Leipzig and University of Tübingen, Germany, AMST Ranshofen, Austria, and University of Toronto, Canada) provide empirical evidence on the relationship between individual vestibulo-ocular eye movement characteristics and spatial orientation aptitudes in expert gymnasts. It is argued, that expert gymnasts who are trained in fast and complex rotational movements have a highly developed, yet individual capability of efficiently orienting in multiaxial movement. However, it is not clear which role the individual level of VOR precision plays therein. The authors utilize an innovative methodological approach for the examination to what extend the individual level of VOR correlates with individual aptitude to cope with multiaxial spatial orientation demands.

Niels Galley, Dirk Betz and Claudia Biniossek (University of Cologne, Cologne, Germany and GESIS Leibniz Institute for the Social Sciences, Cologne, Germany) adress the question why are fixation durations so highly variable? Fixation durations in (everyday) activities can vary between several milliseconds and several seconds. However, the reasons for this large variation have yet to be clarified. The authors present extensive research evidence from more than 1000 subjects, leading to the conclusion that fixation may be a process in time that can be classified into very short fixations, express fixations, cognitive fixations, and very long fixations, whereas each fixation type could potentially serve different behavioral goals.

Kristian Folta-Schoofs, Carina Hilke, Hans-Jörg Bethge and Dieter Felbel (University of Hildesheim, Germany, and AMEOS Clinic, Hildesheim, Germany) refer to the important area of attention deficit hyperactivity disorder and address ADHD-dependent modulations in time perception and distractibility, as well as changes in the velocity profile of saccadic eye movements. Results revealed comparable time reproduction for all examined groups and conditions. The authors could furthermore show, that peak velocity for voluntarily executed saccades varied as a function of children's medication, indicating a pharmacologically effect on brainstem excitation, and thus on saccadic behavior.

Dennis M. Schaffer, Andrew B. Maynor, Benjamin K. Madden, April L. Utt and Ciara N. Adamrovich (The Ohio State University, Mansfield) focus on people's mental representation of thrown objects. The authors highlight, that people tend to mentally represent thrown objects to rise and fall in a parabolic motion. A series of experiments addresses different factors in people's perception of thrown objects. The authors conclude that despite people mentally represent balls thrown away from them to ascend and descend without awareness of how different their perspective view is from physical reality, such regularities may be important for maintaining stability of the visual world.

Sérgio Tosi Rodrigues, Gisele Cristina Bertoloni, Renato Moraes, Ana Maria Forti Barela, Geert Savelsbergh and José Angelo Barela (State University of São Paulo, Bauru, Brazil, University of São Paulo, Ribeirão Preto, Brazil, Cruzeiro do Sul University, São Paulo, Brazil, Research Institute Move VU University, Amsterdam, The Netherlands, and State University of São Paulo, Rio Claro, Brazil) focus on the influence of optical flow information in combination with one's own movement in posture stabilization and grasping. The authors utilize the moving room paradigm in assessing participants grasping behavior under different conditions. The authors found that grasping and movement of the moving room influenced body sway. It can be concluded that postural control may utilize optical flow information in order to maintain body stability.

Laura Pérez Zapata, J. Antonio Aznar-Casanova, Manuel Moreno, Matthias Keil and Hans Supèr (University of Barcelona, Spain, Institute for Brain, Cognition and Behaviour and Catalan Institution for Research and Advanced Studies) examined peoples' precision in matching oriented lines in a 3D environment. The authors conducted a series of experiments adressing the influence of factors such as perspetive or viewing frame on a line matching task. The authors found that task performance could be modulated by viewing perspective as well as the structure of the surronding. The authors argue that the brain may use several spatial transformations related to a given viewing perspective.

Damian Jeraj, Linda Hennig and Thomas Heinen (German Sport University Cologne, Germany and University of Hildesheim, Germany) discuss influencing factors related to the error correction process in sport. The authors argue that in particular visual perspective, visual experience, motor experience, coach-athlete relationship, methodical knowledge and biomechanical knowledge are likely to influence the observation, perception, and detection of movement errors in complex skills.

Andrew Evered, Darren Walker, Andrew Watt and Nick Perham (Cardiff Metropolitan University, Wales, UK) focus on visual perceptual learning in cytopathology. The authors argue that little is known about how the perceptual abilities of cytologists develop. However, a particular set of visual skills may be highly beneficial for cytologists. The authors describe a series of experiments adressing the role of perceptual training in diagnostic behavior. Given the results of their studies, the authors conclude that in particular non-analytical learning strategies should be subjected to further experimental exploration since that could be an innovative technique supporting the acquisition of diagnostic expertise in cytology.

Hirofumi Ida (Jobu University, Japan) reviews the literature on human visuomotor behavior for which computer-simulated displays were used as a tool in the presentation of experimental stimuli. The author refers to studies focusing on topics such as postural control, interceptive action, and biological motion perception. Since stereoscopic presentation techniques are more and more developing, computer-generated stimuli could potentially be an alternative to traditional approaches. It is concluded that researchers should try to recognize the advantages and disadvantages of computer-simulated displays for their own research.

Konstantinos Velentzas, Christoph Schütz and Thomas Schack (University of Bielefeld, Germany) discuss empirical evidence on the effects of using augmented feedback devices in motor learning. The authors conduct an experiment addressing the use of two different head-mounted displays in learning a novel throwing task. Results revealed that both conditions might be beneficial in motor learning as compared to situations without additional feedback. Ideas for further experiments are discussed and practical implications are given.

Luc Tremblay and John de Grosbois (University of Toronto, Canada) address the question why limb and body displacements are encoded in the velocity domain? Since different sensory modalities provide information in different domains the question arises how the sensory-motor system deals with these differences? The authors provide compelling neurophysiological and behavioral evidence for the use of visual and vestibular information in the velocity domain. It is thus argued that the central nervous system converts sensory cues into the velocity domain in order to serve in the execution of perceptual and sensorimotor activities.

Jan M. Hondzinski and Chelsea M. Soebbing (Louisiana State University, Louisiana, United States of America) emphasize the role of visual inputs for the execution of goal-directed movements. The authors argue that performance of precise daily activities relies on the integration of information from different sensory and motor systems, and access to visual inputs strongly influences this precision. This is especially the case when performing pointing movements to targets in the dark as compared to an illuminated environment. The authors discuss recent empirical evidence on differences in reaching to targets between a dark and an illuminated environment as a function of body orientation.

Given the wide range of topics and scientific disciplines, the book "Advances in Visual Perception Research" may be an important source of information for graduate students, researchers and practitioners that study and work in the field of visual perception.

Thomas Heinen
Hildesheim, Germany, January 2015

About the Editor

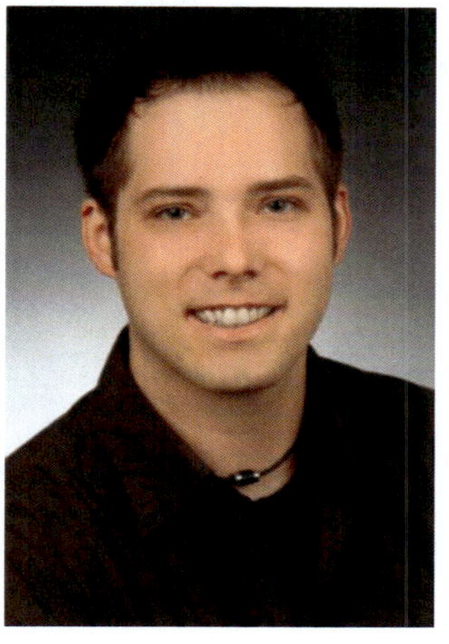

Prof. Dr. Thomas Heinen

Thomas Heinen studied Sport Science at the German Sport University Cologne (Germany) and received his PhD from the German Sport University Cologne in 2006. He currently works as a Professor for Social Science of Sport at the University of Hildesheim. His primary research interests are related to the role of perception and cognition in the selection, control and acquisition of complex skills.

Affiliation Information
Prof. Dr. Thomas Heinen
University of Hildesheim
Institute of Sport Science
Universitaetsplatz 1
31141 Hildesheim
Germany
Email: thomas.heinen@uni-hildesheim.de
Phone: +49 (0) 5121 / 883 - 11914

In: Advances in Visual Perception Research
Editor: Thomas Heinen

ISBN: 978-1-63482-455-2
© 2015 Nova Science Publishers, Inc.

Chapter 1

Visual Processing: The Role of Importance

Ryan Hacklaender[1,2], David Eckert[1] and Christina Bermeitinger[1*]
[1]University of Hildesheim, German
[2]University of Louisville, US

Abstract

In the chapter we focus on the visual processing of "important" things. We understand "importance" in a broad sense and we assume that important things are processed faster or even with specific processing mechanisms. We give a short introduction in terms of an evolutionary perspective. Thereafter, we present in detail two examples of important stimuli. First we focus on motion stimuli. Here, we present an overview of research and results regarding motion processing. Then, we introduce the response priming paradigm as a well suited tool for studying the close relation between perception and action. We describe an experiment using the response priming paradigm and motion stimuli.

Additionally, we mention the distinction of biological and nonbiological motions. Second we consider threatening stimuli. Here we start with the introduction of the so-called Innate Threat Superiority hypothesis. We then summarize evidence supporting and contradicting this hypothesis. After focusing on "importance", we make some concluding remarks on the threat part. At the end of the chapter we provide a short summary and an outlook on future directions.

Keywords: vision; relevance; threat stimuli; motion perception; movement

* University of Hildesheim, Institute of Psychology, Universitätsplatz 1, 31141 Hildesheim, Germany. Email: bermeitinger@uni-hildesheim.de

Introduction

"It has long been an axiom of mine
that the little things are infinitely the most important."
— Arthur Conan Doyle, *The Memoirs of Sherlock Holmes*

As a general introductory claim we will understand "importance" in the broad sense that those things are important to an organism which have the potential to either frustrate or facilitate goal achievement. Important stimuli should be preferentially processed in order to ensure quick and optimal reacting in view of chances or threats regarding goals. According to Darwin (1859), one of the hierarchically highest goals of all organisms, including humans, is to survive. Thus, it seems plausible that organisms are tuned to detect and react to (possibly even with specific processing mechanisms) important things faster than less important things. We will expand upon these general points in the section on an evolutionary perspective of importance. Thereafter, we will present in detail two different types of important (visual) stimuli, i.e., motion and threat stimuli. We close with an outlook including some ideas for future research.

Importance: An Evolutionary Perspective

Evolution has endowed humans with highly developed visual abilities, including visual sensation, perception, and attention (Isbell, 2009). This allows us to deal with a wide range of stimuli present in a visual scene. However, not all stimuli are equal and, due to our limited capacity to react to and/or affect our environment at any given moment, treating them as such could be dangerous or lead to lost opportunities. Therefore, one of the greatest challenges for the cognitive system is to decide which stimuli are worth the most rapid attention and the greatest amount of attention. Through the development of domain-specific and domain-general mechanisms natural selection has provided humans with efficient methods of deciding which stimuli are important and therefore should receive preferential processing.

Domain-specific mechanisms are systems, or modules, in the brain that react to a specific set of information (Chiappe & MacDonald, 2005). This information has been recurrently important and highly stable throughout evolutionary history. Due to the relatively small range of information dealt with by a particular module, activation of that module leads directly and rapidly to a specific set of behaviors. As applied to the system of visual perception, the presence of specific modules would allow for the rapid perception of and attention to patterns of visual sensation that have been consistently important to the survival of humans and our ancestors.

Domain-general mechanisms, on the other hand, are systems in the brain that respond to a large set of information. Domain-general mechanisms can deal with all types of information, including information that has been consistently important over evolutionary time-scales, information that has been important within the lifetime of the individual, and completely novel information (Chiappe & MacDonald, 2005). As domain-general mechanisms respond to a wide variety of information, they also allow for a wide variety of behavioral outcomes. The cost of the increase in response options is that responses are slower than they would be for domain-specific mechanisms, because a decision must be made about which course of action is the most appropriate to take. As applied to the visual perception system, a domain-general mechanism would mean that all information is processed by one system, which determines the importance of the information based solely on learning.

In combination, the visual system uses specific modules and domain general processes to determine which stimuli in a visual scene are most important and therefore should receive preferential processing. Motion perception and attention to threatening stimuli are two areas that seem to clearly show this blend. In the following part, we will present an overview and data on the processing of motion stimuli as the first example for the processing of important stimuli.

Perceiving Motion

Moving or changing things are especially significant indicators that something important is happening. Thus, moving things are able to capture attention and to guide attention and gaze towards the direction in which the movement is made. Perception and discrimination of different kinds of motion represents an essential ability already present in newborns (e.g., Farroni, Massaccesi, Pividori, & Johnson, 2004; Simion, Regolin, & Bulf, 2008; Wickelgren, 1969). When attending to moving things and their goals the observer can get a fast impression of the present situation and can adapt current actions, ensuring appropriate behavior in the given situation. Because movements can be of very high speed, high speeded perceptual and attentional processes are necessary.

The perception of motion is a unique phenomenon and has spurred a quickly developing field of research, especially since the Gestalt-theory (Wertheimer, 1912) and its fundamental thoughts on motion perception. How is it possible for us to perceive motion, and what kinds of mechanisms are responsible for such a feat? What processes and mechanisms give us the ability to quickly react to fast movements, such as catching a ball thrown towards us or the fight-and flight response to a predator approaching? How can the perception of others' movements help us in social interactions? These and other questions are the focus of current research.

There is a considerably large amount of research on processing motion (for a review see Raymond, 2000) coming from single unit recording studies with monkeys and cats (e.g., Albrecht & Geisler, 1991; Treue & Maunsell, 1996), event related potential studies and fMRI studies with humans (e.g., O'Craven, Rosen, Kwong, Triesman, & Savoy, 1997), and studies with lesion patients (e.g., Newsome & Paré, 1988). Additionally, there are some studies with specially designed motion paradigms to investigate influences of attention on motion perception (e.g., Cavanagh, 1992) or specific perceptual phenomena regarding motion perception (e.g., Ramachandran & Anstis, 1983).

In contemporary approaches, perception and action are seen as inseparably connected. In embodied views, for example, there is the general claim that 'perception is for action', or in other words, that the fundamental function of perception is to allow for action (e.g., Chemero, 2006; Gibson, 1979; Warren, 2006). Further, perceived motion is closely related to own actions. First, there is converging evidence that perception of action and performance of action is coded in a common representational code (i.e., *Theory of Event Coding*, Hommel,

Müsseler, Aschersleben & Prinz, 2001) also supposing the same neural basis for action observation and production (e.g., Calvo-Merino, Glaser, Grézes, Passingham, & Haggard, 2005; Decety & Grèzes, 1999; di Pellegrino, Fadiga, Fogassi, Gallese, & Rizzolatti, 1992; Grèzes & Decety, 2001). Second, perception of motion often triggers an own action (e.g., Saygin, Wilson, Hagler, Bates, & Sereno, 2004).

In cognitive psychology there is one tool which seems especially appropriate for the investigation of perceptuomotor processes and thus to study the link between motion perception and motor activations – the response priming paradigm. Given the general view of a close relation between perception and action, it seems noteworthy that this tool is used rather seldom to study perceptuomotor processes with motion stimuli. In the following section we will describe this paradigm in detail.

Response Priming Paradigm

Response priming refers to the finding that a preceding prime stimulus influences the response to a following target stimulus. The typical task in response priming is the classification of basic features like direction or shape of the target stimulus (for a methodological overview on response priming see Schmidt, Haberkamp, & Schmidt, 2011). Response priming was largely investigated using shape and color stimuli (e.g., Eimer & Schlaghecken, 2002). If the influence of the prime – on which no response should be given – on the target can be shown, a priming effect occurred. Generally in response priming experiments, the prime and target stimuli signal either the same response tendencies (e.g., both times pressing the right key; i.e. compatible trials) or different tendencies (i.e. incompatible trials). Comparing compatible and incompatible trials, compatible trials typically lead to faster reactions and fewer errors than incompatible trials. Priming effects are typically calculated as the difference between incompatible and compatible trials, thus, faster reactions in compatible than incompatible trials represent a positive priming effect. However, the prime's influence can be reversed in some cases (i.e., faster reactions in incompatible than compatible trials = a negative priming effect). Research has shown that temporal parameters, namely the SOA (stimulus onset asynchrony; delay between prime and target stimulus onset) play a crucial role in determining both the size and the sign of the priming effect (e.g. Aaron et al., 2003; Bermeitinger, 2013; Eimer, 1999; Eimer & Schlaghecken, 1998, 2002, 2003; Jaśkowski, Bialunska, Tomanek, & Verleger, 2008; Klauer & Dittrich, 2010; Lleras & Enns, 2005).

Response priming effects can be observed even when observers do not consciously perceive the prime or the response predicting prime features (e.g., Fehrer & Raab, 1962; Klotz & Neumann, 1999; Mattler, 2006; Neumann & Klotz, 1994; Schmidt, 2000, 2002; Vorberg, Mattler, Heinecke, Schmidt, & Schwarzbach, 2003, 2004). Here, the response priming effect crucially depends on perceptual features of the mask and the timing of prime, mask, target presentation, and response execution (e.g., Lingnau & Vorberg, 2005; Praamstra & Seiss, 2005; Schlaghecken & Eimer, 2002; for review see e.g., Sumner, 2007). For example, the direction of the priming effect is mainly influenced by the SOA between prime and target, especially when using subliminal prime presentations. Often with short SOAs (below 200 ms), responses to compatible targets are faster than to incompatible targets (i.e., positive priming effect). With longer SOAs a reversed effect, with faster reaction times (RTs) to incompatible than to compatible targets, was observed (i.e., negative priming effect, inverse priming effect, or negative compatibility effect; e.g., Eimer & Schlaghecken, 2002). There is continuous debate on whether this pattern of effects is a result of motor or perceptual mechanisms (e.g., Jaśkowski et al., 2008; Jaśkowski & Verleger, 2007; Klapp & Hinkley, 2002; Mattler, 2005, 2007; Schlaghecken, Klapp, & Maylor, 2009; Sumner, 2007; Verleger, Jaśkowski, Aydemir, van der Lubbe, & Groen, 2004).

In summary, the response priming paradigm is a strong and well suited tool to investigate visual motor control, visual attention, and connections between visual awareness and motor activation.

Advantages of the Response Priming Paradigm

Why could it be beneficial to use the response priming paradigm when studying motion perception, especially compared to experiments in which participants must react directly to moving things? First, response priming as a priming paradigm represents an *implicit* measure – participants do not have to provide an explicit statement on the object being studied. In the case of response priming with motion primes this is the direction of the motion, the kind of motion, visual processing of motion, or activation/inhibition processes elicited by motion. Implicit measures are thought to capture attitudes, traits, habits, processing mechanisms, or the structure of memory in an automatic manner (see De Houwer & Moors, 2007). The core feature of implicit measures is that "the measurement outcome is causally produced by the to-be-measured attribute in the absence of certain goals, awareness, substantial cognitive resources, or substantial time" (De Houwer, Teige-Mocigemba, Spruyt, & Moors, 2009, p. 350). Second, participants have explicit knowledge of neither the (perceived) motion nor of verbal representations of the targets, as long as they can execute a simple discriminative task on the target. This point could be very important in subjects with specific deficits or brain lesions as well as in very young or very old subjects. Third, pre-activations and inhibition processes can be studied without brain imaging methods. That is, on the one hand we can measure early (motor) activations which are triggered by the presentation of the prime but which do not become overt responses. Instead, they influence the following answer and here, we can make those pre-activations visible in terms of slightly relatively faster responses.

On the other hand, inhibition processes can be made visible by relatively slower responses. Fourth, in response priming it is possible to compare compatible as well as incompatible trials with a neutral baseline (i.e., the prime does not imply information on one response). Thus, if someone has respective research questions, it is possible to distinguish effects of facilitation or inhibition. This might also be interesting when thinking about possible applications of the paradigm in clinical studies, for example regarding psychic disorders which are related to more or less specific inhibition problems (e.g., schizophrenia, depression etc.) or in developmental studies, specifically as age is sometimes also related to inhibitory deficits (e.g., Schlaghecken & Maylor, 2005; Lustig, Hasher, & Zacks, 2007).

Response Priming Using Motion Stimuli

Until now there have been just a few response priming experiments in which moving stimuli were used. In the tradition of response priming, Mattler and Fendrich (2007) investigated the influence of moving dots (however, motion was too rapid to be consciously seen) on the response to a subsequently presented second display, also containing moving dots. They presented a prime consisting of a briefly flashed circle of 16 dots that rotated so rapidly that participants were not able to report their direction. This prime was followed by a second circle of 16 dots with a clearly visible clockwise or counterclockwise apparent rotation. Participants' task was to indicate the direction of the target rotation. The result again depended on the prime-target SOA. However, in contrast to the above reported pattern of results, there were inverse effects with short SOAs: with a short SOA (i.e., 38 ms between the beginning of the prime motion and the beginning of the target motion) compatible targets were classified slower than incompatible targets. SOAs from 88 to 238 ms led to positive priming effects, with faster reactions on compatible than incompatible targets. Interestingly, until now there have only been a few experiments using *clearly visible* apparent motions as primes, although most of the motions outside of the experimental context are apparent motions, not subliminal ones. For instance, Sarkheil, Vuong, Bülthoff, and Noppeney (2008) used 3D forms as primes and targets. Prime forms were rotated for 350 ms. Thereafter a blank display was presented for 100 ms (thus, the SOA was 450 ms). Then a rotating form was presented as the target. Primes and targets could be compatible or incompatible regarding form identity and rotation direction (clockwise/counterclockwise). Participants' task was either to classify the form or the motion direction of the target. There was no motion priming effect in RTs and overall in brain activity within selected regions of interest. However, participants made more errors on incompatible than compatible motion priming trials. Recently, Bermeitinger (2013) tested priming effects with moving prime stimuli on static arrow targets. In several experiments, participants responded to the direction of a left or right arrow. Before each arrow, participants saw a row of 11 dots at the center of the screen. These dots were "moved" rightwards, leftwards, to the center, or towards the borders of the screen by shifting each dot some pixels to the right, to the left, towards the center, or towards the border, respectively, after each refresh cycle. The shifting of the dots led to the impression of motion. The sign of the priming effect depended on the SOA between prime and target, although the motion direction of the prime was clearly visible. Essentially, with an SOA of 50 ms, no priming could be observed. With SOAs of 100 and 150 ms, positive priming effects emerged. With SOAs between 250 and 500 ms, negative priming effects emerged. Further experiments showed that the negative effects were also present in very long SOAs of up to 1000 ms (Bermeitinger & Wentura, subm.). This pattern of positive priming effects with short SOAs and negative priming effects with long SOAs appeared whether the SOA was varied between participants or within participants, and independent of prime duration. However, in the first experiments, prime duration and SOA was sometimes confounded. Until now, it is not clear whether the same pattern of a positive priming effect with a short SOA and a negative priming effect with a longer SOA would also occur if SOAs were varied block-wise but within participants, with prime duration held constant for both SOAs. To resolve this confound we conducted the experiment, which we present in the next section in detail.

Experiment

Method

Participants. Overall, 31 students from the University of Hildesheim were tested. We had to exclude 1 participant due to technical reasons. From the remaining participants (*Mdn* = 22 years, range: 19-38; 2 male), 15 started with the 147 ms SOA condition, the other 15 started with the 360 ms SOA condition. Participants had self-reported normal or corrected-to-normal vision and were right-handed except for three who were left-handed. They were paid for their participation or participated in exchange for partial course credit.

Design. A 3 (motion direction: rightwards, leftwards, neutral) x 2 (arrow direction: leftwards, rightwards) x 2 (SOA: 147 vs. 360 ms) x 2 (order of SOA conditions: 147 ms SOA first vs. 360 ms SOA first) design was used. The factors 'motion direction', 'arrow direction', and SOA were varied within participants. The factor 'order of SOA conditions' was varied between participants. In the tradition of priming experiments, the priming effect was computed as the target RT difference between incompatible (dots moved rightwards and the arrow pointed to the left; dots moved leftwards and the arrow pointed to the right) and compatible (dots moved rightwards and the arrow pointed to the right; dots moved leftwards and the arrow pointed to the left) trials.

Material. The same material as in Bermeitinger (2013) was used. Two arrows were used as target stimuli, one pointing to the left and one to the right. The arrows were approximately 3.5 cm in length and 1.0 cm in height. The primes were rows of 10.5, 11, or 11.5 dots. The first row of each priming event consisted of 11 equal-sized dots; each dot was approximately 0.4 cm in diameter. The whole row measured approximately 14.5 cm in length; the distance from one dot to the next dot was approximately 1.0 cm. To instantiate the movement, the dots were shifted from their original position (row number 1 in Figure 1b) in 0.17 cm steps leftwards or rightwards. Thus, after six steps, a dot had reached the original position of its neighboring dot and the movement started again from row number 1. Note, for some steps, it was necessary to present bisected dots at the end or at the middle of a row. Arrows and dots were presented in black on a white background.

Procedure. Participants were individually tested in sound-attenuated chambers or in groups of up to 5 persons at separated workstations. The experiment was run using E-Prime software (version 1.3) with standard PCs and 17'' CRT monitors with a refresh rate of 75 Hz. Stimulus presentation was synchronized with the vertical retrace signal of the monitor. Viewing distance was about 60 cm. Instructions were given on the CRT screen. Participants were requested to quickly and accurately categorize each arrow with regard to its direction (by pressing the right/left key with their right/left index finger for right/left arrows, respectively; response keys were the 3 and 1 key on the numeric pad on which a right or left arrow was pasted, respectively). The sequence of each trial was as follows: first a fixation stimulus (+) appeared at the center of the screen for 1000 ms. It was followed by the first row of dots, which was presented for one refresh cycle (i.e., approximately 13 ms). Then, the next 10 rows of dots were presented for the next 10 refresh cycles, respectively (i.e., resulting in a prime duration of overall 147 ms). (Note, after six refresh cycles, the row sequence started again from row number one.) The prime event was followed immediately by the target in the 147 ms SOA condition or by a blank screen of 213 ms in the 360 ms SOA condition, which was then followed by the target. The target remained on the screen until a response was given. The intertrial interval was 400 ms.

Each participant worked through two experimental parts, one part with the 147 ms SOA, and the other part with the 360 ms SOA. Each part included four blocks with 36 trials each. Each block consisted of 12 compatible trials (6 each with dots moving rightwards or leftwards, respectively), 12 incompatible trials (6 each with dots moving rightwards or leftwards, respectively), and 12 neutral trials (6 each with dots moving outwards or inwards, respectively); half of the trials had right arrow targets, the other half had left arrow targets. There was a short pause after each block. Before the first experimental block of each SOA, there was a practice phase with 12 trials. After the first part, participants could also take a short pause before starting with the second part of the experiment.

Results and Discussion

Mean RTs were derived from correct responses. Outlying RTs that were above 1500 ms, were below 200 ms, or were 1.5 interquartile ranges above the third quartile with respect to the individual distribution (Tukey, 1977) were discarded. Due to these outlier and error criteria, 6.6 % of all trials had to be excluded (2.9 % due to errors). Mean RTs and mean error rates for each condition are shown in Table 1. Mean RTs were subjected to a mixed analysis of variance (ANOVA) with the within-participants factor prime-target compatibility (compatible, incompatible, neutral) and the between-participants factors SOA (147 vs. 360 ms). The factor 'order of SOA conditions' did not interact with any other factor (all $ps > .10$). Therefore, this factor was not included in the analyses reported. Results not subsequently reported were not significant ($p > .05$, two-tailed).

The main effect of SOA was significant, $F(1, 29) = 24.49$, $p < .001$, $\eta_p^2 = .46$. Participants reacted slightly faster in the long than the short SOA. Most interesting, there was a significant interaction of SOA and prime-target compatibility, $F(2, 58) = 20.85$, $p < .001$, $\eta_p^2 = .42$. Further analyses revealed the expected pattern: Participants showed a positive priming effect in the short SOA, $M = 14$ ms, $SD = 14.76$, $t(29) = 5.04$, $p < .001$, and a negative priming effect in the long SOA, $M = -6$ ms, $SD = 19.12$, $t(29) = 1.84$, $p = .04$ (one-tailed).

Table 1. Mean response times (in ms; error rates in % in parenthesis) of the compatible, the incompatible, and the neutral conditions for each SOA (147 vs. 360 ms) condition in a within-subjects design with a blocked presentation of SOA condition

	compatible	incompatible	neutral
147 ms SOA	355 (2.2)	368 (4.2)	357 (3.1)
360 ms SOA	350 (2.5)	344 (2.5)	347 (2.7)

Overall, our results conformed to previous results – we found positive priming effects at the 147 ms SOA and negative priming effects at the longer SOA of 360 ms. However, the motion type we used was rather special and the question arises whether the special kind of motion is relevant for the result. Thus, we conducted further experiments to test another kind of motion using only a single dot which is moved rightwards or leftwards. Here, positive compatibility effects were found even with a relatively long SOA of 360 ms; however, for very long SOAs (800 to 1200 ms), negative effects were found (Bermeitinger & Wentura, subm.). This could be interpreted as evidence that the specific *type* of motion is irrelevant for the occurrence of a negative effect with long SOAs. However, activation and inhibition processes act with another time course in response priming with different motion stimuli.

In direct comparisons, we found no negative effects with static stimuli (Bermeitinger, 2013). (Admittedly, with clearly visible static stimuli, there were some single reports of negative priming effects; e.g., Klauer & Dittrich, 2010; Machado, Wyatt, Devine, & Knight, 2007.) Differences between moving and static primes in response priming were found also with other paradigms (e.g., Raymond, O'Donnell, & Tipper, 1998) and could be explained by several accounts. One account could rely on the assumption that static and dynamic stimuli are processed differently in some respects (e.g., in relation to the distinction of the ventral and dorsal stream of processing, e.g., Cardoso-Leite & Gorea, 2010; Decety & Grèzes, 1999). Another account could assume that activation processes – and, in turn, the need for inhibitory processes – are faster when moving stimuli are used. As the negative effects found with motion stimuli are huge and robust and independent of a lot of factors on which negative effects with static stimuli depend, motion stimuli seem to have a specific impact. We interpret the general finding of (large) positive effects with short SOAs and negative effects with longer and even very long SOAs as evidence that motion stimuli have the impact to trigger activation very fast. This might be due to the high importance of moving stimuli in our environment (which require a fast and appropriate response).The negative effects might reflect the – also fast acting – process of inhibition in those cases in which the fast activation is interpreted or classified as unfounded. This mechanism comes into play to prevent us from uncontrolled acting on each (moving) stimulus.

Biological vs. Nonbiological Motion

Besides the perception of moving objects in general, the perception of biological movements (which are movements carried out by humans and animals, e.g. a predator approaching) seems to be given an even more special role in human information processing (e.g. Beauchamp, Lee, Haxby & Martin, 2003, Grossman & Blake, 2002, Johannson, 1973; 1976, Troje, 2008). It is, potentially, a stunning skill that allows us to retrieve a lot of information from a moving creature in our environment (Dittrich, Troscianko, Lea & Morgan, 1996, Jokisch & Troje, 2003, Kozlowski & Cutting, 1977). This information, in turn, can indicate the appropriate reaction to the creature we perceive.

Motion perception, especially in the case of biological motion, is seen as an important skill for appropriate action responses. How is biological motion perception investigated? One of the first and most important scientific approaches to what we call biological motion perception comes from Swedish psychologist Gunnar Johannson (1973). In the first of his experiments, small light bulbs were attached to the major joints of a human actor dressed in black. By filming that person in front of a black background, only light dots were visible, which, surprisingly, still quickly evoked the impression of a walking figure even though very few light dots were shown. Since then, these point-light displays, which nowadays are often constructed by computer programs (Cutting, 1978), became an effective tool in research of the underlying mechanisms of biological motion perception (Troje, 2008). One can identify a point-light display as a human being very quickly (Johannson, 1975) and one is able to extract characteristic features from point-light walkers like sex (Kozlowski & Cutting, 1977), body size (Jockisch & Troje, 2003), or emotions (Dittrich et al., 1996). Additionally, some information can be identified by young children (e.g., Berthental, 1993) and even new-born babies (e.g., Simion et al., 2008).

Current research in the field of biological motion perception focuses on several of the implications and suggestions of the many stunning findings since Johannson (1973). One of these suggestions is that there is a specific brain area which is responsible for the recognition of biological movements, and especially movements carried out by conspecifics (i.e. humans), and that this area is not completely dependent on earlier stages of visual processing. This suggestion becomes especially plausible in light of findings that show patients with bilateral extrastriate lesions, who thus have a deficit processing moving stimuli (as shown by neuropsychological examinations and MRI), are nevertheless able to report actions in a biological motion display (McLeod, 1996; Vaina, Lemay, Bienfang, Choi & Nakayama, 1990).

Nowadays it is widely accepted that human visual information processing, in general, comprises multiple visual areas. These areas seem to be neuroanatomically organized into two different hierarchical pathways that focus on different elements of the visual scene, like information concerning "what" and information concerning "where" (Ungerleider & Mishkin, 1982), i.e. the ventral and the dorsal pathways. Related to the perception of biological motion, an important difference between the two pathways is that the dorsal pathway (covering mainly dorsal regions of extrastriate cortex) focuses on the analysis of objects' locations and movements (motion based processing of visual information), whereas the ventral pathway (covering ventral cortex parts) is specialized for the analysis of shapes and characteristics of visual objects (object based processing of visual information) (Livingstone & Hubel, 1987). Thus, the dorsal pathway might play an important role in the perception of biological motion. Still, biological motion perception is neuroanatomically special due to the fact that it can operate despite strong impairments in the perception of movements in general (McLeod, 1996; Vaina et al., 1990). The region found to be most responsive to biological motion (mostly studies using fMRI) is the sulcus temporalis superior (STS) (Beauchamp et al., 2003; Grossman & Blake, 2002; Vaina, Solomon, Chowdhury, Sinha & Belliveau, 2001). It is located near areas MT and MST (Grossman et al., 2000), and thus has a strong relation to the dorsal pathway. Studies identifying this sulcus not only showed activation of the STS during the presentation of human movements, but also non-activation while alternative, nonbiological movements were presented (Grossman & Blake, 2002).

In light of these findings, and keeping in mind that our environment is frequently full of moving objects which are often important to us (e.g. living beings, approaching objects), the idea of applying biologically moving stimuli in cognitive paradigms is promising. In recent years, several experiments of traditional cognitive paradigms using dynamic biological stimuli have been conducted, such as the flanker task (Thornton & Vuong, 2004), the cuing paradigm (Shi, Weng, He & Jiang, 2010; Wang, Yang, Shi & Jiang, 2014) and the Simon task (Bosbach, Prinz & Kerzel, 2004). In all cases, biologically moving stimuli significantly influenced task performance.

Güldenpenning and colleagues (Güldenpenning, Koester, Kunde, Weigelt & Schack, 2011) investigated the perception of complex actions in the field of sports. In detail, they were interested to learn whether the availability of a motor representation of a high jump movement (which is obviously a biological stimulus) in skilled athletes can influence the processing of visual information that is related to this representation (complex sports movement of high jump). In order to take into account the suggested automatic activation of motor representation in the observers of the movement, a subliminal priming paradigm with prime and target stimuli being images of high jump movements was used. The images either belonged to the same movement phase or not, and either showed the natural or reversed order of the jump movement. When prime-target pairs reflected the natural order of a high-jump movement, positive priming effects in terms of faster reactions in skilled athletes occurred, indicating an automatic activation of the future aspect of the movement representation.

Research in this field in general strengthens the suggestion of a domain-specific expertise, arisen through performance (Calvo-Merino, Grèzes, Glaser, Passingham & Haggard, 2006), that enables unconscious processing of related stimuli that evoke a static (Kiesel, Kunde, Pohl, Berner & Hoffmann, 2009) or a moving (Calvo-Merino, Glaser, Grèzes, Passingham & Haggard, 2005, Calvo-Merino et al., 2006, Güldenpenning et al., 2011) impression. Thus, these findings are related to suggestions about common representations in perception of action and performance of action (see also above; i.e. a *common representational medium* as supposed by the *Theory of Event Coding*, Hommel et al., 2001), supposing the same neural basis for action observation and production (Decety & Grèzes, 1999; di Pellegrino et al., 1992, Grèzes & Decety, 2001).

Again, we used the response priming paradigm to investigate differences between biological and nonbiological motion (Eckert & Bermeitinger, subm.). In one series of experiments we used point-light walkers as biological motion type and a directional scrambled dot pattern as nonbiological motion type. In other experiments, we used eye gazes as biological motion type and either only the irises from the eye gaze stimuli (without any eye, head etc. information) or control stimuli with the same iris motions but with meaningless strokes and points surrounding them as nonbiological motion type. In short, we found larger priming effects with biological motions than nonbiological motions for SOAs up to approximately 600 ms. With very long SOAs (920 & 1320 ms), there were small positive priming effects of comparable height with biological as well as nonbiological motions. That is, also in response priming we found differences between biological and nonbiological motion – biological motion seems to be processed preferentially and it seems to have larger and faster impact on our motor system than nonbiological stimuli.

Conclusion on the Motion Part

Taken together, the perception of motion is an extremely important ability in human information processing. In cognitive paradigms, the response priming task is a well suited method for investigating motor pre-activations and perceptuomotor associations in general. Here, we found differences between motion and static displays, between different motion types and between biological and nonbiological motions. Motion, in general, seems to be important information for our cognitive system, which is able to trigger activation processes fast and reliably. The largest effects are found with biological motion, which in turn is among the most important social and environmental information for our daily acting. There is a crucial difference in processing between biological and nonbiological movements. Several findings of lesion patients and of neuroimaging studies confirm the suggestion that the perception of biological motion plays a special role, in terms of both functional and structural features.

Perceiving Threats

In the previous section we described differences between static and moving stimuli, as well as between different motion types, in terms of importance. In this section we will extend the argument that importance influences perception using an independent field of psychological research. This research has focused on individuals' abilities to rapidly detect and attend to nonthreatening and threatening stimuli in visual scenes. We will first outline the traditionally predominant hypothesis in this field and briefly review supporting findings. We will then review findings that contradict the predictions of this hypothesis. Finally, we will show how an alternative perspective, focusing on the importance of stimuli to the individual, more completely and parsimoniously accounts for the results of research in this field.

Innate Threat Superiority Hypothesis

Beginning with Gibson in 1979, there has been a push to view visual perception as a process influenced by the environment that individuals live in, and the recurrent properties of these environments that were faced by their ancestors (Öhman, 2007). Following this line of reasoning, the way that an individual perceives the environment, and the stimuli present in it, should enhance that individual's chances of survival and reproduction. We will discuss how this line of reasoning has been applied to the human visual system and has led to particular ideas about which stimuli should receive preference of perception and attention.

Theory

Several papers have been published in recent years arguing that human visual perception has evolved in direct response to the recurring influence of specific threatening stimuli in the ancestral environment (e.g., Penkunas & Coss, 2013a; Rakison & Derringer, 2008). While these papers have focused on the influence of different threats, as we will expand upon below, they share the underlying argument that humans should rapidly detect and attend to the presence of particular threatening stimuli due to natural selection. We here term their argument the Innate Threat Superiority (ITS) hypothesis.

The ITS hypothesis is based on the knowledge that certain stimuli threatened the survival of our ancestors in the past, and the assumption that our ancestors had variable, heritable abilities to detect and attend to these threatening stimuli. Those of our ancestors who were able to rapidly detect the presence of these threatening stimuli were also better able to avoid or escape them, and therefore enhance their chance of survival. Since those individuals were better able to survive, they were also more likely to reproduce and pass along the ability to rapidly detect threatening stimuli.

Below, we will provide more detailed information about the theoretical bases for the ITS hypothesis in visual perception. The ITS hypothesis has been applied to several different groups of threatening stimuli to date. The three groups that have received particular attention are all from the category "animals", namely snakes, spiders, and lions. The first stimuli that we will consider are snakes, as they have been the main focus of research in this area.

Snakes

Snakes have long been creatures of fascination for the human psyche (Öhman & Mineka, 2003). While they have sometimes been seen as creatures of protection and healing, such as in ancient Greece and Egypt (Antoniou, Antoniou, Learney, Granderath, & Antoniou, 2011), they have more commonly been viewed as symbols of danger. This is true for ancient cultures, as evidenced by the story of the fall of Adam and Eve, as well as for modern cultures, as evidenced by the role of snakes in the Harry Potter stories. This negative portrayal in literature and culture likely comes from the fact that snakes have a long history of being dangerous for humans and our ancestors.

The human fascination with snakes has not passed the attention of researchers of human visual perception. Indeed, snakes have become the prototypical 'threatening' stimuli used in research. Not surprisingly, the role of snakes on the influence of the human visual system has also received a great deal of theoretical attention. A paper by Isbell (2006) argued that human visual perception has evolved in direct response to the recurrent presence of snakes in the environment of our ancestors. She argued that this influence has led to our, relatively, exceptional general visual abilities, as well as our ability to rapidly detect snakes in the environment. We will explore two parts of her argument here, as they are particularly relevant to this paper. The first is that our frontal focused vision helps us rapidly detect snakes. The second is that our color vision helps us rapidly detect snakes.

One prominent feature of the human face is our orbital convergence, or the proximity of our eyes to one another. When the eyes are closer to one another, it leads vision to be focused more towards the bottom-center of the visual field, i.e., those stimuli closest to the ground. Isbell (2006) argued that snakes are most dangerous to us when they are in exactly this location. Although snakes are occasionally arboreal and attack from above, or strike from the side, they are most likely to attack us when we accidentally step on them. As we typically look in the direction that we are about to step, this usually puts the snake in the bottom-center of our visual field.

In addition to increased orbital convergence leading to a focus on the area where snakes are at their most dangerous, a higher degree of orbital convergence may also lead to better three-dimensional vision. Having better 3-D vision could allow for a greater discrimination of particular stimuli when several similar looking objects are in one visual scene. This could be particularly important for detecting camouflaged snakes.

As additional evidence, Isbell (2006) compared the human visual features to those of raptors. In support of her argument she pointed out that the degree of orbital convergence varies in raptors. The eyes are closer together on raptors that prey on snakes than raptors that do not prey on snakes. Isbell argued that, similar to humans, the need to detect snakes in visual scenes is what has led to the greater degree of orbital convergence in snake-eating raptors. Although this is only a correlation, it is typical for natural selection to produce convergent evolution of features or behaviors in different evolutionary lines when they face a similar problem (Mayr, 2001), in this case the need to detect snakes.

As well as frontally focused vision due to enhanced orbital convergence, Isbell (2006) also argued that our ability to see and discriminate a variety of colors is due to the selective pressures provided by snakes. In this case, Isbell focused specifically on the influence of venomous snakes. She pointed out that the variable presence of trichromatic color vision in primates correlates with the evolutionary history of cohabitation with venomous snakes. Specifically, trichromatic color vision is an almost ubiquitous feature of Old-World Monkeys, which have consistently shared the environment with venomous snakes. Trichromatic color vision is, however, only present in some of the New-World Monkeys, which have had an interrupted evolutionary history of cohabitation with venomous.

In sum, what Isbell (2006) argued is that snakes, due to the threat they posed to the survival of our ancestors, have significantly influenced the way that modern humans visually perceive the world. We have the long history of cohabitation with snakes to thank for our exceptional general visual abilities, our orbital convergence, and our trichromatic color vision. It follows, then, that snakes should be detected especially rapidly and well in the visual environment, and more so than other, especially nonthreatening (but otherwise comparable), stimuli.

Lions and Spiders and Other Threats, Oh My!

While the theoretical work concerning the ITS hypothesis has mostly focused on the influence of snakes, at least two other potentially dangerous stimuli have received attention as well, namely spiders and lions. Similar to snakes, spiders are creatures that frequently fascinate and frighten humans; and while many spiders are in fact harmless, several species of spiders can be dangerous. Rakison (2009) argued that spiders have consistently posed a danger to humans and our ancestors over the course of evolutionary time, and that those humans who were able to rapidly detect the presence of spiders had a better chance of surviving and reproducing. Similarly, Penkunas and Coss (2013a), argued that lions have been significant predators of humans, and that modern humans should therefore show the ability to rapidly detect these predators in the environment.

Although these arguments have, as of yet, only been applied to snakes, spiders, and lions, there is no theoretical reason that it must be limited to these groups of animals. This form of argument can extend to any group of animals, or perhaps even inanimate stimuli, which occupied the same geographical areas as our ancestors. If a reasonable argument can be made that a certain stimulus acted as a recurrent threat to the survival of our ancestors *and* that the rapid detection of this threat significantly decreased its potential to threaten the survival of an individual, then it follows that rapid visual detection of that particular stimulus may have been selected for in humans. If that is the case, then we should be able to find evidence of these rapid detection benefits in modern humans as well.

Evidence Supporting the ITS Hypothesis

Support for the ITS hypothesis has come from several sources. One of the earliest forms of evidence came from the clinical field, with an interesting observation about phobias. Although many modern stimuli are extremely dangerous to humans, and account for many deaths per year (e.g., cars and guns), many of the most common phobias are to natural stimuli, including stimuli that no longer account for many human deaths (such as spiders and snakes) (Rakison, 2009). Humans may, in fact, be prepared by natural selection to learn to fear certain stimuli that posed a recurrent threat to our ancestors (Seligman, 1971). For example, conditioned fears to ancestral threats, such as snakes, are more easily learned and more difficultly extinguished than conditioned fears to nonthreatening stimuli, such as flowers (Öhman & Mineka, 2003). This can be viewed as indirect support for the ITS hypothesis, as it does not relate specifically to visual perception. Other research more specifically addresses the visual nature of the ITS hypothesis.

Öhman, Flykt, and Esteves (2001) performed several experiments comparing the time required to detect the presence of threatening (snakes and spiders) and nonthreatening (flowers and mushrooms) stimuli in a visual scene. In their experiments, the researchers had subjects view either 2x2 or 3x3 grids on a computer screen which contained either 4 or 9 pictures from the same category or 3 or 8 pictures from the same category and one picture from a different category. The subjects had to flip one switch if all the pictures came from the same category and another switch if one of the pictures came from a discrepant category. The researchers found that when the one discrepant picture was taken from one of the threatening categories, subjects responded faster than when the discrepant picture was taken from one of the nonthreatening categories. The researchers also found that RTs to grids with a threatening discrepant picture did not increase depending on grid size, while RTs to grids with a nonthreatening discrepant picture did increase from 2x2 to 3x3 size grids.

The finding that snakes and spiders are detected faster than nonthreatening stimuli has been replicated several times (e.g., Flykt, 2006). Further research by Penkunas and Coss (2013a) has extended this finding, showing that humans also detect lions more rapidly than nonthreatening stimuli, in this case antelopes. This research, performed with adults as subjects, has been used as evidence in support of the ITS hypothesis.

In addition to performing research with adults, investigations have also focused on younger populations. The reason for using younger populations is to control for the variable of experience. As we age our visual perceptions become increasingly influenced by our life experiences. Therefore, visual detection preferences shown for threatening stimuli in adults may actually be due to experience rather than an innate mechanism for rapid detection of threatening stimuli. If findings could be extended to increasingly younger populations it would better support the argument that the superior detection of threatening stimuli has nothing to do with experience and everything to do with natural selection, thus supporting the ITS hypothesis.

Several investigations have accomplished this extension, showing that children (aged 3-5 years) detect both snakes (LoBue & DeLoache, 2008) and spiders (LoBue, 2010a) more rapidly than nonthreatening stimuli. Attempting to even further remove the role of life experience, research has also tested infants (aged 5-14 months). Rakison and Derringer (2008) showed that infants' looking time was longer towards schematic spiders than towards scrambled spiders, even though looking time towards schematic and scrambled flowers did not differ. Additionally, LoBue and DeLoache (2010) found that infants turned to look at snakes more rapidly than at nonthreatening stimuli.

The research using children and infants attempted to account for the role of experience, showing that the faster detection of threatening stimuli is due to an evolved and innate tendency to do so. Another common way for researchers to strengthen the claim that a behavior is innate is through cross-cultural research. The reasoning behind this is that peoples of different cultures and in different geographical regions are less likely to share the same experiences, but they are still likely to share any innate traits that have been selected for in human ancestry.

In an attempt to make their work cross-cultural, Penkunas and Coss (2013b) tested samples of children in India who live in either a rural or an urban setting. The researchers found that lions were detected faster than antelopes, regardless of the area where the children live. Penkunas and Coss argue that this is further support for the ITS hypothesis and that the detection of threatening predators is due less to experience than to an innate tendency to rapidly respond to stimuli that consistently posed a survival threat to human ancestors.

To this point we have reviewed research that has found faster detection of threatening than nonthreatening stimuli, and that this threat superiority effect is present in children and infants, as well as present across cultures. This research has supported the ITS hypothesis, which is based on the argument that, due to the constant selection pressure, those of our ancestors who had the (innate) ability to rapidly detect and respond to these threats became more likely to survive and reproduce. While this is a sound argument, what most researchers have not addressed is that this argument requires a mechanism for producing this threat superiority. In other words, research must address the question of what it is about the particular threatening stimuli that allows humans to rapidly detect them in visual scenes.

To date, only a limited amount of research has addressed this point. LoBue and DeLoache (2011) attempted to determine what features of snakes led to their rapid detection by humans. Two of the main features that the researchers considered could lead to rapid detection of snakes were bright color patterns and the coiled shape of snakes. In one experiment LoBue and DeLoache found that snakes were detected faster than nonthreatening stimuli even if presented in gray-scale, a result that was independently supported by Hayakawa, Kawai, and Masataka (2011). LoBue and DeLoache did, however, show that snakes were not detected faster than other coiled, but nonthreatening stimuli, while other coiled nonthreatening stimuli were detected faster than non-coiled nonthreatening stimuli. The results of these experiments seem to suggest that the coiled shape of snakes is critical for rapid detection.

Evidence Contradicting the ITS Hypothesis

Although the ITS hypothesis has received a deal of backing in the literature, the support has not been universal or complete. On the contrary, several research findings seem to contradict the central tenets of the ITS hypothesis. We first review evidence that seems to suggest that the threat superiority effect is not, in fact, innate. We then review evidence that suggests that threatening stimuli are *not* always detected more rapidly than nonthreatening stimuli.

One of the main challenges to the ITS hypothesis is to the claim that the rapid detection of threatening stimuli is innate. Instead of the threat superiority effect being due to an innate tendency to detect particular stimuli that posed a recurrent threat in the ancestral environment, it could be that humans detect threatening stimuli more rapidly than nonthreatening stimuli because they have *learned* that particular stimuli can be dangerous. In line with this counter argument to the ITS hypothesis, several researchers have independently shown that, in addition to ancestral threatening stimuli, such as snakes, being detected more rapidly than ancestral nonthreatening stimuli, such as flowers, modern threatening stimuli, such as guns, are also detected more rapidly than modern nonthreatening stimuli, such as toasters (Blanchette, 2006; Brosch & Sharma, 2005; Fox, Griggs, & Mouchlianitis, 2007). Unlike with snakes, it is extremely difficult to make an argument that humans have been naturally selected to rapidly detect the presence of modern threatening stimuli like guns, as there has not been enough passage of time for guns to have created a true selective pressure.

In response to this challenge LoBue, Rakison, and DeLoache (2010) have put forward a modified version of the ITS hypothesis. In their modified version, which we here call the Learned and Innate Threat Superiority (LITS) hypothesis, the authors argue that the threat superiority effect may depend on two separate pathways, one learned and one innate. In support of their argument they cite research using modern stimuli to show that there is clearly a learned component to the threat superiority effect. They also point out that research has shown more rapid detection of ancestral threatening than nonthreatening stimuli in infants (e.g., LoBue & DeLoache, 2010), but that there is only more rapid detection of modern threatening than nonthreatening stimuli in children when the individual observer has had a personal negative experience with the threatening modern object (LoBue, 2010b).

One thing that the ITS and LITS hypotheses have in common is the central argument that threatening stimuli should be detected more rapidly in visual scenes than nonthreatening stimuli. This assumes that threatening stimuli are in some way special due to the potential risk they pose to survival. This argument for a general threat superiority effect has not, however, gone unchallenged. Indeed, several experiments have shown that there are cases when threatening stimuli are *not* detected faster in visual scenes than nonthreatening stimuli.

Lipp, Derakshan, Waters, and Logies (2004) performed a series of experiments testing whether the threat superiority effect reported in the original experiments by Öhman et al. (2001) was due to the threatening nature of snakes and spiders or due to the fact that they were animals, while the nonthreatening stimuli used (flowers and mushrooms) were not. In one experiment Lipp et al. found that cats and horses were detected as rapidly as snakes and spiders when presented as a discrepant picture in an array of pictures of flowers or mushrooms. In another experiment Lipp et al. showed that pictures of animals were detected faster in arrays of flowers and mushrooms than flowers and mushrooms were in an array of animals, and that this was regardless of whether the animals were nonthreatening (cats and horses) or threatening (big cats and wolves).

Additional research has challenged the threat superiority effect using inanimate, but motivationally relevant stimuli. De Oca and Black (2013) tested detection speed for threatening (guns and snakes), neutral (trees and couches), and pleasant (money and food) discrepant stimuli in arrays of neutral (cacti and pots) stimuli. The researchers found that both threatening and pleasant stimuli were detected more rapidly than neutral stimuli. Crucially, they also found that the time it took to detect one of the types of pleasant stimuli (money) was not significantly longer than the time it took to detection the threatening stimuli, when they were presented in the same arrays.

Taken together, the research by Lipp et al. (2004) and De Oca and Black (2013) challenges the ITS and LITS hypotheses. This research shows that threatening stimuli are not always detected and attended to more rapidly than nonthreatening stimuli in visual scenes. Based on this research, we need to consider an alternative way of thinking about this research which does not rely strictly on the role of threat.

Importance

As we have discussed to this point, there have been several arguments put forward to account for the results reviewed above. The ITS hypothesis states that threatening stimuli should be detected faster than nonthreatening stimuli due to past selection pressures of particular stimuli. The LITS hypothesis states that threatening stimuli should be detected faster than nonthreatening stimuli due to past selection pressures of particular stimuli and the pressure to detect stimuli that are learned threats. Additionally, it has been suggested that we should more rapidly detect the presence of animals than inanimate stimuli, due to selection pressures (New, Cosmides, & Tooby, 2007). None of these hypotheses, however, can account for all of the results that we have presented in a coherent and parsimonious way.

As an alternative to the hypotheses presented above, we believe that the combined results reflect that there are multiple influences on visual perception, both bottom-up and top-down (*memory access* is also influenced by top-down settings and/or context information, see e.g., Bermeitinger, Wentura, & Frings, 2011; Barsalou, 1982). Due to these various influences, visual perception and attention is biased towards stimuli that are deemed most important in the visual scene, rather than stimuli that fall into a specific category (i.e., threatening, pleasant, animal, etc.). In order to make our point more clearly, we will revisit four of the results we presented above (summarized in Table 2) and show how they fit into a framework of an importance superiority effect rather than a threat superiority effect.

Table 2. Summary of relevant results showing faster RTs to more important stimuli

Study	Faster RTs to	Slower RTs to
Öhman et al. (2001, Exp. 1)	Snakes & spiders	Flowers & mushrooms
Blanchette (2006, Exp. 1)	Guns & knives	Clocks & toasters
Lipp et al. (2004, Exp. 2a)	Cats, horses, big cats, & wolves	Flowers & mushrooms
De Oca & Black (2013, Exp. 2)	Snakes, guns, & money	Food, trees, & couches

In their original paper on this topic Öhman et al. (2001) showed that humans responded faster to pictures of snakes and spiders when presented in arrays of flowers and mushrooms than vice versa (i.e., flowers and mushrooms presented in arrays of snakes and spiders). While the authors originally argued that this reflected a tendency for the human visual system to prefer threatening to nonthreatening stimuli, we argue that their results reflect the tendency for the human visual system to prefer more important stimuli.

Although most people have not had a personal negative experience with snakes and spiders, stories about snakes and spiders harming or killing humans abound. Most humans, therefore, have learned vicariously that it is important to avoid snakes and spiders because they are potentially dangerous. Flowers and mushrooms can also be very dangerous to humans when ingested, but they cannot act of their own volition to pose a threat to humans. Based on this, it is more important to rapidly perceive, attend to, and possibly respond to the stimuli that can pose an immediate threat to survival, namely snakes and spiders, than to the stationary stimuli which are generally harmless, namely flowers and mushrooms.

This same logic holds for an explanation of the results reported by Blanchette (2006). She found that humans respond faster to guns and knives in arrays of clocks and toasters than vice versa (i.e., clocks and toasters in arrays of guns and knives). Although guns and knives cannot be threatening to a human of their own volition, their presence in the environment usually signals a potential danger, or at least that the individual should be cautious around these stimuli. This is not the case for clocks or toasters, which are only important to us when we seek out their functions (i.e., we want to know if it is breakfast time so we can toast ourselves some delicious Pop-Tarts!).

Our explanations of the results reported by Öhman et al. (2001) and Blanchette (2006) rely on the fact that the threatening stimuli that were responded to more rapidly than the nonthreatening stimuli were more important to the observers because of their threatening nature. In other words, we agree that something being threatening can, and usually is, a very important cue to our visual system. It is, however, not the only important cue, as we will see with the next two examples.

Lipp et al. (2004) showed that humans responded to animals in arrays of non-animals (flowers and mushrooms) faster than vice versa (i.e., non-animals in arrays of animals). This was irrelevant of whether the animals were threatening (such as big cats or wolves) or nonthreatening (such as cats or horses). This result shows that the visual system does not always favor threatening stimuli, but instead favors stimuli that are most important in the visual scene. As we mentioned above, flowers and mushrooms are not so important in visual scenes that they require immediate detection and attention. Big cats, such as lions, and wolves are clearly stimuli that require immediate attention, as they can be potentially threatening. Although this may be less clear with normal cats and horses, they are certainly more important than flowers and mushrooms in a visual scene because they are organisms that can move of their own volition, and therefore can impart important information to the observer. For example, any stimulus that moves of its own accord can be threatening or signal that other threats are present in the environment. They may also signal where shelter or resources are present (New et al., 2007). Additionally, animals that are not predators can be considered as sources of food. Finally, cats and horses are stimuli that we are very familiar with, because of their domesticated status. They can therefore be important to certain individuals because their presence may be pleasant and enjoyable.

Evidence of pleasant and motivationally relevant stimuli being important for the visual system comes from De Oca and Black (2013). They found that money, a pleasant and motivationally relevant stimulus, was responded to faster than trees and couches, and as fast as snakes and guns, when these stimuli were presented in the same arrays (cacti and pots). The rapid detection of money cannot be explained as a preference for threatening stimuli or a preference for animal stimuli. Money is, however, very important in our society, and we have lots of experience telling us that the location and acquisition of money is important.

Considering that De Oca and Black (2013) found faster detection for one pleasurable and motivationally relevant stimulus (money) than the neutral stimuli of trees and couches, one may wonder why they did not find this advantage for the other pleasurable and motivationally relevant stimulus they used, namely food. This may demonstrate the relevance of current states to determining what is important to the visual system. While detecting money may always be important to an individual, locating food is probably only important to the visual system when the individual is hungry. Indeed, research has shown preferential detection of food-related words when subjects were hungry (Mogg, Bradley, Hyare, & Lee, 1998). Level of hunger was not experimentally manipulated in De Oca and Black's study and the subjects in Experiment 1 of their paper reported only low levels of hunger. Already Lewin (1935) assumed that things are motivationally relevant, affectively loaden, and thus individually important if a corresponding state (top-down) is given. Evidence for this also comes from studies on subliminal persuasion. Participants' consumption behavior is only biased into the direction of the subliminally presented stimuli (associated with a specific brand) if they are in a corresponding (top-down) state (for thirst and the subliminal advertisement for ice tea, see e.g., Karremans, Stroebe, & Claus, 2006; for tiredness and the subliminal advertisement for dextrose, see e.g., Bermeitinger, Goelz, Johr, Neumann, Ecker, & Doerr, 2009).

Conclusion on Threat Part

For the visual system to function efficiently it must constantly prioritize certain stimuli in the visual environment over others. Researchers have proposed several hypotheses explaining what types of stimuli should be prioritized, including threatening, pleasant, and animal stimuli. Partial readings of the literature can be used to support any one of these hypotheses. However, when taken altogether, the literature supports instead the argument that the visual system prioritizes those stimuli which are most important to the individual at the moment. The level of importance of a particular stimulus is driven by bottom-up stimulation as well as top-down goals and states.

Conclusion and Outlook

At any given moment the visual system is bombarded with sensations coming from a variety of stimuli. One of the main challenges for the cognitive system is to determine which stimuli require rapid perception and attention as only a limited amount of actions can be performed at any given time. We have argued that stimuli that are more important (for current or general goals), as determined by both domain-specific and domain-general mechanisms, receive preferential processing by the visual system. In support of our argument we showed that motion stimuli are processed more efficiently than static stimuli, and that this is especially true for biological motion stimuli. We have also shown that threatening stimuli are generally attended to more rapidly than nonthreatening stimuli, although nonthreatening stimuli also receive rapid attention when they are pleasant and/or motivationally relevant.

Research in this area is still required to further support and expand upon the argument we have presented here. We will briefly discuss how future research could be beneficial. This research can be broadly placed into one of the following three categories: 1) research that determines new stimuli that may be considered of particular importance, 2) research that manipulates the stimuli being observed, and 3) research that manipulates the mental states/goals of the observer.

The first category is research that attempts to determine new stimuli or information that can be considered as important for the visual system. In this chapter we have focused on motion stimuli and threatening stimuli. These are, however, by no means the only two categories of stimuli that should be considered of high importance to the visual system. For example, it may be that stimuli from other categories (e.g., disgusting) are also considered to be particularly important. Also, stimuli which fall into these categories may differ in their level of importance, and it is important to determine why this may be the case.

The second category is research that attempts to manipulate the stimuli, in order to manipulate their level of importance. One way of achieving this may be to manipulate the positioning of the stimuli. As a specific example, it may be that a gun pointed at the observer is considered more important than a gun pointed away from the observer. Similarly, other aspects of the stimuli can be manipulated. This type of research is especially useful in determining what exactly makes certain stimuli more important than others. Additionally, it might be interesting to find out the underlying features which determine the preferential processing of important stimuli and which processing paths are involved.

Another interesting line of research that falls into this category would be research which combines the aspects we discussed in this chapter, namely motion and threat. While the rapid detection of static threatening stimuli is important, it seems logical that this would be enhanced for threatening stimuli in motion. This may depend on several factors such as perceived distance, style of motion (relaxed or tensed for attack), and direction of motion (towards the observer or away from the observer). This line of research would be particularly informative, as many of the threatening stimuli encountered in the world are frequently encountered while they are in motion, not in a static and discrete scene.

Finally, the third category of future research is that which manipulates the states or goals of the observer. For example, an experiment which experimentally manipulated the importance of nonthreatening stimuli and threatening stimuli would be particularly informative. If nonthreatening stimuli were deemed more important for a particular goal than threatening stimuli, would the nonthreatening stimuli then be detected and attended to more rapidly, where the threatening stimuli were detected more rapidly? Similar manipulations are theoretically possible for motion and static stimuli as well. Such experiments would provide strong support for the hypothesis that importance for the visual system is determined by both the properties of the stimuli in the environment, as well as the states and goals of the observing organism.

We hope that future research in this area will be fruitful in helping us determine which stimuli are considered important, how importance can be manipulated, and how this depends on the mental states and goals of the observer. Such knowledge would be theoretically interesting to researchers of visual perception and attention as well as in motivation research. This knowledge could also be useful for practical applications, especially in instances where it is important to rapidly grab the attention of observers.

References

Albrecht, D.G., & Geisler, W.S. (1991). Motion selectivity and the contrast-response function of simple cells in the visual cortex. *Visual Neuroscience*, *7*, 531-546.

Antoniou, S.A., Antoniou, G.A., Learney, R., Granderath, F.A., & Antoniou, A.I. (2011). The rod and the serpent: History's ultimate healing symbol. *World Journal of Surgery*, *35*, 217-221.

Aron, A.R., Schlaghecken, F., Fletcher, P.C., Bullmore, E.T., Eimer, M., Barker, R., et al. (2003). Inhibition of subliminally primed responses is mediated by the caudate and thalamus: Evidence from functional MRI and Huntington's disease. *Brain*, *126*, 713-723.

Barsalou, L.W. (1982). Context-independent and context-dependent information in concepts. *Memory & Cognition*, *10*, 82-93.

Beauchamp, M.S., Lee, K.E., Haxby, J.V., & Martin, A. (2003). Parallel visual motion processing streams for manipulable objects and human movements. *Neuron*, *34*, 149-159.

Bermeitinger, C. (2013). Response priming with apparent motion prime. *Psychological Research*, *77*, 371-387.

Bermeitinger, C., Goelz, R., Johr, N., Neumann, M., Ecker, U.K.H., & Doerr, R. (2009). The hidden persuaders break into the tired brain. *Journal of Experimental Social Psychology*, *45*, 320-326.

Bermeitinger, C., Wentura, D., & Frings, C. (2011). How to switch on and switch off semantic priming effects for natural and artifactual categories: Activation processes in category memory depend on focusing specific feature dimensions. *Psychonomic Bulletin & Review*, *18*, 579-585.

Berthental, B.I. (1993). Infants' perception of biomechanical motions: Intrinsic image and knowledge-based constraints. In C.E. Granrud (Ed.), *Visual perception and cognition in infancy* (pp. 175-214). Hillsdale, NJ: Erlbaum.

Blanchette, I. (2006). Snakes, spiders, guns, and syringes: How specific are evolutionary constraints on the detection of threatening stimuli? *Quarterly Journal of Experimental Psychology*, *59*, 1484-1504.

Bosbach, S., Prinz, W., & Kerzel, D. (2004). A Simon effect with stationary moving stimuli. *Journal of Experimental Psychology: Human Perception and Performance*, *30*, 39-55.

Brosch, T., & Sharma, D. (2005). The role of fear-relevant stimuli in visual search: A comparison of phylogenetic and ontogenetic stimuli. *Emotion*, *5*, 360-364.

Calvo-Merino, B., Glaser, D.E., Grèzes, J., Passingham, R.E., & Haggard, P. (2005). Action observation and acquired motor skills: An fMRI study with expert dancers. *Cerebral Cortex*, *15*, 1243-1249.

Calvo-Merino, B., Grèzes, J., Glaser, D. E., Passingham, R. E., & Haggard, P. (2006). Seeing or doing? Influence of visual and motor familiarity in action observation. *Current Biology*, *16*, 1905-1910.

Cardoso-Leite, P., & Gorea, A. (2010). On the perceptual/motor dissociation: a review of concepts, theory, experimental paradigms and data interpretations. *Seeing and perceiving*, *23*, 89-151.

Cavanagh, P. (1992). Attention-based motion perception. *Science*, *257*, 1563-1565.

Chemero, A. (2006). *Radical embodied cognitive science*. Cambridge: MIT Press.

Chiappe, D. & MacDonald, K. (2005). The evolution of domain-general mechanisms in intelligence and learning. *The Journal of General Psychology*, *132*, 5-40.

Cutting, J. E. (1978). Generation of synthetic male and female walkers through manipulation of a biomechanical invariant. *Perception*, *7*, 393-405.

Darwin, C. (1859). *On the origin of species by means of natural selection; Or, the preservation of favored races in the struggle for life*. New York: Collier.

De Houwer, J., & Moors, A. (2007). How to define and examine the implicitness of implicit measures. In B. Wittenbrink & N. Schwarz (Eds.), *Implicit measures of attitudes: Procedures and controversies* (pp.179-194). New York, NY: Guilford Press.

De Houwer, J., Teige-Mocigemba, S., Spruyt, A., & Moors, A. (2009). Implicit measures: A normative analysis and review. *Psychological Bulletin*, *135*, 347-368.

De Oca, B.M., & Black, A.A. (2013). Bullets versus burgers: Is it threat or relevance that captures attention? *The American Journal of Psychology*, *126*, 287-300.

Decety, J., & Grèzes, J. (1999). Neural mechanisms subserving the perception of human actions. *Trends in Cognitive Sciences*, *3*, 172-178.

Di Pellegrino, G., Fadiga, L., Fogassi, L., Gallese, V., & Rizzolatti, G. (1992). Understanding motor events: A neurophysiological study. *Experimental Brain Research*, *91*, 176-180.

Dittrich, W.H., Troscianko, T., Lea, S.G.D., & Morgan, D. (1996). Perception of emotion from dynamic point-light displays represented in dance. *Perception*, *25*, 727-738.

Eckert, D., & Bermeitinger, C. (subm.). *Response priming using biological and non-biological movements as primes*. Manuscript submitted for publication.

Eimer, M. (1999). Facilitory and inhibitory effects of masked prime stimuli on motor activation and behavioral performance. *Acta Psychologica, 101*, 293-313.

Eimer, M., & Schlaghecken, F. (1998). Effects of masked stimuli on motor activation: behavioral and electrophysiological evidence. *Journal of Experimental Psychology: Human Perception and Performance, 24*, 1737-1747.

Eimer, M., & Schlaghecken, F. (2002). Links between conscious awareness and response inhibition: Evidence from masked priming. *Psychonomic Bulletin & Review, 9*, 514-520.

Eimer, M., & Schlaghecken F. (2003). Response facilitation and inhibition in subliminal priming. *Biological Psychology, 64*, 7-26.

Farroni, T., Massaccesi, S., Pividori, D., & Johnson, M.H. (2004). Gaze following in newborns. *Infancy, 5*, 39-60.

Fehrer, E., & Raab, D. (1962). Reaction time to stimuli masked by metacontrast. *Journal of Experimental Psychology, 63*, 143.

Flykt, A. (2006). Preparedness for action: Responding to the snake in the grass. *The American Journal of Psychology, 119*, 29-43.

Fox, E., Griggs, L., & Mouchlianitis, E. (2007). The detection of fear relevant stimuli: Are guns noticed as quickly as snakes? *Emotion, 7*, 691-696.

Gibson, J.J. (1979). *The ecological approach to visual perception.* Boston, MA: Houghton Mifflin.

Grézes, J., & Decety, J. (2001). Functional anatomy of execution, mental simulation, observation, and verb generation of actions: a meta-analysis. *Human Brain Mapping, 12*, 1-19.

Grossman, E.D., & Blake, R. (2002). Brain areas active during visual perception of biological motion. *Neuron, 35*, 1167-1175.

Grossman, E.D., Donelly, M., Price, R., Pickens, D., Morgan, V., Neighbor, G., et al. (2000). Brain areas involved in perception of biological motion. *Journal of Cognitive Neuroscience, 12*, 711-720.

Güldenpenning, I., Koester, D., Kunde, W., Weigelt, M., & Schack, T. (2011). Motor expertise modulates the unconscious processing of human body postures. *Experimental Brain Research, 213*, 383-391.

Hayakawa, S., Kawai, N., & Masataka, N. (2011). The influence of color on snake detection in visual search in human children. *Scientific Reports, 1*, 1-4.

Hommel, B., Müsseler, J., Aschersleben, G., & Prinz, W. (2001). The theory of event coding (TEC): A framework for perception and action planning. *Behavioral and Brain Sciences, 24*, 849-937.

Isbell, L.A. (2006). Snakes as agents of evolutionary change in primate brains. *Journal of Human Evolution, 51*, 1-35.

Isbell, L.A. (2009). *The fruit, the tree, and the serpent.* Cambridge, MA: Harvard University Press.

Jaśkowski, P., Bialunska, A., Tomanek, M., & Verleger, R. (2008). Mask- and distractor-triggered inhibitory processes in the priming of motor responses: An EEG-study. *Psychophysiology, 45*, 70-85.

Jaśkowski, P., & Verleger, R. (2007). What determines the direction of subliminal priming. *Advances in Cognitive Psychology, 3*, 181-192.

Johannson, G. (1973). Visual perception of biological motion and a model for its analysis. *Perception & Psychophysics, 14*, 201-211.

Johannson, G. (1976). Spatio-temporal differentiation and integration in visual motion perception. *Psychological Research*, *38*, 379-393.

Jokisch, D., & Troje, N.F. (2003). Biological motion as a cue for the perception of size. *Journal of Vision*, *3*, 252-264.

Karremans, J.C., Stroebe, W., & Claus, J. (2006). Beyond Vicary's fantasies: The impact of subliminal priming and brand choice. *Journal of Experimental Social Psychology*, *42*, 792-798.

Kiesel, A., Kunde, W., Pohl, C., Berner, M. P. & Hoffmann, J. (2009). Playing chess unconsciously. *Journal of Experimental Psychology: Learning, Memory, and Cognition*. *35*, 292-298.

Klapp, S.T., & Hinkley, L.B. (2002). The negative compatibility effect: unconscious inhibition influences reaction time and response selection. *Journal of Experimental Psychology: General*, *131*, 255-269.

Klauer, K.C., & Dittrich, K. (2010). From sunshine to double arrows: An evaluation window account of negative compatibility effects. *Journal of Experimental Psychology: General*, *139*, 490-519.

Klotz, W., & Neumann, O. (1999). Motor activation without conscious discrimination in metacontrast masking. *Journal of Experimental Psychology: Human Perception and Performance*, *25*, 976.

Kozlowski, L.T., & Cutting, J.E. (1977). Recognizing the sex of a walker from a dynamic point-light display. *Perception & Psychophysics*, *21*, 575-580.

Lewin, K. (1935). *A dynamic theory of personality*. New York: McGraw-Hill.

Lingnau, A., & Vorberg, D. (2005). The time course of response inhibition in masked priming. *Perception & Psychophysics*, *67*, 545-557.

Lipp, O.V., Derakshan, N., Waters, A.M., & Logies, S. (2004). Snakes and cats in the flower bed: Fast detection is not specific to pictures of fear-relevant animals. *Emotion*, *4*, 233-250.

Livingstone, M.S., & Hubel, D.H. (1987). Connections between layer 4B of area 17 and the thick cytochrome oxidase stripes of area 18 in the squirrel monkey. *The Journal of Neuroscience*, *7*, 3371-3377.

Lleras, A., & Enns, J.T. (2005). Updating a cautionary tale of masked priming: Reply to Klapp (2005). *Journal of Experimental Psychology: General*, *134*, 436-440.

LoBue, V. (2010a). And along came a spider: An attentional bias for the detection of spiders in young children and adults. Journal *of Experimental Child Psychology*, *107*, 59-66.

LoBue, V. (2010b). What's so scary about needles and knives? Examining the role of experience in threat detection. *Cognition & Emotion*, *24*, 180-187.

LoBue, V., & DeLoache, J.S. (2008). Detecting the snake in the grass: Attention to fear-relevant stimuli by adults and young children. *Psychological Science*, *19*, 284-289.

LoBue, V., & DeLoache, J.S. (2010). Superior detection of threat-relevant stimuli in infancy. *Developmental Science*, *13*, 221-228.

LoBue, V., & DeLoache, J.S. (2011). What's so special about slithering serpents? Children and adults rapidly detect snakes based on their simple features. *Visual Cognition*, *19*, 129-143.

LoBue, V., Rakison, D.H., & DeLoache, J.S. (2010). Threat perception across the lifespan: Evidence for multiple converging pathways. *Current Directions in Psychological Science*, *19*, 375-379.

Lustig, C., Hasher, L., & Zacks, R. (2007). Inhibitory deficit theory: Recent developments in a ,New view‘. In D.S. Gorfein & C. M. McLeod (Eds.), *Inhibition in cognition* (pp. 145-162). Washington, DC: American Psychological Association.

Machado, L., Wyatt, N., Devine, A., & Knight, B. (2007). Action planning in the presence of distracting stimuli: An investigation into the time course of distractor effects. *Journal of Experimental Psychology: Human Perception and Performance, 33*, 1045-1061.

Mattler, U. (2005). Inhibition and decay of motor and nonmotor priming. *Perception & Psychophysics, 67*, 285-300.

Mattler, U. (2006). On the locus of priming and inverse priming effects. *Perception & Psychophysics, 68*, 975-991.

Mattler, U. (2007). Inverse target-and cue-priming effects of masked stimuli. *Journal of Experimental Psychology: Human Perception and Performance, 33*, 83-102.

Mattler, U., & Fendrich, R. (2007). Priming by motion too rapid to be consciously seen. *Perception & Psychophysics, 69*, 1389-1398.

Mayr, E. (2001). *What evolution is.* New York: Basic Books.

McLeod, P. (1996). Preserved and impaired detection of structure from motion by a 'motion-blind' patient. *Visual Cognition, 3*, 363-392.

Mogg, K., Bradley, B.P., Hyare, H., & Lee, S. (1998). Selective attention to food-related stimuli in hunger: are attentional biases specific to emotional and psychopathological states, or are they also found in normal drive states? *Behaviour Research and Therapy, 36*, 227-237.

Neumann, O., & Klotz, W. (1994). Motor responses to nonreportable, masked stimuli: Where is the limit of direct parameter specification. In C. Umiltà & M. Moscovitch (Eds.), *Attention and performance XV: Conscious and nonconscious information processing* (pp. 123-150). Cambridge, Mass.: MIT Press.

New, J., Cosmides, L., & Tooby, J. (2007). Category-specific attention for animals reflects ancestral priorities, not expertise. *Proceedings of the National Academy of Sciences, 104*, 16598-16603.

Newsome, W.T., & Paré E.B. (1988). A selective impairment of motion perception following lesions of the middle temporal visual area (MT). *The Journal of Neuroscience, 8*, 2201-2211.

O'Craven, K.M., Rosen, B.R., Kwong, K.K., Treisman, A., & Savoy, R.L. (1997). Voluntary attention modulates fMRI activity in human MT–MST. *Neuron, 18*, 591-598.

Öhman, A., & Mineka, S. (2003). The malicious serpent: Snakes as a prototypical stimulus for an evolved module of fear. *Current Directions in Psychological Science, 12*, 5-9

Öhman, A. (2007). Has evolution primed humans to 'beware the beast'? *Proceedings of the National Academy of Sciences, 104*, 16396-16397.

Öhman, A., Flykt, A., & Esteves, F. (2001). Emotion drive attention: Detecting the snake in the grass. *Journal of Experimental Psychology: General, 130*, 466-478.

Penkunas, M.J. & Coss, R.G. (2013a). Rapid detection of visually provocative animals by preschool children and adults. *Journal of Experimental Child Psychology, 114*, 522-536

Penkunas, M.J. & Coss, R.G. (2013b). A comparison of rural and urban Indian children's isual detection of threatening and nonthreatening animals. *Developmental Science, 16*, 463-475.

Praamstra, P., & Seiss, E. (2005). The neurophysiology of response competition: Motor cortex activation and inhibition following subliminal response priming. *Journal of Cognitive Neuroscience*, *17*, 483-493.

Rakison, D.H., & Derringer, J. (2008). Do infants possess an evolved spider-detection mechanisms? *Cognition*, *107*, 381-393.

Rakison, D.H. (2009). Does women's greater fear of snakes and spiders originate in infancy? *Evolution and Human Behavior*, *30*, 438-444.

Ramachandran, V.S., & Anstis, S.M. (1983). Displacement thresholds for coherent apparent motion in random dot-patterns. *Vision Research*, *23*, 1719-1724.

Raymond, J.E. (2000). Attentional modulation of visual motion perception. *Trends in Cognitive Sciences*, *4*, 42-50.

Raymond, J.E., O'Donnell, H.L., & Tipper, S.P. (1998). Priming reveals attentional modulation of human motion sensitivity. *Vision Research*, *38*, 2863-2867.

Sarkheil, P., Vuong, Q.C., Bülthoff, H.H., & Noppeney, U. (2008). The integration of higher order form and motion by the human brain. *Neuroimage*, *42*, 1529-1536.

Saygin, A.P., Wilson, S.M., Hagler, D.J., Bates, E., & Sereno, M.I. (2004). Point-light biological motion perception activates human premotor cortex. *The Journal of Neuroscience*, *24*, 6181-6188.

Schlaghecken, F., & Eimer, M. (2002). Motor activation with and without inhibition: Evidence for a threshold mechanism in motor control. *Perception & Psychophysics*, *64*, 148-162.

Schlaghecken, F., Klapp, S.T., & Maylor, E.A. (2009). Either or neither, but not both: Locating the effects of masked primes. *Proceedings of the Royal Society B: Biological Sciences*, *276*, 515-521.

Schlaghecken, F., & Maylor, E.A. (2005). Motor control in old age: Evidence of impaired low-level inhibition. *Journal of Gerontology: Psychological Sciences*, *60B*, 158-161.

Schmidt, T. (2000). Visual perception without awareness: Priming responses by color. In T. Metzinger (Ed.), *Neural correlates of consciousness: Empirical and conceptual questions* (pp. 157-179). Cambridge, Mass.: MIT Press.

Schmidt, T. (2002). The finger in flight: Real-time motor control by visually masked color stimuli. *Psychological Science*, *13*, 112-118.

Schmidt, F., Haberkamp, A., & Schmidt, T. (2011). Dos and don'ts in response priming research. *Advances in Cognitive Psychology*, *7*, 120-131.

Seligman, M. E. (1971). Phobias and preparedness. *Behavior Therapy*, *2*, 307-320.

Shi, J., Weng, X., He, S., & Jiang, Y. (2010). Biological motion cues trigger reflexive attentional orienting. *Cognition*, *117*, 348-354.

Simion, F., Regolin, L., & Bulf, H. (2008). A predisposition for biological motion in the newborn baby. *Proceedings of the National Academy of Sciences*, *105*(2), 809-813.

Sumner, P. (2007). Negative and positive masked-priming–implications for motor inhibition. *Advances in Cognitive Psychology*, *3*, 317.

Thornton, I. M., & Vuong, Q. C. (2004). Incidental processing of biological motion. *Current Biology*, *14*, 1084-1089.

Treue, S, Maunsell. J. H. R., (1996) Attentional modulation of visual motion processing in cortical areas MT and MST. *Nature, 382*, 539–541.

Troje, N.F. (2008). Biological motion perception. In A.I. Basbaum, M.C. Bushnell, D.V. Smith, G.K. Beauchamp, S.J. Firestein, P. Dallos, D. Oertel, R.H. Masland, T.D.

Albright, J.H. Kaas & E.P. Gardner (Eds.), *The senses: A comprehensive references* (Vol. 2, pp. 231-238). New York: Academic.

Tukey, J.W. (1977). *Exploratory data analysis*. Reading, MA: Addison-Wesley.

Ungerleider, L.G., & Mishkin, M. (1982). Two coartical visual systems. In D. J. Ingle, M. A. Goodale, & R.J.W. Mansfield (Eds.), *Analysis of visual behavior* (pp. 549-586). Cambridge, MA: MIT Press.

Vaina, L.M., Lemay, M., Bienfang, D.C., Choi, A.Y., & Nakayama, K. (1990). Intact 'biological motion' and 'structure from motion' perception in a patient with impaired motion mechanisms: A case study. *Visual Neuroscience, 5*, 353-369.

Vaina, L.M., Solomon, J., Chowdhury, S., Sinha, P., & Belliveau, J.W. (2001). Functional neuroanatomy of biological motion perception in humans. *Proceedings of the National Academy of Sciences, 98*, 11656-11661.

Verleger, R., Jaśkowski, P., Aydemir, A., Van der Lubbe, R., & Groen, M. (2004). Qualitative differences between conscious and non-conscious processing? On negative and positive priming effects induced by masked arrows. *Journal of Experimental Psychology: General, 133*, 494-515.

Vorberg, D., Mattler, U., Heinecke, A., Schmidt, T., & Schwarzbach, J. (2003). Different time courses for visual perception and action priming. *Proceedings of the National Academy of Sciences, 100*, 6275-6280.

Vorberg, D., Mattler, U., Heinecke, A., Schmidt, T., & Schwarzbach, J. (2004). Invariant time course of priming with and without awareness. In C. Kaernbach, E. Schröger, & H. Müller (Eds.), *Psychophysics beyond sensation: Laws and invariants of human cognition* (pp. 271-288). Mahwah, NJ: Erlbaum.

Wang, L., Yang, X., Shi, J., & Jiang, Y. (2014). The feet have it: Local biological motion cues trigger reflexive attentional orienting in the brain. *NeuroImage, 84,* 217-224.

Warren, W.H. (2006). The dynamics of perception and action. *Psychological Review, 113*, 358-389.

Werthheimer, M. (1912). Experimentelle Studien über das Sehen von Bewegung. *Zeitschrift für Psychologie, 61*, 161-265.

Wickelgren, L.W. (1969). The ocular response of human newborns to intermittent visual movement. *Journal of Experimental Child Psychology, 8*, 469-482.

In: Advances in Visual Perception Research
Editor: Thomas Heinen

ISBN: 978-1-63482-455-2
© 2015 Nova Science Publishers, Inc.

Chapter 2

Accuracy and Bias in Emotion Perception Predict Affective Response to Relationship Conflict

William J. Brady and Emily Balcetis*
New York University, US

Abstract

Facial expressions of emotions are a communicative tool in relationships. We argue that given expressions' impact on social experiences, individual differences in people's abilities to read others' emotional expressions may predict affective reactions to conflict. We theoretically distinguish between emotion perception accuracy and bias, and describe when these two perceptual abilities apply to the perception of facial displays. We then present data from a preliminary study testing the impact of emotion perception accuracy and bias on affective reactions people have during stages of conflict. While only conflict severity predicted negative affect experience in the stages prior to a fight, bias predicted negative affect during conflict and the ability to recover from conflict. Accuracy predicted negative felt affect after conflict. Implications for the study of emotion perception and relationship quality are discussed.

Keywords: Emotion, facial expression, ambiguous perception, identification, interpretation, regulation, recovery

* 6 Washington Place, Psychology Dept, New York University, New York, NY 10003. Email: emilybalcetis@nyu.edu

Introduction

Recent statistics indicate that 62% of first marriages and non-married cohabitations end within 10 years (Copen, Daniels, Vespa, & Mosher, 2012). While relationship dissolution arises for various reasons, the manner in which couples communicate their emotions to one another and interpret one another's emotions stands as a key predictor of relationship quality and decisions to terminate them (e.g. Gaelic, Bodenhausen, & Wyer, 1985; Gottman & Levenson, 1986; Noller & Gallois, 1986). For instance, couples who are highly inaccurate when interpreting the message and affective tone their partners intend to communicate tend to experience less satisfying relationships (e.g., Noller & Venardos, 1986; Noller & Ruzzene, 1991; Koerner & Fitzpatrick, 2002). Moreover, individuals' self-reported accuracy in judging their partners' emotions predicts relationship dissatisfaction; those who believe themselves to be poor judges of their partners' emotions are less satisfied than others (e.g. Schutte et. al, 2001; Brackett, Warner, & Bosco, 2005; Smith, Heaven, & Ciarrochi, 2008). Given that facial expressions of emotion serve as a primary means of communicating emotions to others (Darwin, 1872/1998; Ekman, Friesen, & Ancoli, 1980; Mayer, DiPaolo, & Salovey, 1990) and the nuanced emotional lives of couples best predicts the longevity of their relationship (e.g. Gottman, 2014), couples' abilities to discern emotions may serve as a distinctive diagnostic tool for assessing relationship quality.

However, challenges remain when using individual differences in emotion perception to describe the quality and foreshadow the future of relationships. For instance, people's self-reported abilities do not necessarily coincide with actually abilities. While people may believe themselves to be precise observers of the emotional states of their partners, such beliefs about the self may in fact be erroneous, particularly when people are motivated to hold certain beliefs about their own skills and intentions (e.g. Dunning, 2010). Moreover, these beliefs in personal abilities to intuit others' emotions do not necessarily measure actual perceptual abilities. Indeed, people with the poorest skills may be least able to intuit how accurate or inaccurate they actually are (e.g. Kruger & Dunning, 1999).

Defining Emotion Perception through Visual Perception

Given that self-reported abilities to understand the emotional lives of one's partner pose complications, we propose that other measures of emotion perception may prove useful when determining the quality of relationships. In particular, we suggest emotion perception be defined through the visual experiences people have when perceiving and interpreting the emotional displays on others' faces. We define emotion perception through visual perception. With this work, we explore measurable differences in the way in which people perceive the facial displays of emotion on others' faces and use specific individual differences in emotion perception to predict the quality of relationships.

Indirect empirical evidence supports our proposition that differences in visual perception of emotional displays may serve as additional predictors of relationship quality. For instance, certain groups of people who experience low levels of satisfaction in their relationships also demonstrate specific patterns of emotion perception. Insecurely attached individuals tend to identify negative emotion expressions more quickly than they identify positive emotion expressions (Niedenthal, Brauer, Robin, & Innes-Ker, 2002; Fraley et. al, 2006), and they report greater relationship dissatisfaction compared to securely attached individuals (Feeny, 2002; Butzer, & Campbell, 2008). Individuals high in neuroticism tend to perceive negative emotions as more intense than positive emotions (Mayer & Salovey, 1988), and they also experience greater relationship dissatisfaction relative to individuals high in extraversion, impulsivity, agreeableness, or conscientiousness (Karney & Bradbury, 1995). Finally, individuals diagnosed with social anxiety disorder tend to perceive negative emotion expressions as more threatening than positive emotion expressions (Phan, Fitzgerald, Nathan, & Tancer, 2006), and also report greater relationship dissatisfaction compared to non-anxious individuals (La Greca & Harrison, 2005). Taken together, these data provide strong, albeit indirect, evidence that visual perception of emotions may be related to relationship quality.

Emotion Perception Accuracy and Bias

Following a rich tradition of interpersonal perception research in social psychology (e.g. Kruglanski, 1989; Kunda, 1990; Kenny & Acitelli, 2001), we suggest that visual perception of emotion can be decomposed into and precisely defined by both emotion perception accuracy and emotion perception bias. These two related, but non-redundant components of the visual perception of emotion may serve to explain unique variation in relationship quality.

Emotion perception *accuracy* is defined as the ability to correctly identify discrete emotions from non-verbal behavior such as facial expressions (Fitness, 2006). Emotion perception accuracy is calculated by comparing the discrepancy between participants' judgments of emotion and a correct judgment of the target. "Correct" identifications can be determined through various means. Some researchers gage accuracy by comparing perceivers' identifications to the discrete emotion as determined by the researcher (e.g. Isaacowitz et al., 2007 for a review), as intended by a target (e.g. Ekman & Friesen, 1971; Salovey & Mayer, 1989), or as indicated by targets' own assessment of their facial expressions when viewing themselves afterwards as if a third-party observer (e.g. Thomas, Fletcher, & Lange, 1997; Koerner & Fitzpatrick, 2002; Zaki, Bolger, & Ochsner, 2009).

Other researchers developed scientific procedures for the standardization of emotion categorization that are used to train third-party coders to determine the correct emotion expression displayed (e.g. Ekman & Friesen, 1976). Through these various methods, emotion perception accuracy reflects the discrepancy between participants' identifications against established correct identifications. In comparison to accuracy, emotion perception *bias* can be defined as a systematic tendency for the perceptual system to privilege certain classes of emotion over others when identifying emotions expressions. Bias can track accuracy in some situations, but in other situations may diverge from accuracy (Kenny & Acitelli, 2001). For example, a negativity bias in which a person tends to identify expressions as negative may increase accuracy in the context of a sad event but decrease accuracy in the context of a happy event. Emotion perception bias is typically measured by comparing the frequency, speed, or intensity with which perceivers categorize facial displays as positive rather than negative. For instance, bias can be measured as discrepancies in reaction time when identifying discrete positive versus negative emotions (Niedenthal et al., 2002). Bias can also be measured as discrepancies in the intensity perceivers ascribe to positive rather than negative emotion expressions (Joorman & Gotlib, 2006). Finally, bias can be measured as a discrepancy in the number of negative versus positive emotions recognized in mixed emotion stimuli (Bouhuys, Geerts, & Gordijn, 1999).

Indeed, individuals vary in the specific emotions they identify in ambiguous displays (Bouhuys et al., 1999), how intense they perceive the emotions (Joorman & Gotlib, 2006), and how complex they perceive them to be (Kellough & Knight, 2012). Rather than noting differences in correct identifications, emotion perception bias quantifies differences in how readily positive or negative emotions come to be consciously experienced. Accuracy and bias may also apply in different instances, as is the case when considering different qualities of facial displays of emotion.

Determinations of accuracy, for instance, require target facial displays afford a correct identification of a discrete emotion, using any of the various methods available. However, not all facial displays of emotion can be discretely categorized. Not all facial expressions assume the properties of a single emotional display. Indeed, natural emotional experiences in and of themselves are vastly complex and heterogeneous (Barrett, Mesquita, Ochsner, & Gross, 2007). For instance, the display of anger and fear share three muscle movements, and surprise shares the same muscle movements as fear, but fear is distinguished by an additional two muscle movements (Ekman & Friesen, 1978). Emotion expressions often send multiple, partially overlapping, or conflicting signals of discrete emotions to the perceiver. As a result, the emotional displays that cross others' faces are complex, multifaceted, and ambiguous. In these cases, determining a correct identification becomes difficult if not arbitrary, as a standard of accuracy is not available. In these instances where accuracy is not applicable, bias still is.

Accuracy and bias are measured in different ways, and can gauge perceptual experiences in response to different classes of expressions. Because they are conceptually distinct, bias may predict unique variation in relationship quality relative to accuracy.

Overview

In order to investigate the importance of emotion perception accuracy and bias in predicting relationship outcomes, we designed a preliminary study to simultaneously measure these perceptual experiences in a normal population of adults to determine the extent to which each predicts unique aspects of relationship quality. We chose to focus on negative affect experienced during a conflict as it is a robust predictor of relationship quality and reliably determines whether relationships survive (Gottman & Levenson, 1992; Carstensen, Gottman & Levenson, 1995; Gottman, Coan, Carrere, & Swanson, 1998). For example, one study found that 50% of couples experiencing a great deal of negative affect divorced within 7 years (Gottman & Levenson, 2000). We used a daily reconstruction method to assist participants in recalling a conflict within their relationship.

This allowed an exploration of the impact of emotion perception accuracy and bias on negative affect experienced at three stages of conflict: before conflict occurred, during conflict, and after conflict ended. In so doing, we could also calculate the impact of emotion perception on regulatory abilities during recovery periods.

Methods

Participants

We recruited participants (N = 310) from Amazon's Mechanical Turk in exchange for 75 cents with the intention of recruiting participants in committed relationships. We excluded data from 37 participants who reported completing the survey by reporting on a conflict with a close friend rather than a committed relationship partner, leaving a final sample of 273 (220 female, 53 male, M_{age} = 35.95, SD = 13.69, age range: 18-74 years). The mean length of relationship was 10.51 years (SD=11.28).

Materials, Measures and Procedure

Measuring Emotion Perception Accuracy

To measure emotion perception accuracy, participants categorized 18 positive and 18 negative posed, non-ambiguous emotion expressions taken from the NimStim stimuli set (Tottenham et. al, 2012; see Figure 1a). Participants indicated whether the face displayed either a positive or negative expression within a 500ms response window.

Participants began each trial by clicking on a button on the bottom of their screen with their mouse, and clicked on a box labeled "positive" or "negative" that appeared on the upper corners of the screen. Between blocks, the location of the labels switched.

Measuring Emotion Perception Bias

To measure emotion perception bias, participants categorized ambiguous emotion expressions. We created ambiguous emotion expressions by blending positive and negative faces of White male and female actors from the NimStim set (Tottenham et. al, 2012) using Abrosoft FantaMorph face morphing software. We blended the positive and negative emotions such that each morphed image contained 50% positive (happiness) and 50% negative (sadness or fear). A separate group of pretest participants (n = 30) reported how intensely negative the expression was (1 = *not at all intense* to 7 = *very intense*). They also reported how intensely positive the expression was using the same scale.

We created a database of 24 ambiguous expressions by selecting photographs that participants rated as both moderately high negative intensity in addition to moderately high positive intensity (see Figure 1b). Moreover, we selected photographs for which the standard deviation of both negative and positive intensity ratings were high. Participants saw 12 different male faces and 12 different female faces; within stimulus gender, they saw 6 morphs of happy and sad and 6 morphs of happy and angry. Participants saw an ambiguous face and categorized it as positive or negative within a 500 ms response window.

Recalling Relationship Conflict

Participants followed a daily reconstruction method (Kahneman, Krueger, Schkade, Schwarz, & Stone, 2004). Participants were randomly assigned to either write in detail about a recent minor conflict or major conflict they experienced with their relationship partner. Participants received instructions to write about three specific episodes that occurred before the conflict began, three that occurred during the conflict, and three that occurred after the conflict subsided.

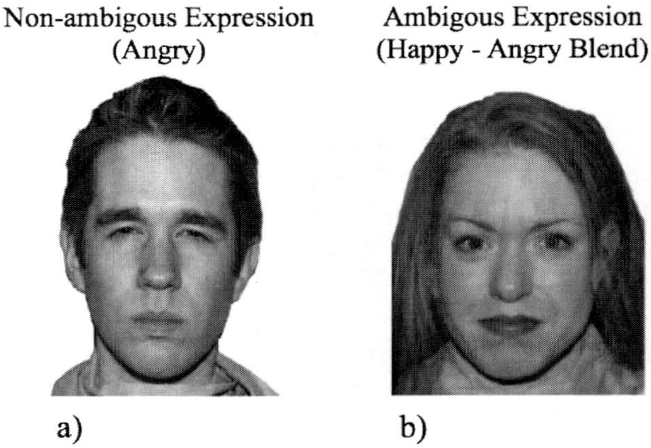

Figure 1. Examples of an (a) unambiguous expression taken from NimStim Set (Tottenham et al., 2012) used in the emotion perception accuracy task and an (b) ambiguous expression we created and used in the emotion perception bias task.

Negative Affect Experienced

We measured the negative affect experienced during conflict by asking participants to report their feelings during each of the nine conflict episodes using the mood subscale of the 9-point Self Assessment Manikin (SAM; Bradley & Lang, 1994). The SAM mood subscale is a non-verbal pictorial array depicting icons that range from a happy, smiling figure to an unhappy, frowning figure; participants selected which of 9 icons bests represented their current affective state. After participants recalled 3 episodes during a particular stage of conflict (e.g. during conflict), they were reminded of each episode individually and reported negative affect during that specific episode using the SAM scale.

Procedure

Participants consented to take part in the online study and then completed a short demographics survey. Next they always completed the emotion perception task, by identifying clear and ambiguous expressions as either positive or negative. Then, participants completed an ostensibly unrelated survey describing a conflict experienced in one close relationship using the daily reconstruction method. During this reconstruction, participants rated how each episode of the conflict made them feel using the SAM mood scale. Finally, participants were debriefed.

Data Analysis

Emotion Perception Accuracy Scores. To create an index of emotion perception accuracy, we calculated the percent of unambiguous faces correctly categorized as positive and the percent correctly categorized as negative faces. We subtracted accuracy rates when categorizing negative faces from accuracy rates when categorizing positive faces. Positive values indicated relatively greater accuracy for positive faces, while negative values indicated relatively greater accuracy for negative faces.

Emotion Perception Bias Scores. To create an index of emotion perception bias, we calculated the number of ambiguous emotion expressions identified as negative and subtracted this from the number of ambiguous emotion expressions identified as positive. Positive scores indicate a relatively greater tendency to interpret ambiguous faces as positive, while negative scores indicate a relatively greater tendency to interpret ambiguous faces as negative.

Relationship Conflict Severity Scores. To create a measure of conflict severity, research assistants coded each of the 9 episodes from the daily reconstruction task for severity of the topic (1 = *not serious at all*, 7 = *extremely serious*). We summed the three conflict severity ratings within each stage of conflict, and then computed the average across these stages to create a single index of the conflict severity. Because we gave participants minimal prompting regarding the type of issue on which they should report, the severity of those conflict topics varied tremendously as illustrated by the severity index (conflict severity range = 1-18, out of possible range of 1-21). For analyses, we elected to use the continuous index of conflict severity.

Negative Affect Scores. To create an index of negative affect experienced before, during and after conflict, we used responses to the SAM scale; we averaged each of the episodic negative affect scores within each conflict stage, creating an index of negative affect experienced during each stage of the conflict. Each stage of the conflict therefore consisted of 3 SAM mood ratings, which we summed.

Results

Descriptives

Relationships among all continuous variables, reported as zero-order correlations, appear in Table 1.

Table 1. Means, standard deviations, and correlations for variables

Variable	*M*	*SD*	1	2	3	4	5	6
1. Conflict Severity	10.20	3.47						
2. Emotion Perception Bias	-.01	12.69	-.116†					
3. Emotion Perception Accuracy	-14.70	0.03	-.071	.250**				
4. Negative Affect – Before	6.00	1.84	.408**	-.116†	-.033			
5. Negative Affect – During	7.11	1.60	.403**	-.159**	-.104†	.504**		
6. Negative Affect – After	5.45	2.23	.401**	-.102†	-.142*	.231**	.398**	
7. Recovery	.71	0.89	-.165**	-.002	-.083	.066	.073	-.174**

$^{\dagger}p < .10$ $^{*}p < .05$ $^{**}p < .01$.

Predicting Negative Affective Experience

Predicting Negative Affect Felt before Conflict

We first tested whether individual differences in emotion perception accuracy or bias predicted negative affect felt before conflict occurred. We regressed the mood index reported before conflict occurred on emotion perception accuracy scores, emotion perception bias scores, conflict severity, and two-way interactions with conflict severity. The model was significant, $R^2 = .17$, $F(5, 267) = 11.20$, $p < .001$. Only conflict severity significantly predicted mood in the moments leading up to conflict, $b = .21$, $SE = 0.03$, $t(267) = 6.98$, $p < .001$. Accuracy did not predict negative mood before conflict, $b = 0.90$, $SE = 3.20$, $t(267) = 0.27$, $p = .79$, nor did bias, $b = -0.01$, $SE = 0.01$, $t(267) = -1.24$, $p = .22$. No interactions between conflict and either bias or accuracy were found, $t(267) = 0.002$, $p = .44$, $t(267) = -.34$, $p = .75$, respectively. People felt worse when in the beginning stages of a more severe, as opposed to less severe conflict.

Predicting Negative Affect Felt during Conflict

We explored whether emotion perception accuracy and bias predict negative affect experienced during conflict. We regressed the mood index reported during conflict on emotion perception accuracy scores, emotion perception bias scores, conflict severity, and 2-way interactions with conflict severity. The model was significant, $R^2 = .17$, $F(5, 267) = 12.61$, $p < .001$. Conflict severity was a significant predictor of negative affect experienced during conflict, $b = 0.18$, $SE = 0.03$, $t(267) = 6.96$, $p < .001$. Emotion perception bias was a marginally significant predictor of negative affect experienced during conflict, $b = -0.01$, $SE = 0.01$, $t(267) = -1.77$, $p = .09$; individuals with stronger negativity biases tended to report greater negative affect during conflict.

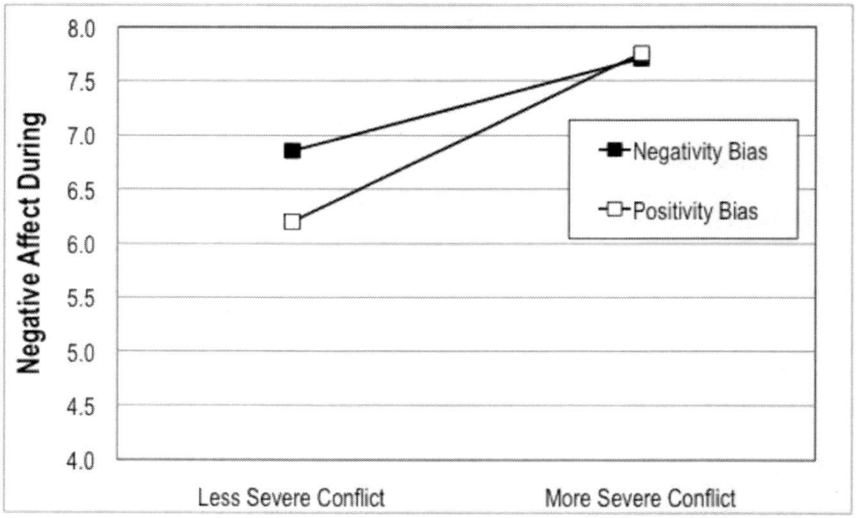

Figure 2. Negative affect experienced during conflict as a function of conflict severity (plotted at -1 SD and +1 SD from mean severity) and emotion perception bias (plotted at +1 SD indicating a positivity bias and -1SD indicating a negativity bias).

The main effect of emotion perception accuracy was not significant, $b = -2.70$, $SE = 2.86$, $t(267) = -0.95$, $p = .35$. The main effect of emotion perception bias was qualified by a significant interaction between emotion perception bias and conflict severity, $b = 0.01$, $SE = 0.02$, $t(267) = 1.93$, $p = .05$. When conflict was less severe, negativity bias predicted more negative affect experienced during conflict than did positivity bias, point slope: $t(267) = -8.50$, $p < .001$. However, when the conflict was more severe, negativity and positivity biases led to the same levels of experienced negative affect, point slope: $t(267) = 0.60$, $p = .55$, see Figure 2. In addition to conflict severity, emotion perception bias rather than accuracy predicted negative affect experienced during conflict.

Predicting Negative Affect Felt after Conflict

We explored whether emotion perception accuracy and bias predict negative affect experienced after conflict. We regressed the mood index reported after conflict on emotion perception accuracy scores, emotion perception bias scores, conflict severity, and 2-way interactions with conflict severity. Because no interactions between conflict severity and bias, $t(267) = 1.18$, $p = .24$, or conflict severity and accuracy were significant, $t(267) = -1.26$, $p = .21$, and as the model with interactions did not account for significantly more variation than the model without them, $\Delta R^2 = .01$, $F(2, 267) = 1.10$, $p = .33$, we reran the model excluding interaction terms.

A model regressing mood index on accuracy, bias, and conflict severity was significant, $R^2 = .17$, $F(3, 269) = 18.90$, $p < .001$. Conflict severity predicted negative affect experienced after conflict, $b = 0.25$, $SE = .04$, $t(269) = 6.98$, $p < .001$. Emotion perception accuracy marginally predicted negative affect, $b = -7.29$, $SE = 3.93$, $t(269) = -1.86$, $p = .065$, such that the more accurately participants could identify negative expressions, the stronger they experienced negative affect after the conflict subsided. Emotion perception bias did not predict negative affect, $b = -0.01$, $SE = 3.93$, $t(269) = -0.52$, $p = .60$. Accuracy and not bias predicted negative affect after conflict.

Predicting Recovery

We created a recovery index by calculating the drop in negative affect experienced after conflict relative to negative affect experienced during conflict (Recovery = $(\text{MoodIndex}_{\text{During}} - \text{MoodIndex}_{\text{After}}) / \text{MoodIndex}_{\text{During}}$). We regressed recovery on emotion perception accuracy, bias, conflict severity, and 2-way interactions with conflict severity. The overall model was significant, $R^2 = .17$, $F(5, 269) = 3.08$, $p = .01$. Accuracy did not predict recovery, $b = -2.25$, $SE = 0.02$, $t(267) = -1.32$, $p = .19$. Bias also did not predict recovery, $b = <.001$, $SE < .001$, $t(267) = .06$, $p = .949$. The interaction between conflict severity and accuracy was not significant, $b = -0.88$, $SE = .55$, $t(267) = -1.60$, $p = .11$.

However, the interaction between conflict severity and bias did predict recovery, $b < .001$, $SE = 0.01$, $t(267) = 2.09$, $p = .04$, see Figure 3. Individuals with a negativity bias in emotion perception showed poorer recovery when conflicts were more severe compared to less severe, simple slope: $b = -0.07$, $t(272) = -5.24$, $p < .001$.

However, individuals with a positivity bias showed resilience, in that their recovery did not depend on the severity of the conflict, simple slope: $b = -0.02$, $t(272) = -1.56$, $p = .12$. Individuals with a positivity bias tended to recover equally well regardless of the severity of the conflict.

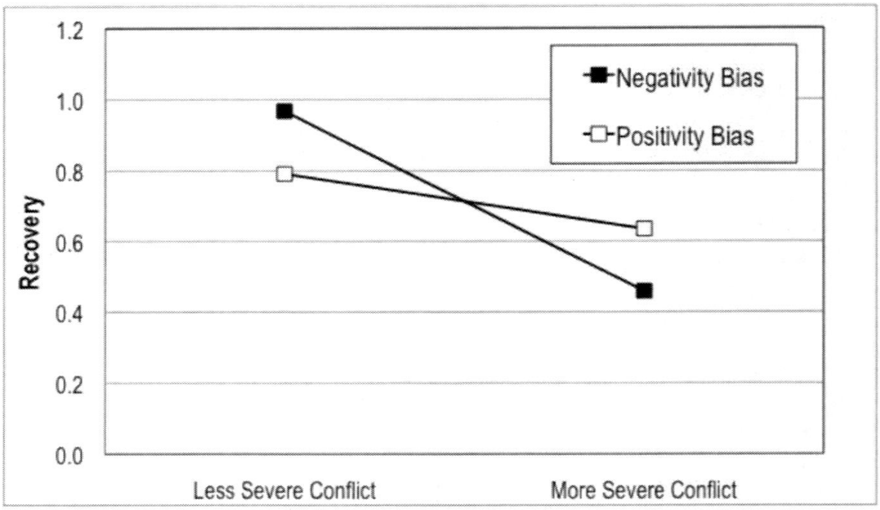

Figure 3. Recovery experienced from during to after conflict as a function of conflict severity (plotted at -1 SD and +1 SD from mean severity) and emotion perception bias (plotted at +1 SD indicating a positivity bias and -1SD indicating a negativity bias).

Discussion

Individual differences in visual perception of emotional expressions affects the health of relationships. A complete understanding of visual experience requires considering both emotion perception accuracy and bias. When expressions are discrete and afford correct identification, accuracy applies. When expressions are comprised of multiple, competing emotional signals, bias applies. With this work we explored whether these two conceptually distinct perceptual processes uniquely affect reactions during different stages of conflict development.

Indeed they do. When entered simultaneously in models of negative affect experienced during conflict, emotion perception bias and not accuracy predicted variation how individuals felt during conflict and their ability to recover from conflict. People with a positivity bias showed resilience; the ability to recover remained stable even in more severe conflicts. These results suggest emotion perception bias may serve as an effective tool for emotion regulation. While the reason for their resilience is unclear in this study, it is possible that people demonstrating a positivity bias in emotion perception may shift attention away from visual cues suggesting negative emotions (e.g. the frown) or may automatically employ successful regulatory strategies, like distraction or reappraisal (cf. Mauss, Bunge & Gross, 2007).

Juxtaposed against these results, emotion perception accuracy rather than bias predicted affective reactions after the conflict ended. People with greater accuracy at identifying negative emotions than positive emotions felt worse after conflict than people who were more accurate at identifying positive emotions. These data are consistent with previous work suggesting that couples experiencing a threat felt dissatisfied with their relationship the more accurately they perceived emotional expressions (e.g. Sillars, Pike, Jones, & Murphy, 1984; Simpson, Oriña & Ickes, 2003). While it remains to be tested, it is possible that individuals who accurately identify negative emotions may be more likely to realize ineffectual attempts at resolution and a partner's residual negative reactions.

Future Research

Bias predicted affective responses during conflict. We conjecture that heightened states of arousal place the perceptual system under stress. Arousal impacts perceptual processing, leading to increased sensitivity for threatening components of environments (Shields, Larson, Swartz, & Smith, 2011) and affecting how negative information, specifically, is perceived (Mathews & Mackintosh, 2004). To fully test this physiological account, future research should map physiological profiles during conflict and test variables that moderate the likelihood of bias or accuracy to better predict affective reactions during conflict development. Adding emotion perception bias, in particular, to models of relationship quality may also promote an ecological approach to understanding responses to conflict. Bias quantifies interpretations of facial displays that lack a correct identification, and exposure to these types of emotional displays may arise far more often than displays of discrete emotions during real social interactions. Emotional displays during conflict are likely quite complex due to the multifarious nature of thoughts, emotions, and reactions people have when arguing. Even outside of arguments, emotional signals are not always clear. Expressions do not necessarily map on to emotional states people experience; happy states are expressed with smiles and sad states are expressed with frowns far less frequently than intuition would suggest (see Russell, Bachorowski, & Fernández-dols, 2003). Bias may serve as an ecologically valid indicator of reactions to conflict given bias' relevance to the expressions to which people are actually more frequently exposed. As models that integrate visual perception of emotion grow, researchers may find that individual differences in emotion perception, the severity of conflict, and the intensity of the affective responses to conflict are reciprocally related. Our data suggest that variation in negative affect experienced during conflict can be predicted from the visual experiences people have when looking at others. Existing research supports other directional effects; people with chronically volatile emotional lives experience conflict as more severe (Kiecolt-Glaser, Newton et al., 1996). Moreover, interpretations of facial expressions as negative may arise through repeated exposure to hostile expressions, given that interpretation of ambiguous visual stimuli can be predicted by the content, recency, and frequency of previous visual experiences (e.g. Bugelski & Alampay, 1961; Balcetis & Dale, 2007; Epstein & Rock, 1960). Although we conceptualized perceptual experiences and conflict severity as predictors of affective reactions to fights, they are likely dynamically related.

Conclusion

Committed relationships buffer against psychological and physiological problems (Coyne & Downey, 1991; Waldron, Hughes, & Brookes, 1996; Holt-Lundstad, Smith, & Layton, 2008), but the consequences of conflict in relationships can be detrimental. Conflict contributes to psychopathological conditions such as depression (Beach et al., 1998), eating disorders (Norre, Van den Broucke, & Vandereycken, 2006), and alcohol abuse (O'Farrell, Choquette, & Birchler, 1991). Our conceptual model distinguishing emotion perception bias and accuracy, and these preliminary data, offer visual perception of emotion as an additional factor that identifies relationships in need of repair. Demarcating couples that experience specific, systematic errors and biases when perceiving emotional expressions may serve useful when designing tools to diagnose, forewarn, and intervene in relationships before they dissolve.

Acknowledgments

We thank Jon Freeman, Zach Ingbretsen, Caroline Christianson, and Jonathan Stahl for assistance creating the study included in this manuscript.

References

Balcetis, E., & Dale, R. (2007). Conceptual set as a top-down constraint on visual object identification. *Perception*, *36*(4), 581-595.

Barrett, L. F., Mesquita, B., Ochsner, K. N., & Gross, J. J. (2007). The experience of emotion. *Annual Review of Psychology*, *58*, 373-403.

Beach, S. R., Tesser, A., Fincham, F. D., Jones, D. J., Johnson, D., & Whitaker, D. J. (1998). Pleasure and pain in doing well, together: an investigation of performance-related affect in close relationships. *Journal of Personality and Social Psychology*, *74*(4), 923-938.

Bouhuys, A. L., Geerts, E., & Gordijn, M. C. (1999). Depressed patients' perceptions of facial emotions in depressed and remitted states are associated with relapse: a longitudinal study. *The Journal of Nervous and Mental Disease*, *187*(10), 595-602.

Brackett, M. A., Warner, R. M., & Bosco, J. S. (2005). Emotional intelligence and relationship quality among couples. *Personal Relationships*, *12*(2), 197-212.

Bradley, M. M., & Lang, P. J. (1994). Measuring emotion: the self-assessment manikin and the semantic differential. *Journal of Behavior Therapy and Experimental Psychiatry*, *25*(1), 49-59.

Bugelski, B. R., & Alampay, D. A. (1961). The role of frequency in developing perceptual sets. *Canadian Journal of Psychology/Revue Canadienne de Psychologie*, *15*(4), 205-211.

Butzer, B., & Campbell, L. (2008). Adult attachment, sexual satisfaction, and relationship satisfaction: A study of married couples. *Personal Relationships*, *15*(1), 141-154.

Carstensen, L. L., Gottman, J. M., & Levenson, R. W. (1995). Emotional behavior in long-term marriage. *Psychology and Aging*. *10*(1). 140-149.

Copen, C. E., Daniels, K., Vespa, J., & Mosher, W. D. First marriages in the United States: Data from the 2006–2010 National Survey of Family Growth. National health statistics reports; no 49. Hyattsville, MD: National Center for Health Statistics. 2012.

Coyne, J. C., & Downey, G. (1991). Social factors and psychopathology: Stress, social support, and coping processes. *Annual Review of Psychology*, *42*(1), 401-425.

Darwin, C. (1998). *The expression of the emotions in man and animals*. Oxford University Press.

Dunning, D. (2010). *Social motivation*. New York: Psychology Press.

Ekman, P., & Friesen, W. V. (1971). Constants across cultures in the face and emotion. *Journal of Personality and Social Psychology*, *17*(2), 124-129

Ekman, P., & Friesen, W. V. (1976). Measuring facial movement. *Environmental Psychology and Nonverbal Behavior*, *1*(1), 56-75.

Ekman, P., & Friesen, W. V. (1978). *Manual for the Facial Action Coding System*. Consulting Psychologists Press.

Ekman, P., Friesen, W. V., & Ancoli, S. (1980). Facial signs of emotional experience. *Journal of Personality and Social Psychology*, *39*(6), 1125-1134.

Epstein, W., & Rock, I. (1960). Perceptual set as an artifact of recency. *The American Journal of Psychology*, *73*(2), 214-228.

Feeney, J. A. (2002). Attachment, marital interaction, and relationship satisfaction: A diary study. *Personal Relationships*, *9*(1), 39-55.

Fitness, J. (2006). The emotionally intelligent marriage. In J. Ciarrochi, J. P. Forgas, & J. D. Mayer (Eds.), Emotional intelligence in everyday life (2nd ed., pp. 129–139). New York: Psychology Press.

Fraley, R., Niedenthal, P. M., Marks, M., Brumbaugh, C., & Vicary, A. (2006). Adult attachment and the perception of emotional expressions: Probing the hyperactivating strategies underlying anxious attachment. *Journal of Personality*, *74*(4), 1163-1190.

Gaelick, L., Bodenhausen, G. V., & Wyer, R. S. (1985). Emotional communication in close relationships. *Journal of Personality and Social Psychology*, *49*(5), 1246-1265.

Gottman, J. M. (2014). *What predicts divorce?: The relationship between marital processes and marital outcomes*. Psychology Press.

Gottman, J. M., & Levenson, R. W. (1986). Assessing the role of emotion in marriage. *Behavioral Assessment*, *8*(1), 31-48.

Gottman, J. M., & Levenson, R. W. (1992). Marital processes predictive of later dissolution: behavior, physiology, and health. *Journal of Personality and Social Psychology*, *63*(2), 221-233.

Gottman, J. M., & Levenson, R. W. (2000). The timing of divorce: Predicting when a couple will divorce over a 14-year period. *Journal of Marriage and Family*, *62*(3), 737-745.

Holt-Lunstad, J., Smith, T. B., & Layton, J. B. (2010). Social relationships and mortality risk: a meta-analytic review. *PLoS Medicine*, *7*(7), e1000316.

Isaacowitz, D. M., Löckenhoff, C. E., Lane, R. D., Wright, R., Sechrest, L., Riedel, R., & Costa, P. T. (2007). Age differences in recognition of emotion in lexical stimuli and facial expressions. *Psychology and Aging*, *22*(1), 147-159.

Joormann, J., & Gotlib, I. H. (2006). Is this happiness I see? Biases in the identification of emotional facial expressions in depression and social phobia. *Journal of Abnormal Psychology*, *115*(4), 705-714.

Kahneman, D., Krueger, A. B., Schkade, D. A., Schwarz, N., & Stone, A. A. (2004). A survey method for characterizing daily life experience: The day reconstruction method. *Science*, *306*(5702), 1776-1780.

Karney, B. R., & Bradbury, T. N. (1995). The longitudinal course of marital quality and stability: A review of theory, methods, and research. *Psychological Bulletin*, *118*(1), 3-34.

Kellough, J. L., & Knight, B. G. (2012). Positivity effects in older adults' perception of facial emotion: The role of future time perspective. *The Journals of Gerontology Series B: Psychological Sciences and Social Sciences*, *67*(2), 150-158.

Kenny, D. A., & Acitelli, L. K. (2001). Accuracy and bias in the perception of the partner in a close relationship. *Journal of Personality and Social Psychology*, *80*(3), 439-448.

Kiecolt-Glaser, J. K., Newton, T., Cacioppo, J. T., MacCallum, R. C., Glaser, R., & Malarkey, W. B. (1996). Marital conflict and endocrine function: Are men really more physiologically affected than women?. *Journal of Consulting and Clinical Psychology*, *64*(2), 324-332.

Koerner, A., & Fitzpatrick, M. (2002). Nonverbal communication and marital adjustment and satisfaction: The role of decoding relationship relevant and relationship irrelevant affect. *Communication Monographs*, *69*(1), 33-51.

Kruger, J., & Dunning, D. (1999). Unskilled and unaware of it: how difficulties in recognizing one's own incompetence lead to inflated self-assessments. *Journal of Personality and Social Psychology*, *77*(6), 1121-1134.

Kruglanski, A. W. (1989). The psychology of being "right": The problem of accuracy in social perception and cognition. *Psychological Bulletin*, *106*(3), 395-409.

Kunda, Z. (1990). The case for motivated reasoning. *Psychological Bulletin*, *108*(3), 480-498.

La Greca, A. M., & Harrison, H. M. (2005). Adolescent peer relations, friendships, and romantic relationships: Do they predict social anxiety and depression?. *Journal of Clinical Child and Adolescent Psychology*, *34*(1), 49-61.

Mathews, A., & Mackintosh, B. (2004). Take a closer look: emotion modifies the boundary extension effect. *Emotion*. *4*(1), 36-45.

Mauss, I. B., Bunge, S. A., & Gross, J. J. (2007). Automatic emotion regulation. *Social and Personality Psychology Compass*, *1*(1), 146-167.

Mayer, J. D., & Salovey, P. (1988). Personality moderates the interaction of mood and cognition. *Affect, Cognition and Social Behavior*, 87-99.

Mayer, J. D., DiPaolo, M., & Salovey, P. (1990). Perceiving affective content in ambiguous visual stimuli: A component of emotional intelligence. *Journal of Personality Assessment*, *54*(3-4), 772-781.

Niedenthal, P. M., Brauer, M., Robin, L., & Innes-Ker, Å. H. (2002). Adult attachment and the perception of facial expression of emotion. *Journal of Personality and Social Psychology*, *82*(3), 419-433.

Noller, P., & Gallois, C. (1986). Sending emotional messages in marriage: Non-verbal behaviour, sex and communication clarity. *British Journal of Social Psychology*, *25*(4), 287-297.

Noller, P., & Ruzzene, M. (1991). Communication in marriage: The influence of affect and cognition. In G. O. Fletcher, & F. D. Fincham (Eds.), *Cognition in Close Relationships* (pp. 203-234). New York: Psychology Press.

Noller, P., & Venardos, C. (1986). Communication awareness in married couples. *Journal of Social and Personal Relationships*, *3*(1), 31-42.

Norre, J., Van den Broucke, S., & Vandereycken, W. (2006). *Eating Disorders and Marital Relationships*. London: Routledge.

O'Farrell, T. J., Choquette, K. A., & Birchler, G. R. (1991). Sexual satisfaction and dissatisfaction in the marital relationships of male alcoholics seeking marital therapy. *Journal of Studies on Alcohol and Drugs*, *52*(5), 441-447.

Phan, K. L., Fitzgerald, D. A., Nathan, P. J., & Tancer, M. E. (2006). Association between amygdala hyperactivity to harsh faces and severity of social anxiety in generalized social phobia. *Biological Psychiatry*, *59*(5), 424-429.

Russell, J. A., Bachorowski, J. A., & Fernández-Dols, J. M. (2003). Facial and vocal expressions of emotion. *Annual Review of Psychology*, *54*(1), 329-349.

Salovey, P., & Mayer, J. D. (1989). Emotional intelligence. *Imagination, Cognition and Personality*, *9*(3), 185-211.

Schutte, N. S., Malouff, J. M., Bobik, C., Coston, T. D., Greeson, C., Jedlicka, C., ... & Wendorf, G. (2001). Emotional intelligence and interpersonal relations. *The Journal of Social Psychology*, *141*(4), 523-536.

Shields, M. R., Larson, C. L., Swartz, A. M., & Smith, J. C. (2011). Visual threat detection during moderate- and high-intensity exercise. *Emotion*, *11*, 572–581.

Sillars, A. L., Pike, G. R., Jones, T. S., & Murphy, M. A. (1984). Communication and understanding in marriage. *Human Communication Research*, *10*(3), 317-350.

Simpson, J. A., Oriña, M. M., & Ickes, W. (2003). When accuracy hurts, and when it helps: a test of the empathic accuracy model in marital interactions. *Journal of Personality and Social Psychology*, *85*(5), 881-893.

Smith, L., Heaven, P. C., & Ciarrochi, J. (2008). Trait emotional intelligence, conflict communication patterns, and relationship satisfaction. *Personality and Individual Differences*, *44*(6), 1314-1325.

Thomas, G., Fletcher, G. J., & Lange, C. (1997). On-line empathic accuracy in marital interaction. *Journal of Personality and Social Psychology*, *72*(4), 839-850.

Tottenham, N., Tanaka, J. W., Leon, A. C., McCarry, T., Nurse, M., Hare, T. A., ... & Nelson, C. (2009). The NimStim set of facial expressions: judgments from untrained research participants. *Psychiatry Research*, *168*(3), 242-249.

Waldron, I., Hughes, M. E., & Brooks, T. L. (1996). Marriage protection and marriage selection—prospective evidence for reciprocal effects of marital status and health. *Social Science & Medicine*, *43*(1), 113-123.

Zaki, J., Bolger, N., & Ochsner, K. (2009). Unpacking the informational bases of empathic accuracy. *Emotion*, *9*(4), 478-487.

In: Advances in Visual Perception Research
Editor: Thomas Heinen

ISBN: 978-1-63482-455-2
© 2015 Nova Science Publishers, Inc.

Chapter 3

Automated Vector-Based Gaze Analysis for Perception-Action Diagnostics

Ralf Kredel*, André Klostermann and Ernst-Joachim Hossner
University of Bern, Switzerland

Abstract

Research on decision making and perception-action coupling in sports often employs video-based mobile eye-tracking systems. However, technical and methodological limitations of currently available commercial systems impair the utilization of those systems according to scientific standards so that gathered data should be interpreted with caution. In this chapter, an automated vector-based system architecture overcoming such limitations is introduced and its performance and accuracy are evaluated. Furthermore, two application scenarios are outlined and, finally, possibilities for future extension are discussed.

Keywords: Gaze analysis, vector-based eye-tracking, perception-action coupling, decision making, sports, implementation, automation, evaluation

Introduction

Over the last decade, research on expert performance has focused on the identification of perceptual-cognitive skills underlying anticipation and decision making in sports (for a review, see Mann, Williams, Ward, & Janelle, 2007). In this vein, two approaches have prevailed that either indirectly or directly examine differences in gaze behavior in video-

* University of Bern, Institute of Sport Science, Alpeneggstr. 22, 3012 Bern, Switzerland. Email: ralf.kredel@ispw.unibe.ch

based anticipation tasks. On the one hand, potentially crucial visual information is spatially or temporally occluded for testing effects on decision making. On the other hand, gaze behavior is directly analyzed by recording eye movements, which are mapped onto a head-fixed scene camera image (for an overview see Farrow & Abernethy, 2007).

However, a surprisingly small number of studies, e.g. Mann, Abernethy, and Farrow (2010), has pursued the second approach of analyzing gaze behavior with mobile eye-tracking equipment in real world settings so far, albeit the setting's adjacence to reality is considered crucial with respect to studying perception-action coupling (Williams, Davids, & Williams, 1999, p. 170). This deficit might be attributed to technical and methodological limitations. First, most mobile eye-tracking systems only allow for very restricted mobility since participants either are directly connected to recording devices containing heavy battery packs or need to stay close to a desktop computer, as the length of cabling is limited. Second, spatial accuracy of the results is low since the rater-based mappings of the gaze positions to areas of interests are more rough guesses than objective measurements, and errors are further amplified in dynamic situations by inevitable eye tracker movements with respect to the eye. Third, because of the imperfect collocation of the eye and scene cameras (parallax error: Evans, Jacobs, Tarduno, & Pelz, 2012), only a limited depth range is mapped accurately on the scene video stream so that, if not specifically accounted for in the algorithm, spatial analyses of gaze shifts from peripersonal to extrapersonal space should be considered as highly challenging. Fourth, most mobile eye-tracking systems only offer a low temporal resolution, so that thorough analyses of gaze kinematics seem impossible, since saccadic eye movements are fast and highly dynamic (Nyström & Holmqvist, 2010). Fifth and finally, due to the large amount of manual frame-by-frame analysis involved in video-based methods, most studies comprise a small number of participants and trials only, raising the question whether reliability for generalization is assured to a sufficient degree.

Consequently, in order to overcome the problems just mentioned, a technological and methodological shift seems to be needed which is based on measuring gaze behavior by light-weight and non-obstructive eye-tracking systems with high temporal and spatial resolution not suffering from parallax error, while keeping both, stimuli and responses, similar to the real-world demands. Furthermore, in order to guarantee data quality, regular automated checks during data collection need to be implemented in the eye-tracking software, informing the experimenter about the current calibration quality and indicating a need for recalibration. Last, the highly subjective and tedious manual data analysis needs to be replaced by an automated, objective data-to-stimulus assignment process, which would facilitate the analysis of high numbers of participants and trials. Therefore, in the following, the implementation of an eye-tracking and gaze-analysis system fulfilling these criteria will be introduced. Afterwards, experimental system evaluations, application scenarios and possibilities for future extensions of the system will be described.

System Design

To allow for a complete automation of the eye-tracking and analysis process, a methodological shift from video-based capturing to a mathematical representation of gaze seems appropriate (as already proposed by Duchowsky, 2003). With this shift from the direct mapping of the gaze orientation to a gaze position in a video image – as done in classical mobile eye-tracking systems – towards a vector-based representation of gaze, the parallax error, which quantifies the dependence of the measurement's spatial accuracy on the gaze depth relative to a calibration plane, can be eliminated. This is due to the change from determining the gaze position in a video frame towards a mapping procedure where the calculated gaze vector is intersected with the positions of various objects of interest in different depth ranges. In this alternative approach, because of the collocation of the eyeball center and the origin of the gaze vector, different object distances do not exert influence on spatial accuracy of the gaze any longer. Beyond, the mathematical representation makes an additional scene camera dispensable for analysis, opening up the possibility to further reduce the overall weight of the eye-tracking system and allowing for more suitable gaze analyses in highly dynamic sport settings.

More specifically to our setup, the implemented eye tracker hardware consists of a reduced version of the EyeSeeCam developed by Kohlbecher, Bartl, Bardins, and Schneider (2010). Instead of having a scene camera and calibration lasers, the eye tracker is only composed of a single infrared camera, mounted directly on the goggles' frame, which renders the system very lightweight (Figure 1, left panel). Due to the camera's Firewire interface, in its current version, participants need to wear a small bum bag with an optical repeater (UniBrain Glass Optical Fiber Repeater-800), necessary for the extension of the Firewire connection to the control laptop, and its power supply.

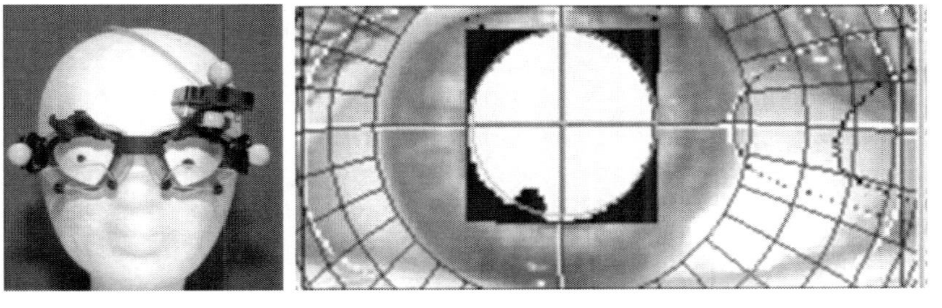

Figure 1. Left panel: Lightweight, monocular EyeSeeCam. Right panel: Extracted pupil center and overlaid eyeball model.

From a mathematical point of view, the gaze vector originates at the center of the eyeball and its orientation is expressed by a rotation matrix, a rotation vector or a quaternion, with respect to a neutral gaze orientation (as already proposed by Haslwanter, 1995). This orientation is calculated by measuring the displacements of the extracted pupil center in the video image plane with respect to a neutral position gazing straight ahead and by using a model of the eyeball, which maps these planar displacements to orientation angles.

As eyeball size and position with respect to the eye tracker cameras are individually different, a calibration routine for the eyeball model is needed in order to estimate these parameters. In our case, this parameter estimation is done by the calibration routine of the EyeSeeCam software (as described in-depth by Kumar, Kohlbecher, & Schneider, 2009), which runs on a control laptop (MacBook Pro, OS X). By processing the obtained video stream (i.e., edge detection, binarization, ellipse fitting and center estimation) and analyzing the planar displacements of the pupil center over a calibration recording, in which the participant needs to repeatedly fixate five different target dots with 8.5° horizontal and vertical spacing (five-point-calibration pattern), the scale factors of the eyeball model are estimated (Figure 1, right panel). After successful calibration, the EyeSeeCam software provides horizontal and vertical eye rotation angles in real-time. Additionally, the calculated angles are mapped on two ports of an analog output card as voltage signals, which can be accessed by third party devices, e.g., by a data acquisition system (DAQ). As the EyeSeeCam system was developed with the real-time control of a gaze-driven camera in mind, low latency of the system was an important design requirement (Schneider et al., 2009). Therefore, the latency from camera input to extraction of the eye rotation angles amounts to 5ms only, while the overall latency from camera input to analog output of the eye rotation angles is reported to be less than 16.5ms (Kohlbecher et al., 2010). In our setting, this low latency is particularly important when taking possible gaze-training applications into account or applications with gaze-driven visual stimuli.

In order to calculate the origin and direction of the gaze vector with respect to a world or laboratory frame of reference while allowing for unconstrained head movements, not only the individually varying neutral gaze orientation and the current eye orientation need to be tracked during calibration and measurement, but also the position of the eyeball's center in space. Assuming that the eyeball center is rather rigidly positioned inside the head and that the eye-tracking goggles remain rigidly attached to the head, a motion capturing system tracking the goggles' position and orientation suffices to fulfill this task. Ideally, the system would support real-time streaming of the acquired data to allow for an easy-to-use online calibration routine without restriction of the head position during the calibration phase. In our setup, we use a 10-camera Vicon T20-System (Oxford Metrics) for this tracking task. Equipped with an additional DAQ interface, which synchronously samples the output ports of the eye tracker's analog card, the Vicon system provides the possibility to access kinematic marker data and analog data in real-time via Ethernet socket connections. Eye rotation angles as well as the goggles' position and orientation and, optionally, further body kinematics are accessible in real-time and can be processed online, e.g., by a Matlab (The Mathworks) script or other custom software. In our case, we implemented a Matlab-based user interface, which simplifies the management and storage of the individual neutral gaze orientations, controls the calculation of the gaze intersection point with the projection screen and renders a graph containing these gaze points on the projection screen. Details of the system's functionality and of the mathematical calculations can be found in Kredel, Lienhard, Klostermann et al. (2011).

Constrictively, one has to mention that assuming a rigid attachment of the eye-tracking goggles to the head is only valid in static situations and as long as no manual touch alters the goggles' position with respect to the head. This precondition, however, can inherently not be assured during normal handling and even less during highly dynamic sport tasks. Therefore, the proposed eye-tracking system needs to constantly monitor the validity of the calibration and eyeball center position with respect to the measured position and orientation, ideally by automated tests during data collection (between experimental trials).

Due to our system's online capabilities, we are able to display stimuli with respect to the current head position and orientation on a large-scale projection screen, which is used to display the five-point-calibration pattern or to adjust the individually varying neutral gaze orientation. As we are also able to display the intersection point of the projected gaze vector with the projection screen (*screen gaze*), we can ask the participants to fixate specific dots on the calibration pattern while evaluating the distance of the screen gaze to the point of the calibration pattern, in other words, we can manually monitor the current accuracy of the system and decide whether recalibration is necessary or not. As this, until now, is still a manual process, we additionally use static fixation points between experimental trials, which gives the opportunity to automatically quantify movements of the goggles with respect to the head (*slippage*) and to calculate correction matrices to account for this systematic error on a trial-by-trial basis. Summing up, the basic functionality of the implemented system can be characterized as follows (see Figure 2): In order to calculate a gaze vector in space, the current orientation of the eye with respect to an individual neutral gaze orientation needs to be tracked, which is done by the EyeSeeCam. To allow for unrestricted head movements, a synchronous acquisition of the eyeball center's reference frame is necessary, specifying its position and orientation in space with respect to a global frame of reference. This can be done with a synchronous acquisition of the eye-tracking goggles' position and orientation by a Vicon system. An extension of this head tracking functionality by additional markers for, e.g., a biomechanical model of the moving participant allows for synchronous recording of gross-scale motion, which, in turn, is relevant to detect movement initiation times or to calculate additional measures related to the motor response. As, in practice, the goggles are not rigidly fixed to the head, online verification of the current tracking and calibration accuracy and, ideally, automated correction routines to account for any slippage have to be implemented between experimental trials.

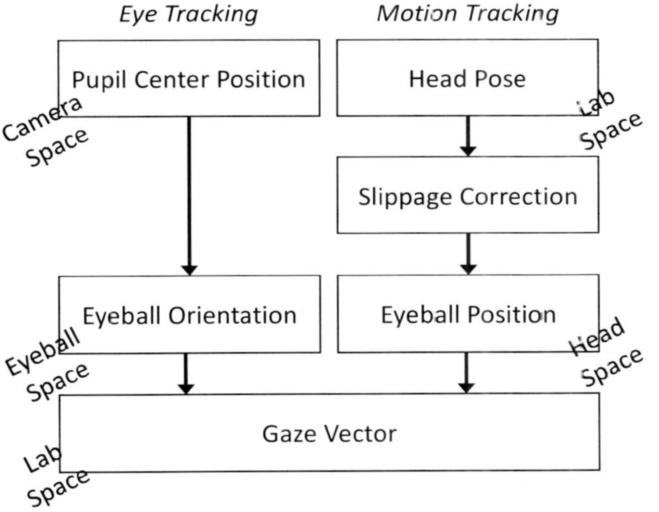

Figure 2. The process of the gaze-vector calculation. The eye tracker records the pupil center in camera space. On the basis of the parameters acquired during calibration, the eye-tracking system calculates eye orientation angles with respect to the eyeball center. By assuming that the eyeball center is rigidly positioned inside the head (or at least that the slippage can be estimated), the head pose in space, simultaneously tracked by the motion capturing system, and a fixed translational offset fully specify the current eyeball position and orientation in lab space. Combined with the eye orientation angles, a gaze vector in space can be calculated.

Evaluation of Performance and Measurement Accuracy

Since the quality of the EyeSeeCam parameter estimation method was unknown and additional error factors for the gaze estimation could have originated from the integration of the tracking system, the overall system's accuracy had to be determined. To this purpose, different calibration and tracking scenarios were analyzed in four experiments with 12 (6 females, 6 males) sport science students of the University of Bern. In the first experiment, effects of the fixation sequence and of the overall calibration duration on the accuracy of the parameter estimation were addressed. With the second experiment, effects of different eye-tracking camera positions on gaze accuracy were checked, and the third and fourth experiment aimed at determining the accuracy of the recalibration procedure and the dynamic accuracy of the gaze vector.

In all experiments, participants were positioned at 3 meters distance from the large-scale projection screen (3 x 2 meters) wearing the EyeSeeCam with additional retroreflective markers tracking its position and orientation in space (see Figure 1, left panel). Participants were instructed to fixate the five displayed dots, which were projected with an 8.5° inter-point distance onto the screen based on the current head pose (five-point-calibration-pattern). As dependent variables, the mean directional errors as well as the mean RMS error of the screen gaze versus the point positions of the displayed 5-point calibration pattern over a 30 seconds measurement interval subsequent to the calibration period were calculated. Manipulation order was counter-balanced and participants repeated each measurement ten times.

In the first experiment, the duration of the calibration routine as well as the sequence order was manipulated. The duration of the calibration routine before parameter estimation was started lasted either 3000 or 6000 valid fixation samples, i.e., measurement points with eye rotation speeds smaller than 5°/s. In sequence "short", the order of fixations was always from the middle dot to the outer dots in a counter-clockwise succession whereas in sequence "long", participants were instructed to fixate the dots in an order, which induces longer saccades compared to the other sequence (see Figure 3).

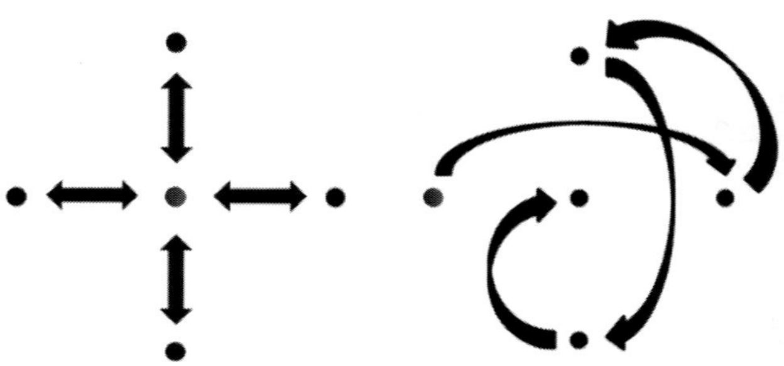

Figure 3. Left panel: Sequence "short", inducing short saccades. Right panel: Sequence "long", inducing long saccades.

The lowest error scores were found for the 3000-samples-short-sequence condition (see Figure 4; $M = 0.86°$, $SE = 0.01°$) with a magnitude, which is comparable to other mobile eye-tracking systems (manufacturer data sheets usually state about 0.5°-1.0° accuracy). However, a great proportion of this error originated from a systematic error in the estimated gaze position. This systematic error could be caused by a mismatch of the actual and measured screen positions, by an offset in the display of the calibration stimuli or by the limiting fact, that the current system configuration used the left eye for gaze estimation only, while the dominant eye of 65-70% of the population is the right eye and therefore might dominate the current gaze location (Roth, Lora, & Heilman, 2002). Irrespective of the actual cause, correcting for this systematic error by subtracting the average directional offset over all conditions, resulted in an RMS accuracy of 0.29° (SE = 0.01°) for the 3000-samples condition (short: M = 0.28°, SE = 0.01°; long: M = 0.30°, SE = 0.01°) and of 0.36° (SE = 0.02°) for the 6000-samples condition (short: M = 0.35°, SE = 0.02°; long: M = 0.37°, SE = 0.02°). Consequently, due to the smaller remaining errors, the 3000-samples-short-sequence condition was chosen for future calibrations.

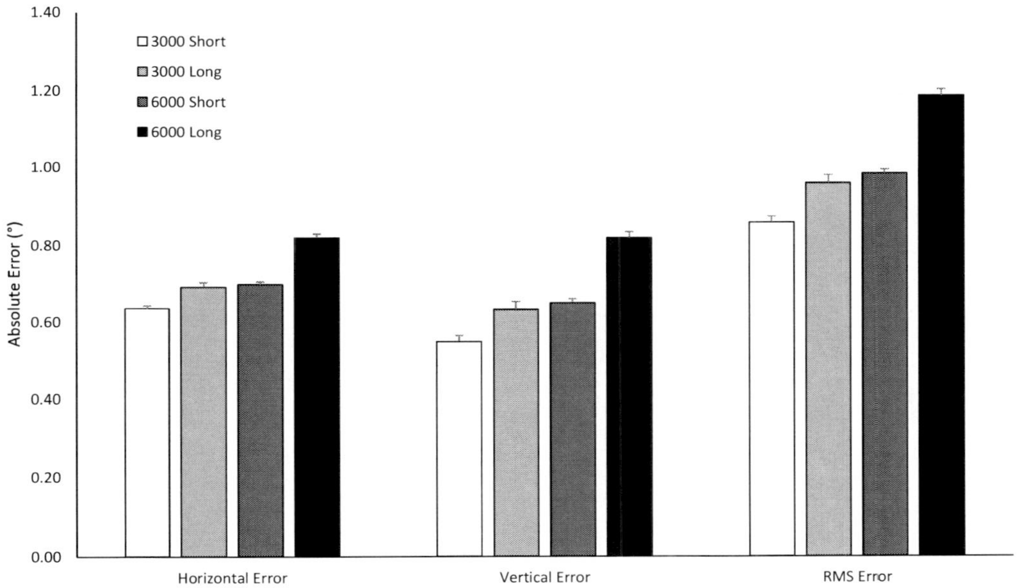

Figure 4. Absolute gaze error (horizontal, vertical and RMS; M and SE) as a function of two durations of the calibration routine (3000 vs. 6000) and two sequences (short vs. long saccades) in Experiment 1.

In the second experiment, the position of the eye-tracking camera was manipulated, putting the pupil center during neutral gazing either into the center, into the upper third or towards the right of the video frame. This manipulation accounts for possible effects of position-dependent lens distortions onto the accuracy of eye orientation estimates. Even if horizontal and vertical components differ for the right position of the camera compared to the two other conditions (see Figure 5), only minor RMS accuracy differences between different eye-tracking camera positions with respect to the neutral gaze direction were found, indicating that – as long as the pupil is roughly centered in the video stream – the effect of lens distortion on gaze accuracy seems to be negligible.

In the third experiment, it was analyzed how slippage of the goggles affects gaze estimation accuracy and to what extent an automated recalibration procedure reduces the resulting error. In order to simulate the effects of the goggles' slippage, after the initial calibration, participants were asked to shift the goggles either up or down with respect to their eyes in such a way that the pupil was still completely visible over the 5-point calibration routine. Afterwards, participants had to fixate a static dot centered on the projection screen. Applying a dispersion-based fixation algorithm (cf., Nyström & Holmqvist, 2010), the longest fixation during the display of the dot was extracted and the difference vector between the dot and the current fixation location, the *slippage vector*, was calculated, which, in turn, was used to calculate a rotation matrix. By applying this matrix, the neutral gaze orientation matrix could be corrected in order to adjust the following gaze estimates, which were used to calculate the remaining absolute horizontal, vertical and RMS errors. After a further calibration recording, the shifting process was repeated to the opposite direction.

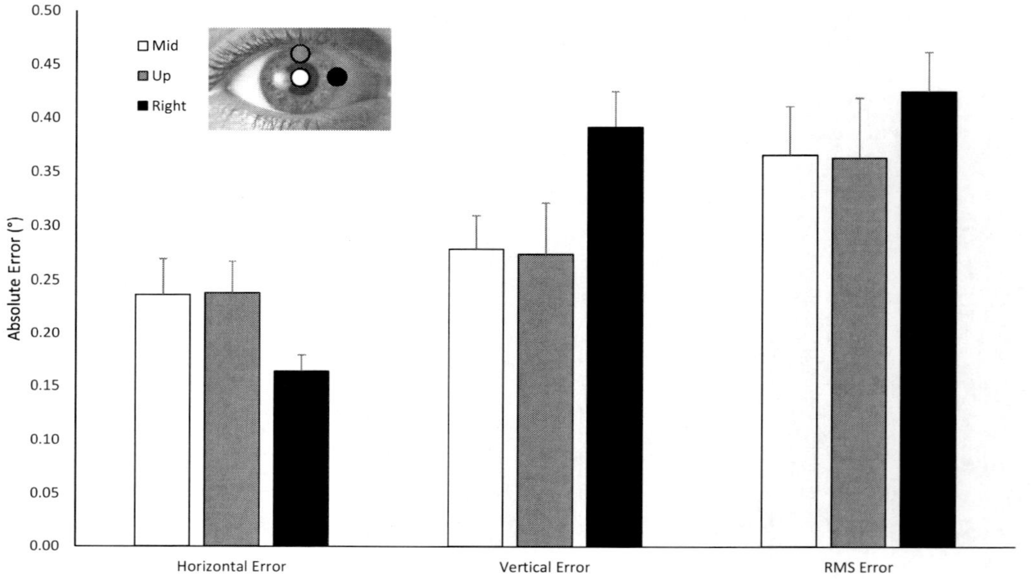

Figure 5. Absolute gaze error (horizontal, vertical and RMS; *M* and *SE*) as a function of camera positions with respect to the eye (Mid, vs. Up vs. Right) in Experiment 2.

The mean arc length of the slippage vector for the “Up”-condition was 15.95° (*SE* = 1.48°) and 25.04° (*SE* = 1.07°) for the “Down”-condition, while the horizontal slippage was 2.47° (*SE* = 0.27°) and 0.85° (*SE* = 0.45°), respectively. After applying the recalibration routine, the residual RMS errors were 0.57° (*SE* = 0.06°) for the “Up”-condition and 0.66° (*SE* = 0.06°) for the “Down”-condition (Figure 6, see also the horizontal and vertical errors). In sum, the recalibration routine can be classified as successful, even if the current implementation does not reach the accuracy of an initial calibration. However, as time consumption for fixating a static dot between experimental trials is minimal and sometimes even a standard procedure, the implemented slippage correction proofs its feasibility for application, especially as the resulting accuracy is well inside accuracy ranges reported for commercial mobile eye-tracking systems.

In the fourth experiment, it was analyzed how movements of the participants affect measurement accuracy. For this purpose, after calibration of the eye tracker, participants were asked to perform either running or jumping moves on the spot for 30 seconds while fixating static dots displayed on the projection screen. Errors were analyzed before and after the movement interval. Descriptively, the mean RMS estimation error increased from 0.16° (*SE* = 0.03°) to 1.28° (*SE* = 0.09°) after the motion phase (Figure 7).

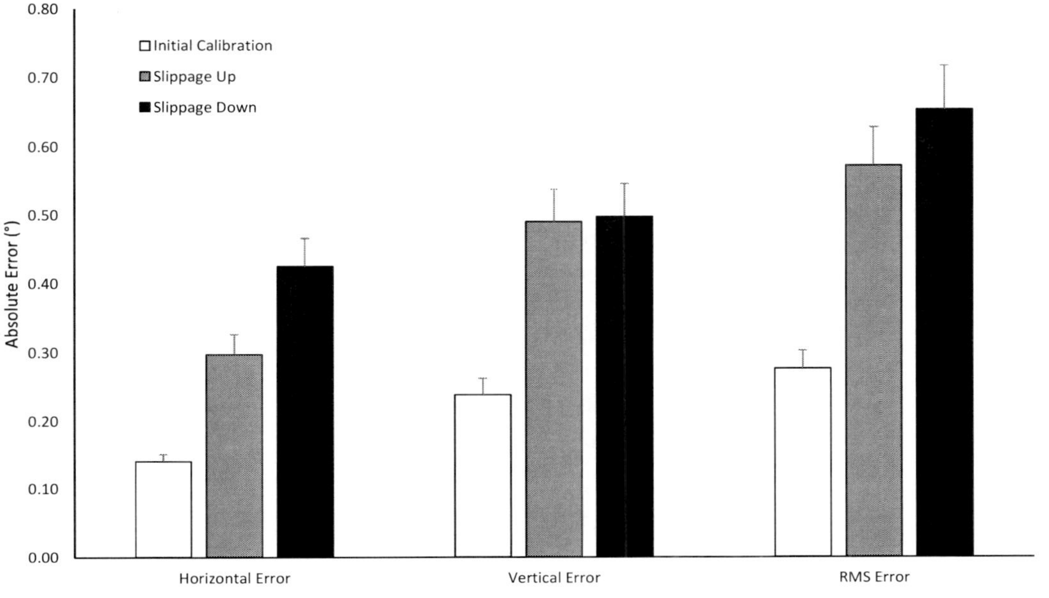

Figure 6. Absolute gaze error (horizontal, vertical and RMS; *M* and *SE*) after initial calibration as well as after slippage of the goggles (Up vs. Down) and application of the proposed *slippage vector* recalibration algorithm in Experiment 3.

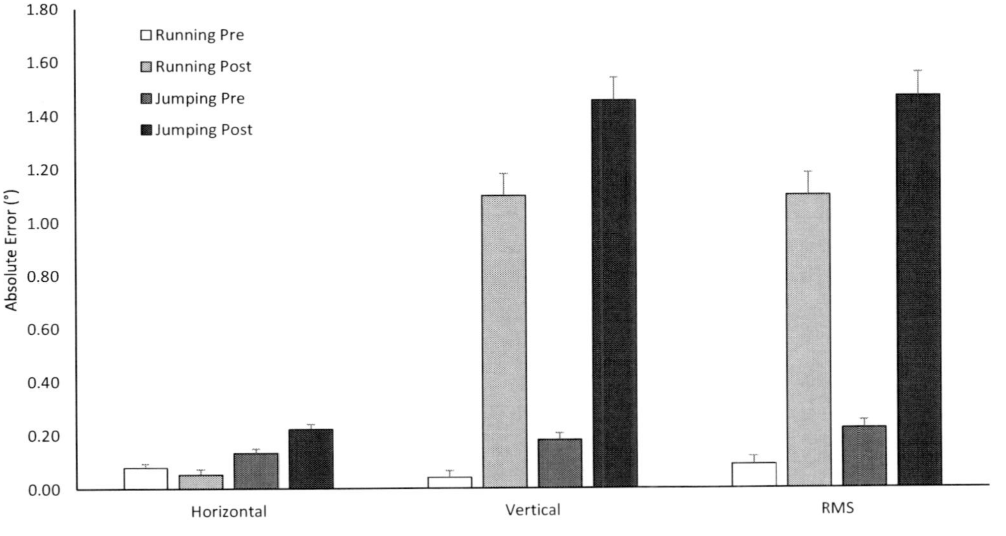

Figure 7. Absolute gaze error (horizontal, vertical and RMS; *M* and *SE*) as a function of movement type (Running vs. Jumping) and of measurement (Pre vs. Post) in Experiment 4.

This increase was mainly caused by the vertical error (M = 1.17°, SE = 0.04°). By separating the two tasks, it seems that movements with higher peak accelerations (jumping) caused higher slippage angles and, therefore, larger errors in gaze estimation than smoother movements (running). However, the achieved average estimation accuracy of 1.28° (SE = 0.09°) confirmed the applicability of the system in dynamic situations – and this even without applying the previously analyzed *slippage vector* recalibration method (which would reduce the errors even further).

In sum, it can be stated that the validation tests confirmed the applicability of the implemented eye-tracking system for static as well as dynamic lab tasks. With accuracies of 0.28° RMS error in static and 1.28° (uncorrected) RMS error after dynamic movements the system was well within reported accuracy ranges for commercial mobile eye trackers, especially as the providers of commercial systems are usually reporting static accuracy only. On top, the implemented slippage vector recalibration procedure was proven to significantly reduce errors caused by slippage of the goggles relative to the head (from up to uncorrected 25° reduced to 0.62° RMS error on average).

Application Scenarios

The implemented and validated system can be applied in a variety of scenarios. As the complexity of the gaze-assignment process may significantly differ over these scenarios, in the following, two use cases will be presented with an either poorer or richer assignment procedure. After a short introduction into the particular field of research, special attention will be directed towards the methods of analysis. The first use case is targeted more towards basic and the second one more towards applied research.

Scenario 1: Basic Research on Quiet-Eye Mechanisms

Originally found in applied sport settings, a gaze strategy called the "quiet eye" (QE) has become a "hot topic" over the last years in sport science research. The QE is defined as the final fixation or tracking gaze before movement initiation (Vickers, 1996). Since the search for functional mechanisms behind this phenomenon constitutes a main research question of our group, an experimental paradigm was developed that allows for independent manipulations of the QE duration in order to address certain characteristics that might explain its functionality for motor performance and learning (cf. Klostermann, Kredel, & Hossner, 2013, 2014). Typically, this is done in a precision task in which retro-reflective balls must be thrown as precisely as possible at targets that are presented on a large screen (see Figure 8). Since participants execute the throwing movement in accordance to an external pacing rhythm, the onset of the QE can be manipulated by presenting the target either earlier or later with respect to movement initiation.

Emphasizing research methodology, we used the integrated gaze analysis system described above to automatically evaluate the gaze data gathered during the experimental trials. By tracking not only the head pose, but additionally the hand and ball position in space and synchronizing the data recording with stimulus onsets on the screen, we were able to automatically identify not only the moment of the movement initiation, ball release and impact, but also the onset, offset and the location of the QE (applying a dispersion-based fixation detection algorithm introduced by Nyström & Holmqvist, 2010). The completely automated process enabled us to conduct 12 QE-related experiments with on average 22 participants and 200 trials over the last 3 years with minimal manpower, i.e., with only one person involved in the analysis phase.

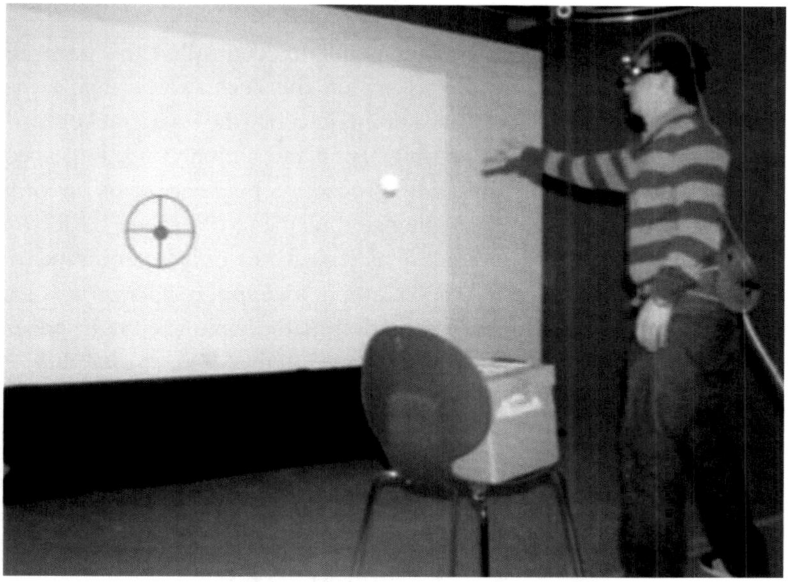

Figure 8. Experimental paradigm for QE research. The participant is wearing the integrated eye tracker and performs an underhand throw with a retro-reflective ball at a target presented at the life-sized screen.

A further basic research direction within our group aims towards the exploration of the functionality of peripheral vision, in particular, how gaze anchoring can help to track multiple objects simultaneously. Beyond the application of the integrated gaze analysis system, in this setting, the introduced vector-based approach can easily be extended towards a mapping of different stimulus locations to foveal, para- and perifoveal conical areas around the central gaze vector so that the gaze analysis is enriched by taking the peripheral information distribution into account. First results within this research direction are described by Vater, Kredel and Hossner (2015).

Scenario 2: Applied Research on Gaze Strategies in Volleyball Defense

In more applied research settings, the gaze analysis system typically has to cope with more dynamic behavior of the participants. This was particularly true in investigations on decision making and gaze strategies in beach-volleyball defensive actions. In the respective experiment (Hossner, Klostermann, Kredel, Schläppi-Lienhard, & Vater, 2015), 16 female and 16 male Swiss Elite players as well as 16 female and 16 male Swiss Near-elite players were subjected to 12 videos with 20 attacking scenes each (10 diagonal smashes, 5 cut shots,

5 line shots in randomized order). The scenes were presented from the perspective of a defense player on a large projection screen. In half of the videos participants were required to react as they would do on the field (action condition), whereas the other half of the videos was temporally occluded (occlusions: -40 ms, -120 ms, -200 ms, -280 ms before ball-hand contact) and participants had to name the attack variant (occlusion condition). Under both conditions, decision accuracy as well as gaze was recorded. Further, in the action condition, movement initiation time was calculated on the basis of participants' body kinematics by using the Vicon motion-capture system.

During data acquisition, the experimenter manually controlled the gaze accuracy after each block of 20 trials. If the accuracy was within the acceptable range (smaller than 2° average RMS error), the next block was started, if not, the eye tracker calibration was repeated. As participants moved very dynamically in the action condition, special attention had to be directed towards the recalibration procedure between trials in order to assure accurate and reliable gaze data. As a consequence, the above described basic *slippage vector* recalibration procedure was refined in such a way, that not only the current trial's fixation distance to the fixation dot was taken into account, but a *slippage function* was estimated over consecutive trials and used for an offline correction of the gaze vector. In general, it can be stated that this approach increased the recalibration quality and its stability against noise significantly as fixation position outliers were eliminated by repeated measures for the *slippage function* estimation.

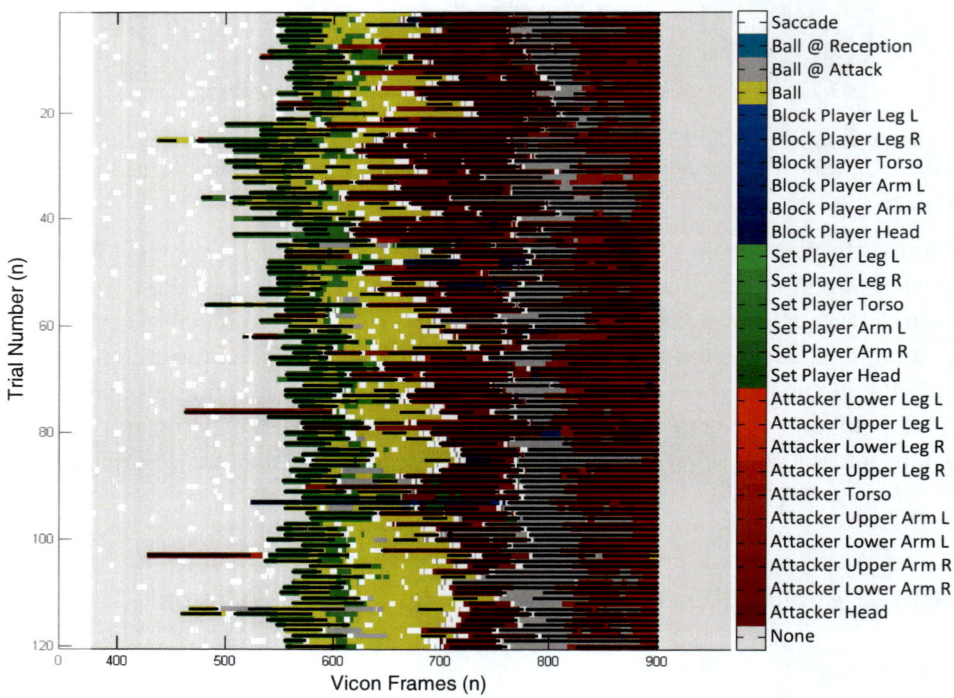

Figure 9. *Gaze Assignment Plot* (GAP) as a novel visualization solution for gaze data of a single participant. Gaze patterns of different trials (vertical axis) are displayed over time (horizontal axis), while the thin black lines represent fixations (spatially static gaze within 1° area). White spaces represent saccades and colors indicate mappings of the gaze vector to different cue regions.

During data collection, each participant was subjected to approx. 90 minutes video material of attacking scenes. Taking this immense amount of data points into account (220 gaze samples per second), a further challenge was the development of a feasible visualization for the descriptive analysis of the captured gaze data. To this regard, *Gaze Assignment Plots* were introduced (GAP, see Figure 9). In each row of the plot, the gaze pattern of one experimental trial is displayed over time. The trials can be aligned with common events, e.g., with the ball-hand contact of the attacker (corresponding to frame 900 in Figure 9). The assignment of the foveated cue region was automated by calculating the Euclidean distance between the gaze vector position and each stimulus position on the screen for each time step and selecting the cue with minimal distance to the gaze vector.

In the GAP, the color represents the mapping to these different cue regions in such a way that white colored areas represent saccadic eye movements, light gray areas are gaze positions outside the screen and the other colors map relevant body segments of the opponents or the ball position on the basis of a nearest-neighbor approach (for details, see legend on the right of Figure 9).

As additional information, thin black lines over the colored gaze patterns represent fixations, which are defined as spatially static gaze within 1° area for longer than 100ms. For the automated identification of the fixations, we use a dispersion-based algorithm and for the saccadic eye movements an adaptive threshold velocity-based algorithm (Nyström and Holmqvist, 2010). After having all (in Figure 9: 120) trials temporally aligned to each other, individual gaze variables can be aggregated automatically and, in turn, subjected to further statistical analyses.

Conclusion and Outlook

After having identified the main limitations of the current state-of-the-art in mobile gaze analysis hindering the broader use of eye-tracking, our aim was to overcome these limitations by using light-weight and non-obstructive eye-tracking equipment with high temporal and spatial resolution and by applying a vector-based gaze analysis procedure with regular automated checks between data collection trials, an automated recalibration procedure and an objective data-to-stimulus assignment process. Within this chapter, the design of the system was described, its functionality and accuracy was evaluated in static and dynamic settings and it applicability was illustrated by two representative use cases. The validated system proved its feasibility to analyze larger amounts of data in mobile settings while keeping accuracy levels high. As the markedly subjective fixation and saccade detection and stimulus assignment processes in video-based mobile eye-tracking have been eliminated, the objectivity of the analysis process was significantly increased and the time effort for analysis could be reduced considerably. On this basis, the introduced system allows to aggregate gaze behavior of larger samples sizes in mobile settings, hereby significantly improving the reliability for generalization.

Even if the accuracy of the system in dynamic situations is already comparable to commercial mobile eye-tracking systems, the proposed *slippage vector* recalibration procedure can further reduce the remaining errors and increase accuracy and reliability of the system. However, as this procedure uses fixation dots in between-trial intervals, the reliability of the procedure is heavily depending on the attention paid by the participants. That is why we currently enhance this procedure towards an online estimation of a *slippage function* over consecutive trials. Another limitation is the current offline implementation of the analysis process rather than a direct online correction and data-to-stimulus assignment. As this online feature is mandatory for gaze feedback, e.g., in gaze training interventions, a further current development focuses on the implementation of online filters and on the reduction of computing time for the gaze estimation and analysis routines. Additionally, it is obvious that the postulated similarity of the test to the real situation might be reduced by the fact that participants are enforced to perform in a lab setting due to the tracking requirements of the head or camera pose. However, as motion tracking systems are becoming more and more flexible and usable in unrestricted spaces (e.g., using local positioning systems or fused 9DOF-IMU sensors), in the near future, the proposed vector-based approach seems to become applicable even outside the lab under on-field or even under competition conditions.

To conclude, we think that our proposed vector-based gaze estimation and analysis procedure enables researchers within the field of perception-action diagnostics to reliably estimate gaze patterns in static as well as dynamic settings with minimal manpower required for data collection and, in particular, for data analysis. Thus, the procedure might offer a useful approach for further disentanglement of crucial mechanisms in perception-action research.

References

Duchowsky, A.T. (2003). *Eyetracking methodology, theory and practice*. London: Springer.

Evans, K.M., Jacobs, R.A., Tarduno, J.A., & Pelz, J.B. (2012). Collecting and analyzing mobile eye-tracking data in outdoor environments, *Journal of Eye Movement Research*, *5*, 1-19.

Farrow, D., & Abernethy, B. (2007). Wahrnehmung von Expertinnen und Experten im Sport: Einige Kernfragen und -probleme [Expert perception in sports: Some key questions and problems]. In N. Hagemann, M. Tietjens, & B. Strauß (Eds.), *Psychologie der sportlichen Höchstleistung* (pp. 71-92). Göttingen, Germany: Hogrefe.

Haslwanter, T. (1995). Mathematics of three-dimensional eye rotations, *Vision Research*, *35*, 1727-1739.

Hossner, E.-J., Klostermann, A., Kredel, R., Schläppi-Lienhard, O., & Vater, C. (2015). *Decision making and gaze strategies in beach volleyball defense: On expertise and the maximization of information*. Manuscript in preparation.

Klostermann, A., Kredel, R., & Hossner, E.-J. (2013). The "Quiet Eye" and motor performance: Task demands matter! *Journal of Experimental Psychology: Human Perception & Performance*, *39*, 1270-1278.

Klostermann, A., Kredel, R., & Hossner, E.-J. (2014). The quiet eye without a target: The primacy of visual information processing. *Journal of Experimental Psychology: Human Perception & Performance*, *40*, 2167-2178.

Kohlbecher, S., Bartl, K., Bardins, S., & Schneider, E. (2010). Low-latency combined eye and head tracking system for teleoperating a robotic head in real-time. In C. H. Morimoto, I. Istance, A. Hyrskykari, & Q. Ji (Eds.): *Proceedings of the 2010*

Symposium on Eye-Tracking Research and Applications (ETRA '10) (pp. 117-120). New York: ACM.

Kredel, R., Lienhard, O., Klostermann, A., Koedijker, J., Michel, K., & Hossner, E.-J. (2011). Perceptual skill identification in a complex sport setting, *BIO Web of Conferences*, *1*, 51.

Kumar, N., Kohlbecher, S., & Schneider, E. (2009). A novel approach to video-based pupil tracking. Paper presented at the IEEE International Conference on Systems, Man and Cybernetics 2009. Retrieved September 4, 2014, from IEEE Xplore.

Mann, D.L., Abernethy, B., & Farrow, D. (2010). Action specificity increases anticipatory performance and the expert advantage in natural interceptive tasks. *Acta Psychologica*, *135*, 17-23.

Mann, D.T.Y., Williams, A.M., Ward, P., & Janelle, C.M. (2007). Perceptual-cognitive expertise in sport: A meta-analysis. *Journal of Sport and Exercise Psychology*, *29*, 457-478.

Nyström, M., & Holmqvist, K. (2010). An adaptive algorithm for fixation, saccade, glissade detection in eye-tracking data. *Behavior Research Methods*, *42*, 188-204.Roth, H.L., Lora, A.N., & Heilman, K.M. (2002). Effects of monocolar viewing and eye dominance on spatial attention. *Brain*, *125*, 2023-2035.

Schneider, E., Villgrattner, T., Vockeroth, J., Bartl, K. Kohlbecher, S., Bardins, S., Ulbrich, H., & Brandt, T. (2009). EyeSeeCam: An eye movement-Ddiven head camera for the examination of natural visual exploration. *Annals of the New York Academy of Sciences*, *1164*, 461-467.

Vater, C., Kredel, R., & Hossner, E.J. (2015). *Detecting single-target changes in multiple object tracking: The case of peripheral vision*. Manuscript in preparation.

Vickers, J.N. (1996). Visual control when aiming at a far target. *Journal of Experimental Psychology: Human Perception & Performance*, *22*, 342-354

Williams, A.M., Davids, K., & Williams, J.G. (1999). *Visual perception and action in sport*. London: Taylor & Francis.

In: Advances in Visual Perception Research
Editor: Thomas Heinen

ISBN: 978-1-63482-455-2
© 2015 Nova Science Publishers, Inc.

Chapter 4

Comparing Vestibulo-Ocular Eye Movement Characteristics with Coaches' Rankings of Spatial Orientation Aptitudes in Gymnasts

***Christoph von Laßberg*[*1,2], *Karl A. Beykirch*[3,4] and *Jennifer L. Campos*[3,5,6]**

[1]Institute for General Movement Sciences and Training Methodology, University of Leipzig, Germany
[2]Medical Clinic, Department Sports Medicine, University of Tübingen, Germany
[3]Max Planck Institute for Biological Cybernetics, Tübingen, Germany
[4]AMST Systemtechnik GmbH, Ranshofen, Austria
[5]Toronto Rehabilitation Institute, Toronto, Canada
[6]University of Toronto, Department of Psychology, Toronto, Canada

Abstract

Visual orientation during head- and self-motion without retinal image slips requires efficient gaze stabilizing oculomotor functions that support unblurred retinal function. These mechanisms are driven by different sensor systems, such as vestibular afferents (vestibulo-ocular reflex - VOR) or retinal afferents (optokinetic reflex - OKR) to generate reflexive eye movements that continuously compensate for 3-dimensional head motions in space. High-level athletes trained in sports that involve fast and complex rotational movements (i.e., gymnasts) have a highly developed capability of efficiently orienting while executing such complex movements. This spatial orientation ability can, to a certain extend be learned. However, one´s intrinsic aptitude for easily coping with such multiaxial orientation challenges seems to be specific to each individual. It is not clear

[*] Medical Clinic, Department Sports Medicine, University of Tübingen, Germany. Email: cvl-lassberg@t-online.de

which role the individual level of VOR precision plays within the possible factors that determine such individual aptitudes. The aim of the present study is to examine to what extend the individual level of VOR correlates with individual aptitude to cope with multiaxial spatial orientation challenges as required in gymnastics. For this we used a method to evaluate the individual aptitude for multiaxial spatial orientation during actively performed maneuvers in competitive gymnasts by exploiting the accumulated expertise of coaches. We directly compared these expert-rating measures to individual VOR characteristics. The results indicate relationships between these ratings and the response of the vertical VOR in gymnasts.

Keywords: Gymnastics, eye movements, vestibulo-ocular reflex, multiaxial rotations

Introduction

Eye movements represent the computational output from multiple sensory inputs, their context-specific weighting and additional influences from motor learning and cognition. Therefore, the study of eye movements is a highly relevant approach to better understand general principles of interactions between perceptual and motor control mechanisms in humans. The most studied eye movements in awake individuals are those that serve to stabilize objects in the environment on the retina to avoid blurred vision. We refer to these as "environment-referenced eye movements" (EREMs). We further distinguish EREMs as being either compensatory, to compensate for head movements in space by keeping the eyes stable in space, compared to non-compensatory, if they do not stabilize the eyes in space. Compensatory eye movements use sensory feedback about the head's motion to reflexively move the eyes in the opposite direction. When the sensory system is the inertial-motion sensor in the inner ear, the vestibular system, the result is termed the vestibulo-ocular reflex (VOR[1]). When vision itself uses large-field optical motion to stabilize the eyes, it is referred to as the optokinetic reflex (OKR), which keeps the large-field image stable on the retina. Head motion that would require too large an eye movement results in a fast, resetting motion, interspersed with the slow compensatory motion. This sawtooth-formed motion is called *nystagmus*, whether it is produced by VOR or OKR. Both vestibularly driven (VOR) and visually driven (OKR) eye movements can result in nystagmus. Nystagmus due to OKR is also called optokinetic nystagmus (OKN).

Whether or not the head is in motion, the volitive tracking of an object that moves relative to the head is accomplished with the smooth pursuit eye movement system. Smooth pursuit function keeps the object of interest on the central, high-resolution area of the retina, the fovea. Another kind of eye movement occurs when the object of interest is not yet on the fovea and the eyes need to be redirected to the new focus of attention. Such a fast motion of the eyes causes blurring of the image, so they move as quickly and accurately as possible to minimise loss of vision. This intentional redirection of the eyes is known as a saccade.

Much less studied are additional eye movement reflexes most likely induced by proprioceptive stimuli, for example, the cervico-ocular reflex (COR), the trunk-ocular reflex (TOR) or the arthrokinetic response (AKN). Their functions are closely related to movements

[1] For further explanations of the VOR and how it is measured: see methods.

of the head (COR), the trunk (TOR), the upper extremities (AKN), and the lower extremities ("leg induced response") respectively.

In general, the measurement of eye movement function is typically done with standardized tests during passive movements of the whole body or parts of it. This approach has the advantage that eye movements can be precisely measured under standardized movement conditions across different subjects. However, the main disadvantage is that passive tests do not represent the *real context* of human movement that is normally *actively* performed by the subject. Actively performed movements however could include interactions with further reflexive systems or cognitive influences that are not apparent during standardized passive tests.

Therefore, in a recent study we investigated oculomotor function, for the first time under highly complex conditions: During *actively* performed multiaxial free-flight elements (multiple twisting somersaults) in high level gymnasts (von Laßberg, Beykirch, Mohler, & Bülthoff, 2014). In contrast to standardized measurements during *passive* movements, during these measurements a phenomenon was observed that has not been described before. Specifically, during the fast body rotations in the flight phase, all gaze stabilizing and EREM functions (VOR, OKR, Smooth pursuit etc.) were completely suppressed, and no nystagmus was observed. Instead, the eye movements were *co-directed* with the body movements during this phase. We therefore called this phenomenon "spinal motor coupled eye movements". They were marked by small circular eye movements that were correlated with small circular hip- and body-movements (hula movements) that are unconsciously performed by the athletes to support the longitudinal body rotations. However, just before the landing phase, these non-compensatory "spinal motor coupled eye movements" stopped, and the eye movements changed their direction to focus on the landing area using the known compensatory (gaze stabilizing) oculomotor functions to support the necessary visual control for a safe landing (for example see: von Laßberg et al., 2014; video 3).

This phenomenon led to the conclusion that eye movements during *actively* performed rotational movements can be completely different from eye movements during *passive* rotational movements, in support of the most efficient, active, *new-orientation* in space. These seem to be supported by a co-direction of eye movements and body movements, undisturbed by any reflexive *stabilizing* functions. The requirement of a *new-orientation* however ends at the moment the counteracting requirements of EREMs (focussing the environmental structures for landing) become dominant again. In that moment, the compensatory (gaze stabilizing) eye movement functions were reactivated.

We therefore concluded (von Laßberg et al., 2014) that eye movements of subjects that need to efficiently cope with *multiaxial new-orientation* are marked by two counteracting eye movement requirements: 1) the phase of spinal motor coupling to support an efficient multiaxial movement (non-compensatory) and 2) the phase of efficient compensatory eye movements to support the visual fixation of environmental structures before landing (EREM). Presumably, the latter phase in particular requires a very high level of precision to sufficiently perceive the environmental structures, even after very fast and complex rotational movements. This may be consistent with the results of other studies that describe the purpose of smooth pursuit and optokinetic reflexes during somersault movements, in particular, to provide sufficient visual control to ensure safe landings (e.g. Davlin, Sands, & Shultz, 2001; Heinen, 2011; Hondzinski & Darling, 2001; Lee, Young, & Rewt, 1992; Luis & Tremblay, 2008).

Therefore, we postulated that the EREMs (environment referenced eye movements, i.e. VOR, OKR, Smooth pursuit etc.) in gymnasts needs to be more accurate, compared with persons who are not used to such complex multiaxial maneuvers.

In our own studies (von Laßberg et al., 2012), we found support for this assumption by showing significantly higher performance of the *smooth pursuit function* in gymnasts compared to controls, which was additionally related to the training schedule (after a 3-week break of training the smooth pursuit level had significantly decreased again within the athletes group).

Several studies have been published concerning vestibular function and the *VOR* in people specifically accustomed to *rotational loads*. Such studies mostly referred to questions related to VOR adaptation and its effects regarding human spatial orientation and visual control. To facilitate comparison, such investigations usually involve standardized, *passively* induced rotational motions. Whereas the phenomenon of habituation of the VOR in populations experienced with rotational loads has been well documented (e.g. Ahn, Lee, Kim, & Lee, 2000; Schwarz & Henn, 1989; Baloh, Henn, & Jäger, 1982; Clement, Tilikete, & Courjon, 2008), their relationships with the accuracy of VOR characteristics (VOR gain [quotient of eye velocity/stimulus velocity] and temporal phase shift to the stimulus; also see methods) seem to be inconsistent and not completely clear. For instance, previous work has investigated differences in vestibular functioning between novices and expert fighter pilots (Aschan, 1954; Lee, Kim, & Park, 2004; Schwarz & Henn, 1989) or figure skaters (Alpini, Botta, Mattei, & Tornese, 2009; Tanguy, Quarck, Etard, Gauthier, & Denise, 2008a, 2008b), all of whom experience high rotational loads more frequently than the average person. However, discrepancies exisit in the literature and thus, the effects of such experiences on measures such as the VOR gain seem not entirely clear. For instance, Lee et al. (2004) demonstrated that the VOR gains in fighter pilots were significantly higher than non-pilots for frequencies that were higher than 0.04 Hz, yet Tanguy et al. (2008a) report significantly lower gain values among figure skaters compared to controls. In contrast, Clement et al. (2008) described no changes in VOR-gains after a specific vestibular training (velocity steps) of normal healthy persons. Some authors assume that these diverging kinds of rotational VOR adaptations are caused by highly context specific cues (e.g. Tanguy et al., 2008b), even though the detailed mechanisms responsible for such contrary findings are not completely identified. Prior investigations specifically involving gymnasts, however, have shown that gymnasts do *not* seem to react differently to interventions such as *galvanic* vestibular stimulation compared to non-gymnasts (Balter, Stokroos, Akkermans, & Kingma, 2004). In our own prior studies (von Laßberg, 2007) we also did not observe significant differences in *rotational VOR* characteristics observed between gymnasts and non-athlete controls. However, in both groups we found high *interindividual* differences of the VOR characteristics. Even though VOR measures can be affected by factors including attention and cognitive influences (e.g. Melvill Jones, Berthoz, & Segal, 1984; Shelhamer, Robinson, & Tan, 1992), it is known that VOR gains naturally differ substantially between individuals (e.g. Schalén, 1980). Therefore the question arose, whether a higher individual VOR gain could be a factor that generally enhances the individual aptitudes to spatially orient during complex multiaxial movements, and so the individual VOR level could be one determining factor associated with whether certain indviduals choose or are successful at activities that require such specific abilities. This could be also one reason for the fact that in some studies with populations accustomed to rotational loads (e.g. dancers, figure skaters etc.) different VOR results have been found (compared to controls), because the subjects possibly are able to better cope with such loads and therefore had a higher affinity to such sports or activities. So, the factor of a pre-selection did possibly influence the results of such studies. To further investigate if such factors of a VOR pre-determination for spatial orientation abilities exist, the aim of the present study was to compare individual VOR characteristics with general spatial orientation aptitudes. As a necessary prerequisite for such comparisons, we needed a method to estimate these general aptitudes for "spatial orientation abilities". Due to the fact that these aptitudes are very complex to measure and because of their multiple (conscious and non-conscious) components, we decided not to use any specific test at any specific measurement time, but a more global evaluation method to build an inter-individual relative ranking score concerning this complex quality of the gymnasts, based on their coaches long term experience with the subjects over month and years. Based on this evaluation system the spatial orientation abilities of the gymnasts should be finally compared to their VOR characteristics, measured during standardized controlled rotational loads. This approach provide a first insight into whether any relationships exist between the individual´s VOR characteristics and their individual abilities to spatially orient during complex movements.

Methods

Participants

Gymnasts

Competitive male gymnasts were recruited from the National Training Centre for Artistic Gymnastics in Stuttgart. They were comprised of a group of D-Level gymnasts (n=9; age 10-13 years; training schedule 20 hours a week). The D-Level is defined as a selection of the best area, or state junior gymnasts. Overall, the gymnasts included in this study all competed in each of the six male Olympic gymnastics apparatuses (floor exercise, high bar, parallel bars, vault, pommel horse and rings). Gymnasts were chosen only if there were at least two or three participating coaches who had extensive experience working with them.

Expert Evaluators of the Gymnasts´ Spatial Orientation Aptitudes

Three coaches were required to have worked with the participating gymnasts for at least one year and for 10 hours per week minimum. These criteria were used to ensure that the coaches were proficient at evaluating individual gymnasts' abilities and were highly familiar with different aspects of their gymnastic aptitudes. Because there are naturally only very few gymnasts and coaches available who satisfy all of the aforementioned criteria, sample sizes were relatively small. The coaches had been working professionally for 15 to 20 years. The group was evaluated by *Coach 1*, who was himself a previous world gymnastics champion from the former USSR. *Coaches 2 and 3* had 15 and 20 years of experience respectively coaching junior elite gymnasts.

VOR-Measurements

Background of VOR Measurements

The function of the VOR is to support dynamic gaze stabilization driven by vestibular afferents (see: introduction). Measuring VOR characteristics is a well-known approach used to judge the health of vestibular functions in clinical and physiological research. VOR function is mostly described by VOR-gain and VOR-phase. The *phase* is defined as the temporal shift (in degrees) between stimulus and response. Therefore a phase close to zero indicates a nearly ideal VOR compensation. The *gain* is defined as the quotient of eye-velocity and head velocity during accelerations. The maximum VOR gain value is 1, in which case there is complete coincidence between head movements and the compensating eye movements (without any slip). Therefore (in contrast to the phase) a *high* gain value (close to 1) indicates the best VOR compensation. In most cases, however, baseline measures of VOR-gain are typically lower than 1 due to the fact that additional mechanisms of stabilizing eye movements are used to augment the VOR (e.g. the optokinetic reflex (OKR); see introduction). Therefore, when measuring only the *VOR component* of oculomotor response, measures must take place in the dark to exclude the effects of retinal afferents (e.g. driven by OKR or smooth pursuit). Therefore, the most common standard stimuli used to measure rotational VOR gain and phase characteristics best are sets of sinusoidal whole body rotations around determined axes (horizontal or vertical) in the dark. We decided to also use these standardized tests.

Stimuli and Apparatus

All VOR-tests were executed using a whole body motion simulator located at the University of Tübingen, Germany (Figure 1). The Tübingen Vestibular Research Simulator (TVRS, see Bechert & Koenig, 1996; Koenig, Westermann, Jager, Sell, Bechert, Fetter, & Dichgans, 1996) was used to precisely stimulate the vestibular system of participants using computer controlled rotational movements about different axes.

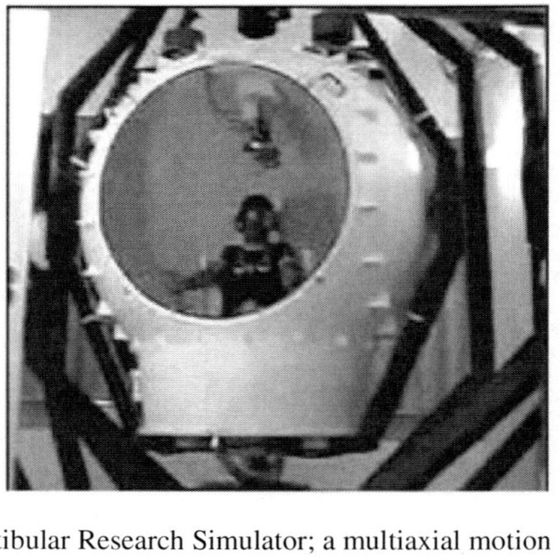

Figure 1. The Tübingen Vestibular Research Simulator; a multiaxial motion simulation device.

Standardized sinusoidal rotation tests were conducted in both the horizontal and vertical plane. All tests consisted of one continuous set of 5 oscillations for each trial, which varied in direction, frequency and maximum velocity (see Table 1). A 30 second pause was introduced between each of the trials. The rotation axis was adjusted exactly to the middle of the head. During all tests the head was fixed in a U-shaped head rest to exclude deviations from the programmed accelerations by extraneous head movements and to exclude additional influences of cerviculo-ocular reflex (COR; see introduction). The participants were instructed to keep their eyes opened and to look straight ahead into the dark during the tests.

Table 1. VOR-Test scheme

Description of rotational whole body accelerations during the VOR tests				
Kind of movement	Direction	F (Hz)	Vmax (°/s)	Label
Sinusoidal rotations	Left / right	0.4	25	Hor1
		0.2		Hor 2
		0.1		Hor 3
		0.1	50	Hor 4
		0.1	100	Hor 5
	Backward / forward	0.4	25	Vert 1
		0.2		Vert 2
		0.1		Vert 3
		0.1	50	Vert 4
		0.1	100	Vert 5

Collection and Processing of Oculomotor Data

Oculomotor data was collected and processed via a videonystagmography system (2D VOG, version 3.2, created by SensoMotoric Instruments [SMI]). In addition to the internal system functions of the SMI software, custom software written using the LabVIEW development environment (created by National Instruments) was used to calculate the oculomotor parameters. All signals were recorded at 50Hz and the signals were upsampled to create a version that was filtered with 21-tap-finite-impulse response digital low-pass filter (42Hz cutoff) that was optimized for noise reduction and preservation of critical fast components dynamics. Fast nystagmus components were removed and replaced with interpolated values. The fast component removal software used a phase space plot of response versus stimulus to remove phase and interactively put boundaries around the slow component plot. Values outside the boundaries were removed. Statistical analyses of the noise of the residuals from the best-fit of the slow component response to the stimulus were used to allow for an objective evaluation of the interactive choices. The gain values were obtained from a cross-spectral density of slow component responses to the stimulus at the frequency of the stimulus. Using the analysis software, it was possible to calculate the average VOR gain and phase, and use this for further statistical analyses. The described evaluation procedure is one of the most popular and well-established methods in the field of oculomotor research (Baloh, Langhofer, Honrubia, & Yee, 1980; Leigh & Zee, 2006).

Expert Evaluation of Individual Spatial Orientation Aptitudes

We developed a very straightforward, relative ranking system in which each coach was asked to rank the gymnasts with whom he/she was highly familiar. This simply required the coaches to rank the gymnasts based on their spatial orientation aptitudes in a variety of common gymnastics manoeuvres (5 different categories of aptitudes; see below). Rather than restricting the evaluation to one particular instance in time (i.e. one testing session), as is often done, the coaches´ evaluations were based on their wealth of information obtained over a long period of time.

When ranking the gymnasts, the coaches were instructed not to evaluate the grade of performance of specific elements but to evaluate the gymnasts' *intrinsic aptitudes* for a particular skill-set. While some gymnasts can achieve a high level of performance through hard work and perseverance, for others it comes more naturally or effortlessly. In other words, coaches were asked to consider the extent to which a category of manoeuvres was "effortless" for some gymnasts in such a way that a demonstrated natural ability was exhibited. Other gymnasts, who might be able to perform the manoeuvres quite well and are highly skilled, may have to work hard to achieve or maintain that high level of performance. For that reason the coaches' evaluations were not based on *one particular evaluation session*, but rather from their *accumulated knowledge* gained from working closely with each gymnast over many months or years. It was this *intrinsic* quality that the coaches were asked to judge. This type of qualitative assessment provides an element of evaluation that has been very difficult to capture using previous methods. While other measures have been very effective at achieving a more detailed level of analysis, few have been able to capture the more global, all-encompassing description of complex spatial orientation abilities revealed here.

So, the goal of the coaches' evaluations was not to provide a detailed breakdown of very specific movement elements or to quantify different elements of a particular manoeuvre. Instead, the goal was to rank the gymnasts qualitatively as a function of their overall aptitude for particular manoeuvres in a more global sense (compare also: Hodges, Regehr, McNaughton, Tiberius, & Hanson, 1999).

Five Categories of Aptitudes for Evaluation

By drawing on their extensive experiences with each gymnast and their repeated exposure to a gymnast's performance on particular manoeuvres, the coaches were asked to assess a gymnast's general aptitude *for five particular categories*. All categories of the manoeuvres that were evaluated were very common and familiar to both the coaches and the gymnasts.

This selection of manoeuvres also captured a broad range of different movement types that systematically varied in the types of vestibular stimulation involved. These manoeuvres were specifically selected because of their dependence on perceived self-orientation. The tasks were specifically chosen as a way of sampling from different types of otolith and semicircular canal stimulation.

This was done to more carefully evaluate the specific capabilities of different vestibular inputs and to understand the relationship of these inputs to the VOR. In order to select from different types of vestibular stimulation, both quasi-static postures and dynamic movements of varying complexity were evaluated. Specifically, three of the five chosen manoeuvres were quasi-static balance regulation tasks (e.g. handstands) and the remaining two were tasks that require dynamic movement regulation during multiaxial whole body rotations during flight (e.g. multiple twisting somersaults) and during hang or support positions, as well (e.g. combined multiaxial rotations around any fixed or quasi-fixed axes; e.g. high bar, parallel bars etc.). Each aptitude is described in detail below.

Quasi-Static Balance-Regulation Tasks

Aptitude 1: Ability to Balance during One-Leg Stands

Aptitude 1 represents all quasi-static regulation tasks performed in one-leg standing positions. In addition to kinaesthetic and other regulatory sensory/motor systems, the vestibular and visual systems, in particular, are used to detect even slight deviations from vertical in order to support a stable standing position.

Aptitude 2: Ability to Balance during Handstands with a Fixed Support

This aptitude is, in general, similar to Aptitude 1, but occurs during a much more difficult manoeuvre that is not typically experienced during daily life. Specifically, it involves balancing in an inverted position on the hands (i.e. maintaining a handstand). Again, visual and vestibular information are critical to performing this task, while there are additional inputs from kinaesthetic information provided by the upper extremities.

Aptitude 3: Ability to Balance during Handstands on a Mobile System

Again increasing in complexity, this aptitude is similar to Aptitude 2, except that the handstand must be maintained on a surface that is moving (e.g. the rings). This position is controlled more by the shoulder and hip angle and by keeping the hands as close as possible to the vertical centre of body mass.

Multi-Axial Spatial Orientation Tasks

Different otolith-ocular influences occur during multi-axial rotations for free-flight conditions compared to hang or support conditions. Specifically, during free-flight (all kinds of somersaults) the centre of body mass moves on a parabolic flight curve and the head rotates around it. Therefore, during free-flight rotations, there are high centrifugal forces on the otoliths. In contrast to this, during hang or support conditions the otoliths and proprioceptive afferents detect higher or lower gravitational and centrifugal forces depending on the actual body position relative to the apparatus and to the earth's vertical while rotating around externally fixed axes.

Aptitude 4: Multi-Axial Rotations during Free- Flight Elements

To control multi-axial rotations during free-flight elements, the specific role of the different types of vestibular processing is not yet clear. It is possible that the acceleration loads on the semicircular canals can help to estimate self-rotation velocity and to interpret the actual position in space. Otolith information could help to interpret the rotational velocity as a function of the centrifugal acceleration components. However, otolithic loads are consistently exerted cranially even in an upright body position during free flight rotations. This is caused by centrifugal acceleration during the flight phase where the axis of rotation is at the centre of body mass that is moving itself on a parabolic flight curve (following the earth gravity). Therefore earth gravity cannot be detected by the otolith signals during somersaults.

Aptitude 5: Multi-Axial Rotations during Hang or Support Positions

Compared to Aptitude 4, multi-axial rotational movements during hang or support positions differ fundamentally as a function of their otolithic loads, depending on the actual rotation axis in relation to the body. Rotations around an external axis (e.g. rotations with superposed longitudinal axis rotations during giant swings on high bar or on parallel bars) can even cause opposite otolithic loads compared to those around the center of body mass experienced during free-flight conditions. Whereas during free-flight phases the otolithic load is consistently directed cranially even during upright positions (relative to the earth vertical), a similar upright body position during a swing on the high bar or on the parallel bars results in a downward directed otolithic load, caused primarily by gravitational and additional centrifugal forces. However, in contrast to *long hang swings*, there is only a minimal centrifugal component to the otoliths during *swings in support positions* (e.g. on parallel bars) because the axis of rotation (shoulders) is very close to the vestibular organs during support swings.

Ranking of the Gymnast´s Aptitudes across the Five Categories

The overall evaluation task introduced here was intentionally developed to be very simple and intuitive. Essentially the coaches were simply asked to rank each of the gymnasts from 1 (best) to 9 (worst) for each of the five aptitudes. For instance, each gymnast was ranked relative to each other for their overall ability to balance during one-leg stands (Aptitude 1), etc.

It was possible for a coach to assign the same ranking value to more than one gymnast if the gymnasts' aptitudes for a category of manoeuvres were equal. The coaches were informed that, if a particular ranking was too difficult to assign, that they should note this on their evaluations; however, no such annotations were recorded. A ranking evaluation sheet was given to all of the coaches, with the request that the ranking scores be estimated very carefully and independently from the other coaches, and be returned within one week.

The different ranking scores of each of the coaches were finally summed as a way of determining an *overall ranking score* for each gymnast and for each aptitude. These overall ranking scores should be finally compared to the VOR parameters of the ranked gymnasts (for further details: see "VOR measurements").

Methods Used to Evaluate the Effectiveness of the Expert Ranking System

In order for these evaluations to be useful, there are several criteria that must be met. First, it would be very important for different coaches to provide similar rating scores across gymnasts.

In other words, by demonstrating high inter-rater reliability, this would strengthen this rating system as an effective measurement tool and suggest an absence of biases by particular coaches. Further, if an overall bias towards a particular gymnast across all manoeuvres was present across coaches (i.e. if one gymnast was considered "the best" and another was considered "the worst" overall), there would be no differences in ratings across the different aptitude categories. If, however, some gymnasts were shown to demonstrate a natural self orientation ability for one type of manoeuvre and other gymnasts for different manoeuvres, this would demonstrate a more careful and systematic expert evaluation.

Thus, in order to determine whether using this expert ranking system is an effective and stable tool for evaluating general spatial-orientation skills, the criteria of inter-rater reliability and global consistency or sensitivity were judged as follows.

Inter-Rater Reliability

Inter-rater reliability provides a measure of the degree of independence of a test from its user. Specifically, it looks at the extent to which the expert evaluators agreed on their rankings. This was determined by calculating the Kendall-W coefficient of concordance.

Global Consistency or Sensitivity

In order to determine the sensitivity of the method used here, the correlations between the rankings of individual aptitudes with each of the other aptitudes were calculated (Spearman correlation coefficient). If an individual gymnast's ratings were identical across aptitudes (e.g. if one gymnast was always ranked first for every aptitude and another gymnast was always ranked last), this might indicate that the coaches' rankings might have been biased by external variables (e.g. results from competitions, interpersonal affinities or conflicts, etc.).

However, if high correlations were not observed across aptitude comparisons for each gymnast, this would indicate that the gymnast was being ranked higher or lower depending on the specific aptitude, thus reflecting a more systematic and careful evaluation.

Statistical Analysis of Cross Correlations between Rankings and VOR Parameters

For a general descriptive analysis, the mean (M) and standard deviation (*SD*) of the VOR data across all test conditions were calculated. We then evaluated whether any relationships exist between the individual VOR values of the gymnasts and their aptitudes ranking scores. To do this we calculated the Spearman's correlation coefficient of VOR gains and phases for each of the five tests in horizontal and vertical plane (see Table 1) for each gymnast. Due to the fact that lower ranking values indicated higher aptitudes (e.g. a rank of 1 = best), *negative correlations* with VOR *gain* indicate that higher gains (representing more ideal VOR compensation) were related to higher spatial orientation aptitudes.

Positive correlations with VOR *phases,* however, indicate that lower phase shifts (representing more ideal VOR compensation) were related to higher spatial orientation aptitudes. In other words, the hypothesis that spatial orientation abilities correlate with a high VOR accuracy would be reflected by negative correlations with gains and positive correlations with phases.

Results

Evaluation Method

Inter-Rater Reliability

Because of the fact that one of the three coaches worked primarily with the gymnasts on the trampoline (thus focussing on multi-axial free-flight skills), this coach only judged Aptitude 4. All of the other aptitudes were judged by the remaining 2 coaches. Table 2 summarizes the inter-rater reliability measures for the rankings of the gymnasts. The results show a high level of agreement between the rankings of the coaches in all cases (M = 0.90).

Table 2. Matrix of coefficient of concordance (Kendall W) relating to the different aptitudes of the gymnasts. One coach was primarily focused on training on the trampoline and did not feel competent enough to judge the other manoeuvres with sufficient accuracy. Therefore he did not take part in these evaluations

Coefficient of concordance (Kendall-W) of coaches rankings					
	Aptitude 1	Aptitude 2	Aptitude 3	Aptitude 4	Aptitude 5
Coaches	n = 2	n = 2	n = 2	n = 3	n = 2
Coefficient	.909	.970	.958	.771	.873
p-value	.060	.040	.045	.013	.073

Global Consistency or Sensitivity

Significant correlations between the aptitude rankings of the quasi-static balance tasks were observed (see Table 3). Specifically, Aptitudes 1 and 3 were significantly correlated, as were Aptitudes 2 and 3. The same was true for the multi-axial spatial orientation aptitudes, such that Aptitude 4 and 5 were highly correlated. There were also significant correlations observed between Aptitude 2 (handstand with fixed support) and Aptitudes 4 and 5 (multi-axial spatial orientation tasks). Figure 2 demonstrates the overall ranking scores of the five aptitudes for all gymnasts.

Table 3. Spearman correlation matrix of the aptitudes 1 - 5. Significant values are printed in bold

Correlations between the aptitudes (Spearman; r_s^*)					
	Aptitude 1	Aptitude 2	Aptitude 3	Aptitude 4	Aptitude 5
Aptitude 1		r_s=.591	**r_s=.928**	r_s=.338	r_s=.610
Aptitude 2	r_s=.591		**r_s=.723**	**r_s=.833**	**r_s=.946**
Aptitude 3	**r_s=.928**	**r_s=.723**		r_s=.588	r_s=.662
Aptitude 4	r_s=.338	**r_s=.833**	r_s=.588		**r_s=.795**
Aptitude 5	r_s=.610	**r_s=.946**	r_s=.662	**r_s=.795**	

* r-values > 0.7 are printed in bold.

Overall, the results show evidence of a systematic differentiation of gymnasts' rankings based on the different types of aptitudes that were evaluated. This indicates that the expert rankings were most likely not exclusively determined by globally assigning a certain gymnast to a certain rank across the different aptitudes (e.g. oriented on external factors like competition results etc.). These results, therefore, argue against the idea that the coaches simply considered, for example, the number of overall awards a gymnast had won and consistently used this criterion to rank them across all aptitudes. Take for example the rankings for Aptitudes 4 and 5, which could differ largely for one individual gymnast. For instance, gymnast B1 was ranked as the first for Aptitude 4 (multi-axial orientation during free-flight elements), but only on the fourth place for Aptitude 5 (multi-axial orientation during hang or support elements).

Some differences were even larger between other tests. For example gymnast K3 was ranked as fourth for Aptitude 1 (one-leg stand) but as the last for Aptitude 2 (handstand) and also for Aptitude 4 (multi-axial orientation during free-flight elements).

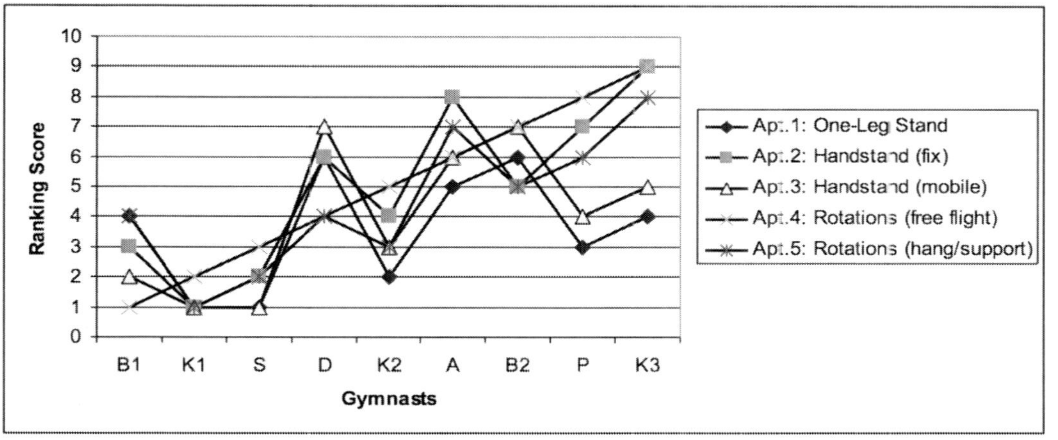

Figure 2. Overall ranking for Aptitudes 1-5 for each of the gymnasts. The order of the gymnasts were sorted according to the rankings of Aptitude 4 (multiaxial free-flight elements). Therefore the development of Aptitude 4 shows a linear ascent that the other Aptitudes are related to.

Summarized, the findings presented here demonstrate highly consistent relative ratings across the coaches. Considering that coaches made their ratings entirely independently of one another and did not use conventional or familiar evaluation methods, their agreement in rankings demonstrates the high consistency with which this simple rating task was performed. Further, because the rankings differed as a function of the different aptitudes, this provides support for the idea that the coaches were not simply ranking gymnasts overall as the "best" or the "worst" of the group, but instead were sensitive enough to judge individual variations among the group.

Comparison of Individual Spatial Orientation Aptitudes (Expert Evaluation) with VOR Characteristics

Descriptive Results of the VOR Measurements

The descriptive results of the general VOR characteristics gave some basic information about the trends between the different test conditions and between horizontal vs. vertical tests within this group of gymnasts.

Concerning to the mean values of the horizontal VOR-gains the tests did not show notable differences across the five rotational test conditions. In the vertical plane, however, the mean values showed a "concave-shaped" development across the five test conditions (see Figure 3). The highest values were observed in test 1 (with also higher gains than in the horizontal plane), followed by test 2, than 3 (with the lowest values). In tests 4 and 5 the gains were raising again and nearly reached the values of test 1.

Generally, the individual gain values in the horizontal plane showed lower variability across the whole group and within intra-individual development over the five test conditions compared to the vertical gain values. In particular, in the vertical plane highly stable intra-individual gain levels were observed across the different test conditions (Figure 3).

The mean values of the phases and in most cases also the individual phase development across the five test conditions show a phase advance associated with increasing rotational amplitudes and velocities of the sinusoidal cycles, both in the horizontal and vertical plane. The mean values in test 1 (smallest amplitude, lowest peak velocity) show the highest phase lags (most negative values); the mean values of test 5 (largest amplitude; highest peak velocity) show a clear shift to a phase lead with highest positive values. The inter-individual bandwidth around zero appears a bit higher in the horizontal than in the vertical phases.

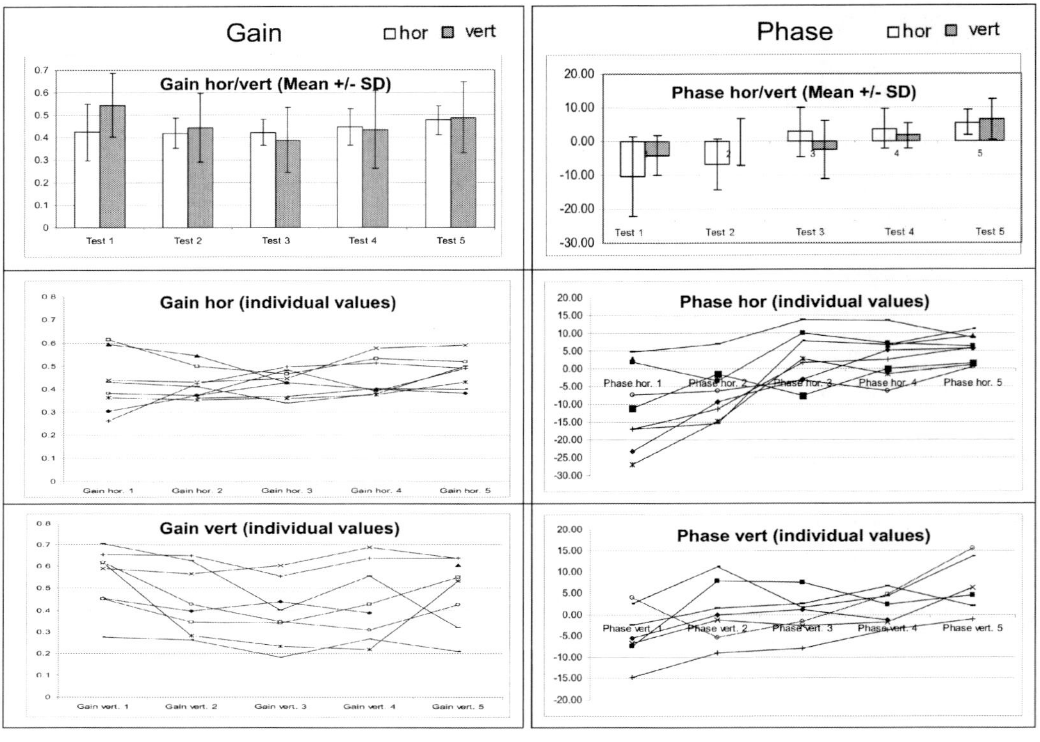

Figure 3. Overview: Descriptive analysis of VOR gain and phase characteristics. Top row: Mean values ±1 standard deviation for gain and phases (horizontal and vertical) across the 5 test conditions. Second row: Individual development of gain and phase values (horizontal) across the 5 test conditions. Bottom row: Individual development of gain and phase values (vertical) across the 5 test conditions. Note: Caused by artefacts some singular values are missing in the graphs.

Cross Correlation of the Expert Evaluation Scores with Individual VOR Characteristics

With respect to the relationship between VOR *gains* and the expert rankings, the results for the *vertical* rotation tests revealed some negative correlations with the rankings. There was a slight tendency for higher correlations concerning the Aptitudes 4 and 5 (i.e. the multi-axial orientation tasks). Lower correlations were observed with regards to the quasi-static orientation tasks (Aptitudes 1-3; compare Table 4). With regards to the *horizontal* rotation tests, however, *no* correlations between the ranking scores and the VOR gain values were observed.

With respect to the relationship between VOR *phase* values and the expert rankings, for the vertical tests, high correlations with the 5 aptitudes were only observed for test 5. However, *no* valuable correlations were found for all the other tests, in either the vertical or horizontal planes. This result did not differ when we calculated using with the *absolute* phase values (absolute difference from zero, independent of a phase lag or phase lead).

Table 4. Correlation matrix comparing aptitude scores with VOR gain and phase values (Spearman)

Correlations between the aptitudes (Apt.) and the VOR gain and phase values (r_s)*						
	Parameter	Apt. 1	Apt. 2	Apt. 3	Apt. 4	Apt. 5
Test 1 hor	Gain hor. 1	0.546	0.095	0.410	0.024	0.252
	Phase hor. 1	0.084	-0.217	-0.118	-0.2	-0.042
Test 2 hor	Gain hor. 2	0.394	-0.377	0.093	-0.527	-0.210
	Phase hor. 2	0.265	-0.095	0.265	-0.262	-0.119
Test 3 hor	Gain hor. 3	0.304	0.083	0.244	0.067	0.142
	Phase hor. 3	-0.41	-0.5	-0.41	-0.095	-0.357
Test 4 hor	Gain hor. 4	0.590	0.024	0.590	-0.071	0.000
	Phase hor. 4	-0.076	-0.35	-0.168	-0.183	-0.176
Test 5 hor	Gain hor. 5	0.283	-0.305	0.197	-0.254	-0.323
	Phase hor. 5	-0.186	-0.367	-0.328	-0.283	-0.176
Test 1 vert	Gain vert. 1	-0.663	-0.500	-0.663	-0.647	-0.548
	Phase vert. 1	-0.169	0.548	-0.169	0.595	0.524
Test 2 vert	Gain vert. 2	-0.473	-0.571	-0.473	-0.786	-0.679
	Phase vert. 2	0.337	0.286	0.337	0.429	0.357
Test 3 vert	Gain vert. 3	0.108	-0.167	0.108	-0.619	-0.286
	Phase vert. 3	0.265	0.167	0.255	0.333	0.286
Test 4 vert	Gain vert. 4	0.073	-0.679	0.073	-0.821	-0.786
	Phase vert. 4	0.255	0.286	-0.255	0.464	0.357
Test 5 vert	Gain vert. 5	0.206	-0.429	0.000	-0.595	-0.443
	Phase vert. 5	0.691	1.000	0.691	0.893	0.964

* r-values > ±0.6 are underlined.

Discussion and Conclusion

The Expert Relative Ranking Method

In this study we used a method to evaluate spatial orientation aptitudes in competitive gymnasts that uses the highly specialized and accumulated expertise of coaches. The thousands of hours that a coach has experienced observing his/her athletes creates an extremely rich and multifaceted information source that is often not exploited. This form of "tacit" knowledge is difficult to quantify or articulate, but rather, reflects the implicit learning that occurs as a function of extensive experience (Cote, Salmela, Trudel, Baria, & Russel, 1995; Nash & Collins, 2006). In the past, coaches' practical intelligence has remained untapped as a resource for evaluating global performance aptitudes in high-level athletes or other expert populations. However, measures such as the relative ranking method used here provide several unique advantages to supplement more traditional measures. For instance, overall rankings provide an opportunity to assess general, intrinsic aptitudes that are often difficult to quantify compared to detailed deconstructions of specific task performance on one particular occasion. This is also a problem that has been expressed in other fields when trying to evaluate skills related to, for example, musicality or artistic abilities where discrete elements are difficult to separate from each other when evaluating overall talent. The advantages of performing these types of more global assessments have, in fact, been demonstrated in fields such as medical education where expert examiners are asked to judge the clinical skills of medical students. Specifically, the Objective Structured Clinical Examination (OSCE) measure asks the examiner to both provide a detailed checklist of specific skill performance and a separate overall, global score on their general competence. Studies have shown that it is, in fact, the global performance score that correlate more closely with level of expertise and amount of experience rather than the detailed scorecard ratings (Hodges, Regehr, Hanson, & McNaughton, 1998; Hodges et al., 1999).

The ranking system introduced in the current study also provides access to the wealth of knowledge possessed by highly experienced expert coaches in a way that does not require them to formally articulate their decision-making process. Nash and Collins (2006) nicely illustrate the role of tacit knowledge in the development of coaching abilities. They describe how coaches often react based on their "gut feelings" without the ability to explain exactly what led them to their decisions or behaviours. It is also indicated that this type of knowledge is one that is difficult or impossible to share through teaching or instruction, but rather must be obtained through direct personal experiences. Finally, it is suggested that as the level of coaching expertise develops, the knowledge becomes less structured and increasingly abstract. Overall, this appears to allow experts to more easily detect patterns of behaviour, which leads to greater flexibility and faster recognition (see Nash & Collins, 2006 for a comprehensive review).

Descriptive VOR Results

The "concave shaped" development of the mean values in the vertical gain across the five test conditions could be explained by the fact that the information provided by the otolith signals (indicating the direction of earth gravity) during tests in the earth *vertical* plane can be additionally integrated and therefore help to enhance VOR accuracy (e.g. Leigh & Zee, 2006,). In contrast to this, during rotations in earth *horizontal* plane the otolith information remains stable and can *not* be used for additional vestibular perception. This higher sensitivity in the vertical plane was marked as a function of frequency on the one hand (test 1-3) and of sinusoidal amplitude on the other hand (test 3-5).

Both gain and phase values show a high inter-individual variability that is marked by a more intra-individual stability across the five test conditions. This is graphically demonstrated by the fact that the lines of the intra-individual development across the tests are oriented in a more parallel fashion than undirectionally crossed with each another (compare Figure 3).

Comparing Expert Ranking Scores to VOR Responses

As described in the introduction there are many studies that report a *reduction* or even *suppression* of the VOR response induced by rotational habituation or by specific cues during rotational loads. However, in contrast to the *smooth pursuit function* (compare: von Laßberg,

Beykirch, Campos, & Krug, 2012) there is no clear evidence that a direct *enhancement* of the individual VOR level can be induced by repeated rotational loads or by a specific rotational training.

The most notable results reported here, however, are slight relationships that were observed comparing the individual VOR characteristics to the relative ranking data. Specifically, some vertical VOR values were correlated with the ranking scores. Essentially, this seems to suggest that for the gymnasts, under the most demanding conditions, vertical VOR appears to relate to aptitude. Specifically, higher gain values were seen in the gymnasts ranked as being better (lower ranking score) relative to their comparable gymnast peers at their level. Again, it must be noted that the relationships between VOR characteristics and aptitudes ranking reported here are based on VOR patterns measured during naïve *passive* motion conditions and therefore do not represent what exactly happens during actively performed movements. However the VOR values during standardized stimuli, as used in the present study, represent the natural level of individual VOR functions best.

While the correlation between a high VOR accuracy and ranking reported here might seem contradictory to the phenomenon of a total *suppression* of the VOR during the fast rotation phase in actively performed multiaxial somersaults (von Laßberg et al. 2014; see introduction), this may relate to the adaptive nature of adjusting oculomotor functions to the needs of the specific task constraints (e.g. total *suppression* of EREM by the function of "spinal motor coupled eye movements" vs. *re-activation* of EREM for efficient visual control before landings [von Laßberg et al., 2014]). For a most efficient function of the re-activation of VOR after total suppression, the results presented here seem to support the hypothesis that higher individual VOR accuracies could be a factor that helps to better orient during that critical phase to ensure a safe landing (or regrasping bars etc. during a routine). However, there were several findings that introduced possible avenues to pursue for future research.

For instance, correlations were only observed for *vertical* VOR gain components rather than horizontal. While the cause of the directional bias in this case is not entirely clear, there is some evidence that unidirectional VOR biases are observed for certain types of athletes (e.g. Alpini et al., 2010; Tanguy, 2008b). Gymnasts are mainly exposed to rotations in the *vertical* plane. Pure rotations in the earth-horizontal plane are rare in gymnastics. In contrast to some few compository elements, like short pirouettes in women´s gymnastics, such elements do not exist in men´s artistic gymnastics. Longitudinal axis rotations appear mostly as superimposed rotational components during rotations in the vertical plane. Therefore, a higher VOR level in the vertical plane may relate to more sport specific advantages (and therefore better rankings).

Further, the correlations between vertical VOR gains and expert rankings were mostly higher for the multi-axial aptitudes than for the quasi-static balance regulation tasks. It could be argued that the VOR is more closely associated with multi-axial rotations than with quasi-static balance tasks because during such fast and dynamic whole body movements an extraordinary precision of visual control is necessary to control safe landings (or re-.grasp movements to bars after flight-elements etc.). In contrast, the eye movement control during more static tasks (such as the balance weighted aptitudes) might be more closely related to OKR and smooth pursuit functions that are known as to be most relevant in slow head movements, whereas the VOR has the highest relevance in fast head rotations (Leigh & Zee, 2006). Additionally, balance aptitudes could be much more closely related to other sensory inputs such as kinaesthetic or tactile afferents than to mechanisms of oculomotor stabilization.

This would fit to prior measures that have suggested that gymnasts demonstrate a greater ability to restabilize their posture after their balance has been perturbed or when stabilizing visual information has been manipulated (Gauthier, Thouvarecq, & Larue, 2008; Gauthier, Thouvarecq, & Vuillerme, 2008; Krug, von Laßberg, & Muehlbauer, 2002; Perrin, Perrin, Boura, Uffhotz, & Conraux, 1989; Vuillerme, Danion, Marin, Boyadjian, Prieur, Weise, & Nougier, 2001).

Concerning the observed *phase* values in the current study, a particularly interesting result is the consistent development across the five test conditions from an initial *phase lag* in the tests with low amplitudes to an increasing *phase lead* in the tests with high amplitudes in nearly all the participants. The phase lag during the short oscillations could be associated with the test conditions that gymnasts were less familiar with (short oscillations of about 30°), in comparison to test five, which had the largest amplitudes (about 340°) and peak velocities that the gymnasts are more experienced with (even though these are still much slower than the most experienced rotational velocities during twisting somersaults or similar elements with about 400 to more than 1000°/s).

The result, that only the phase values of test five were marked by high correlations with the rankings, whereas no correlations were found in the other tests, could also be due to the fact that gymnasts are specifically used to larger rotational amplitudes rather than to shorter oscillations. Another explanation could be that during the longer duration of the sinusoidal cycles and the higher amplitudes, the phase could be better adapted to the present conditions than in the tests with only short cycle durations and small sinusoidal amplitudes.

Overall, it appears as though there is no simple relationship between level of expertise in rotationally-demanding activities and VOR characteristics. Rather, it appears as though having an increased/decreased VOR may be adapted in a more flexible manner depending on the demands of the task. In some scenarios a suppression of VOR can be advantageous to support other reflexive systems such as the "spinal motor coupled eye movements" (von Laßberg et al. 2014). These are assumed to be driven by the more proprioceptively induced oculomotor reflex systems (such as COR, TOR, leg induced response etc.) to support a most efficient new-orientation of the body in space without being disturbed by any counteracting gaze stabilizing functions. Further, in some situations sensory conflicts might be present (e.g. between visual and vestibular afferents) and therefore, there may be also a functional advantage to suppressing specific elements of a signal that is not consistent with other signals. For example, during a double somersault there is a continuous centrifugal otolith signal directed cranially regardless whether the body is in an upright position or in an inverted position (this relates to moving on a parabolic flight curve). Consequently, these ambiguous otolith signals cannot be used to correctly interpret the body position under such circumstances and therefore it might actually be more advantageous to suppress these signals in favour of other sensory signals (e.g. visual). Novice individuals, who have not yet learned which sensory signals should be weighted higher or lower during particular circumstances, may not react as effectively.

We therefore assume that there are two counteracting factors that determine spatial orientation abilities. 1) The individual sensitivity (level) of the VOR system as a prerequisite that supports a high precision for EREM functions that are necessary for visual control when needed to control landings, re-grasps of a bar after flight elements etc. This function does not seem to be training dependent but more influenced and determined by individual factors. 2) The ability to suppress VOR in situations when it is necessary for most efficient movement performance (when stabilizing functions would disturb the movements). During such movement phases all body and gaze stabilizing functions (including the VOR) would inhibit highly efficient movement performance that needs an efficient co-directed new-orientation of eye, head, and all body segments without being disturbed by stabilzing functions. As described in our study during multiaxial flight elements (von Laßberg et al. 2014) we postulate that both functions are necessary, yet they have different (and even counteracting) functions for the context-specific needs during multiaxial whole body movements. So it seems that not only the individual precision of any specific sensory systems is mainly responsible for functional spatial orientation abilities, even though their highly efficient functions are essential prerequisites to enable multiaxial spatial orientation.

The additional ability of adequate context specific activation and deactivation (suppression) of different reflexive systems, and the adequate situational weighting and functional judgement of different sensory signals during movements are also factors that must be learned to cope with, to get able to efficiently orient during complex multiaxial movements. This multimodal and complex ability cannot be measured by passive tests - it will remain a domain of the "tacit knowledge" of highly experienced raters. Eventhough the method we used within this study is based on a subjective estimation of humans, no other (more objective) tests will be able to sufficiently replace this unique ability of human estimation. The results of correlations in individual vertical VOR levels with these expert evaluations provide a first empirical indication that there *could* exist relationships between individual VOR level and spatial orientation aptitudes. So, further studies are necessary to examine whether similar results can be found in future investigations.

Acknowledgments

The study was supported by the "Bundesinstitut für Sportwissenschaft" (National Institute of Sport Science), Germany. Our thanks go to Prof. Dr. Jürgen Krug at Institute of General Kinesiology and Athletics Training, University of Leipzig, for his support, to the Hertie Institute for Clinical Brain Research in Tübingen for using the TVRS, and to the gymnasts and coaches of the National Gymnastics Training Center "KunstTurnForum" in Stuttgart for their cooperation.

References

Ahn, S.C., Lee, C.Y., Kim, D.W., & Lee, M.H. (2000). Short-term vestibular responses to repeated rotations. *Journal of Vestibular Research, 10*, 17-23.

Alpini, D., Botta, M., Mattei, V., & Tornese, D. (2009). Figure ice skating induces vestibulo-ocular adaptation specific to required athletic skills. *Sport Sciences for Health, 5(3)*, 129-134.

Aschan, G. (1954). Response to rotatory stimuli in fighter pilots. *Acta Otolaryngologica,43 (S116)*, 24-31.Baloh, R.W., Henn, V., & Jäger, J. (1982). Habituation of the vestibulo-ocular reflex with low-frequency harmonic acceleration. *American Journal of Otolaryngology, 3,* 235-241.

Baloh, R.W., Langhofer, L., Honrubia, V., & Yee, R.D. (1980). On-line analysis of eye movements using a digital computer. *Aviation Space Environment Medicine, 51(6),* 563-567.

Balter, S.G.T., Stokroos, R.J., Akkermans, E., & Kingma, H. (2004). Habituation to galvanic vestibular stimulation for analysis of postural control abilities in gymnasts. *Neuroscience Letters, 366 (1),* 71-75.

Bechert, K., & Koenig, E. (1996). A search coil system with automatic field stabilization, calibration, and geometric processing for eye movement recording in humans. *Neuro-Ophthalmology, 16 (3),* 163-170.

Clement G., Tilikete C., & Courjon J.H. (2008). Retention of habituation of vestibulo-ocular reflex and sensation of rotation in humans. *Experimental Brain Research,* 190, 307-315.

Cote, J., Salmela, J., Trudel, P., Baria, A. & Russel, S. (1995). The coaching model: a grounded assessment of expert gymnastic coaches´ knowledge. *Journal of Sport & Exercise Psychology, 17*(1), 1 - 17.

Davlin, C.D., Sands, W.A., & Shultz, B.B. (2001). The role of vision in control of orientation in a back tuck somersault. *Motor Control*, 5(4), 337–346.

Gauthier, G., Thouvarecq, R., & Larue, J. (2008). Influence of experience on postural control: Effect of expertise in gymnastics. *Journal of Motor Behavior, 40 (5),* 400-408.

Gauthier, G., Thouvarecq, R., & Vuillerme, N. (2008). Postural control and perceptive configuration: Influence of expertise in gymnastics. *Gait & Posture, 28 (1),* 46-51.

Heinen, T. (2011). Evidence for the spotting hypothesis in gymnasts. *Motor Control,* 15(2), 267–284.

Hodges, B., Regehr, G., Hanson, M., & McNaughton, N. (1998). An objective structured clinical exam in psychiatry: a validation study. *Academic Medicine, 73*, 910-912.

Hodges, B., Regehr, G., McNaughton, N., Tiberius, R., & Hanson, M. (1999). OSCE checklists do not capture increasing levels of expertise. *Academic Medicine, 74,* 1129–1134.

Hondzinski, J.M., & Darling, W.G. (2001). Aerial somersault performance under three visual conditions. *Motor Control,* 5 (3), 281–300.

Koenig, E., Westermann, H., Jager, K., Sell, G., Bechert, K., Fetter, M., & Dichgans, J. (1996). A new multiaxis rotating chair for oculomotor and vestibular function testing in humans. *Neuro-Ophthalmology, 16 (3),* 157-162.

Krug, J., von Laßberg, C., & Muehlbauer, T. (2002). Load effects of fast longitudinal rotations. In: Gianikellis, K.E., editor. Proceedings of XXth International Society of Biomechanics in Sports. Cáceres, Spain. ISBS – Conference Proceedings Archive, pp. 535–538.

Lee, M.Y., Kim, M.S., & Park, B.R. (2004). Adaptation of the horizontal vestibuloocular reflex in pilots. *Laryngoscope, 114 (5),* 897-902.

Lee D.N., Young D.S., & Rewt D. (1992). How do somersaulters land on their feet? *Journal of Experimental Psychology and Human Perception Performance,* 18(4): 1195–1202.

Leigh, R.J., & Zee, D.S. (2006). The Neurology of Eye Movements. Fourth Edition. Oxford University Press. Inc.

Luis, M., & Tremblay, L. (2008). Visual feedback use during a back tuck somersault: evidence for optimal visual feedback utilization. *Motor Control,* 12(3), 210–218.

Melvill Jones, G., Berthoz, A., & Segal, B. (1984). Adaptive modification of the vestibulo-ocular reflex by mental effort in darkness. *Experimental Brain Research, 56*, 149-153.

Nash, C., & Collins, D. (2006). Tacit knowledge in expert coaching: Science or art? *Quest, 58 (4),* 465-477.

Perrin, P., Perrin, C., Boura, M., Uffhotz, H., & Conraux, C. (1989). Posturographie statique et dynamique. Application à une population de jeunes sportifs. *Annales Otolaryngologie, 106*, 463 – 471.

Shelhamer, M., Robinson, D.A., & Tan, H.S. (1992). Context-specific adaptation of the gain of the vestibulo.ocular reflex in humans. *Journal of Vestibular Research, 2*, 89-96.

Schalén, L. (1980). Quantification of tracking eye movements in normal subjects. *Acta Otolaryngologica,*90, 404-413.

Schwarz, U. & Henn, V. (1989). Vestibular habituation in student pilots. *Aviation Space Environment Medicine, 60 (8),* 755-761.

Tanguy, S.G., Quarck, G.M., Etard, O.M., Gauthier, A.F., & Denise, P. (2008a). Vestibulo-ocular reflex and motion sickness in figure skaters. *European Journal of Applied Physiology, 104 (6),* 1031-1037.

Tanguy, S.G., Quarck, G.M., Etard, O.M., Gauthier, A.F., & Denise, P. (2008b). Are otolithic inputs interpreted better in figure skaters? *Neuroreport, 19 (5),* 565-568.

Vuillerme, N., Danion, F., Marin, L., Boyadjian, A., Prieur, J.M., Weise, I., & Nougier, V. (2001). The effect of expertise in gymnastics on postural control. *Neuroscience Letters, 303 (2),* 83-86.

von Laßberg, C. (2007). Okulomotorische Orientierungsregulation bei multiaxialen Ganzkörperrotationen (Oculomotor control during multiaxial whole body rotations). Köln, Germany: Sportverlag Strauß.

von Laßberg, C., Beykirch, K.A., Campos, J.L., Krug, J. (2012). Smooth pursuit eye movement adaptation in high level gymnasts. *Motor Control,* 16(2), 176–194.

von Laßberg, C., Beykirch, K.A., Mohler, B.J., Bülthoff, H.H. (2014). Intersegmental eye-head-body interactions during complex whole body movements. *PLoS ONE*, 9(4), e95450. doi:10.1371/journal.pone.0095450.

In: Advances in Visual Perception Research
Editor: Thomas Heinen

ISBN: 978-1-63482-455-2
© 2015 Nova Science Publishers, Inc.

Chapter 5

Fixation Durations - Why Are They So Highly Variable?

Niels Galley[1], *Dirk Betz*[2,3,*] *and Claudia Biniossek*[2,3]
[1]University Cologne, Center for Anatomy, Cologne, Germany.
[2]GESIS – Leibniz Institute for the Social Sciences, Cologne, Germany.
[3]University of Cologne, Institute of Sociology and Social Psychology, Cologne, Germany

Abstract

Fixation duration is the time during which the eyes rest on an object in the surroundings. Fixation lasts approximately 250 milliseconds (ms) but often is shorter or longer. It is usually defined as the time between the end of one saccade and the beginning of the next one. Usually we fixate on something in our surroundings consciously. However, fixation duration can vary between several milliseconds, which is too short for conscious control, and several seconds. The reasons for this large variation are not obvious. In this book chapter we look at eye movement data collected with an electrooculogram (EOG) from a large population. A total of up to 1131 subjects performed several tasks, for example looking at a picture, tracking a moving spot, solving an intelligence test (Raven matrices) or closing the eyes, a situation in which saccades do not pause. Particularly, we reinforce the view of fixations as a mental or cognitive process that can be separated into several partitions. For example, in the past the so-called *express fixations* in the range of less than 100 ms to approximately 150 ms were assigned to a special group of short fixations and were controversial. These shorter fixation durations as well as ones that last for seconds do occur, and these *very short* or *very long* fixation durations have seldom attracted the interest of researchers. Visual processes and mental processes can be more or less connected. In this book chapter we try to determine some reasons for the obvious high variability of fixation durations, which occur in both the closely and loosely connected modes of the visual-motor and the cognitive system.

* Corresponding author: GESIS – Leibniz Institute for the Social Sciences, Unter Sachsenhausen 6-8, 50667 Cologne, Germany. Email: dirk.betz@gesis.org.

Keywords: eye movement, visual processes, express fixation, fixation duration, saccades, mental processes, electrooculogram (EOG)

Introduction – Why Are Fixation Durations So Different?

In the EOG of a child (see Figure 1) twelve saccades and subsequent fixations can be seen. The child was looking at a table of Raven Matrices (Raven, Court, & Raven, 1978) and trying to figure out which of the six alternatives shown at the bottom correctly filled in the gap at the top.

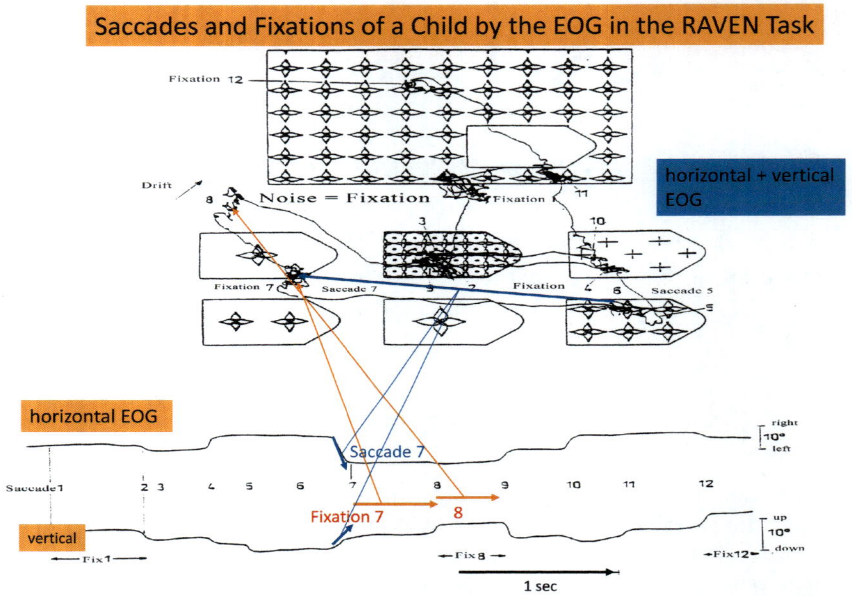

Figure 1. In the lower field have the horizontal and the vertical EOG of a child who looked at the *Raven* table (in the upper field) and tried to decide which of the six alternatives correctly filled the gap in the upper figure. The two-dimensional EOG is spatially overlayed on the figure, which represents fixations as tangles and saccades as straight lines.

Fixation 1 lasts 800 ms, during which the eyes rest on the gap at the bottom of the pattern, which is to be filled with the correct option. Saccade 2 goes down to the second option, and the eyes only rest there for approximately 100 ms. Then, saccade 3 goes horizontally to the third alternative with a fixation of approximately 400 ms. The eyes of the child move further along the lower pattern with the six alternatives to fill the gap until saccade 11 again reaches the upper pattern. After saccade 12 and its accompanying fixation duration 12, which had a duration of 300 ms, the child gave the correct answer by pointing to 'alternative 6'. Interestingly the eyes hadn't rested on alternative 5, and one can speculate if the child had overlooked this choice or excluded this false choice using peripheral vision when the gaze rested at nearby alternatives 6, 2, 4 or 1.

As one can see in Figure 2, most fixations of adults on a *Raven* task designed for adults are shorter. The *median* for the easier to solve tables was 230 ms, and the median for the more difficult tables was 260 ms.

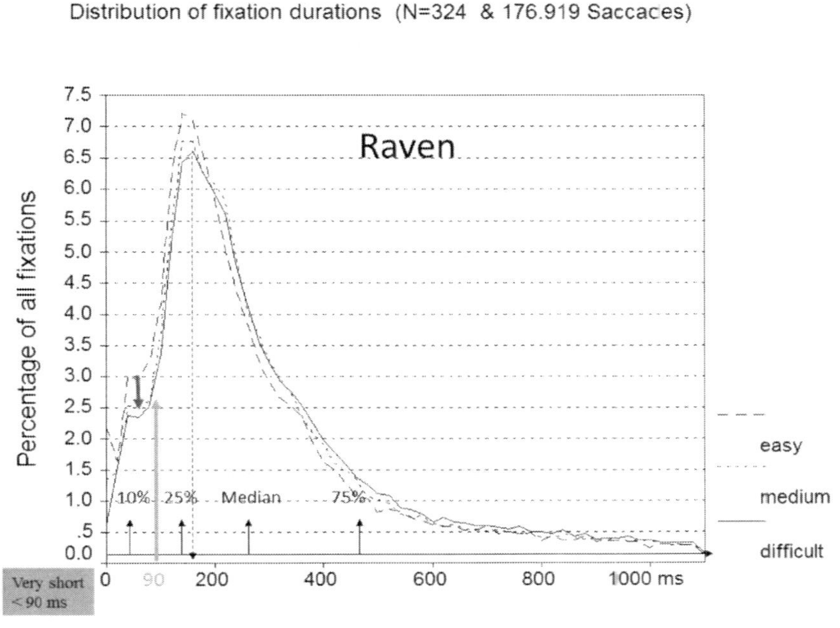

Figure 2. Three frequency curves for fixation durations (in milliseconds = ms) for a subpopulation of 324 students who solved ten *Raven* tables of increasing difficulty. There is a small shift to longer fixation durations when looking at the more difficult *Raven* tables.

The skewed distribution curves show that most of the adult fixations are shorter than those of the child: the *modal* value is 190 ms. However, because there are many long to very long fixations, the median (approximately 250 ms), which is the most used descriptive value of the central tendency, was higher than the most frequent value, which is also known as the modal value. Thus, the modal value seems to be the most obvious choice to describe the distribution curves, instead of the median, which is the more common choice in the literature. It is unnecessary to emphasize that the *mean* value is not appropriate to characterize values of fixation duration, because this description of the central tendency is very dependent on some very high values, which always occur. Nevertheless the mean is often used in the literature (Schweigert, 2003), most likely after the range of too short and too long fixations are eliminated.

It seems obvious from these figures that the reasons for the variability of fixation duration are not evident at first glance but must be deduced from factors that have a measurable effect on duration. Figure 2 shows three distribution curves for fixation duration: one comes from the easy to solve *Raven* tables, one comes from the difficult to solve tables and one comes from those of moderate difficulty. The three curves are *shifted* a *little bit to the right for longer durations*. This is an indication of *one small* factor, which is responsible for different fixation duration values: *the more difficult the task for the subject, the longer the eyes remain on the fixated object.*

Another feature of these three curves seems noteworthy: in the area of very short fixations, roughly less than 90 ms, there are fewer values if the task is more difficult (marked by the red arrow). This is a typical effect of the *inhibition of irrelevant behavior*. More mental effort indicates longer fixations not only by inhibiting the release of the next saccade but also by specifically impeding very short fixations. This can be an effect of *concentration,* which seems to induce a shift to more conscious, late operations and less spontaneous, early ones. The difficulty of the task and the induced mental effort of the subject seem therefore two small factors among many other probable factors that influence fixation duration.

In Figure 1, the child's eyes rest between 100 and approximately 800 ms. In contrast, if a robotic device had scanned this pattern, there would be a very uniform rate. Perhaps some of the child's *internal mental processes* need different lengths of time before the eyes are allowed to move to the next position. However, can there be a *thinking process* that lasts only 100 ms? For example, in such a manner: '*Alternative 3 cannot be the right answer*'. Surely, 'No' should be the answer to this question. This seems to be too short a time to *recognize* the visual object, *to decide something* and then to *initiate another look.* One has to mention that with each shift of the gaze the subject has two tasks: The first is to analyze the stimuli in the central vision and the second is to decide where in the periphery to look next. A new saccade is presumptively not generated until the object(s) falling on the fovea had been sufficiently analyzed. Then, one has to select which object in the visual scene should be looked at next. Some basic analysis needs to be carried out in the near or far periphery to allow for a desirable selection. Thus, very short fixations of <90 ms seem to have no opportunity to be controlled by conscious cognitive operations. Longer fixations in the range of 'express fixations' - as the range between 90 and 150 ms is called – have very little time for cognitive operations, so they will presumptively go to *expected locations* or otherwise foreseen locations. However, what sort of control processes can be assumed for this very short duration behavior of 80 or 70 ms? We will return to this point later on. Now it seems necessary to explain how to measure the exact time of such short fixation durations.

How to Measure Fixations?

To measure fixation duration one has to identify the *saccades* that flank fixation and bring the eyes (and then the visual centers in the brain) into powerful contact with a new object because the fovea is the retinal place where this new object is projected. The fovea has the highest spatial resolution, and its central representation has preferential access to consciousness. For example, it is seldom consciously recognized that most objects in our peripheral vision are doubles.

Saccades are movements of the eyes with very high velocities that are flanked by rests of the eyes, so the human inspector has no difficulties identifying saccades even in a noisy signal such as the electrooculogram (EOG), because these rests are seen as plateaus before and after abrupt changes. We used EOG in our research on fixations. As seen in Figure 3, saccades in the EOG look like large stairs if they were responses (green beams) to the target jumps or like small stairs between jumps.

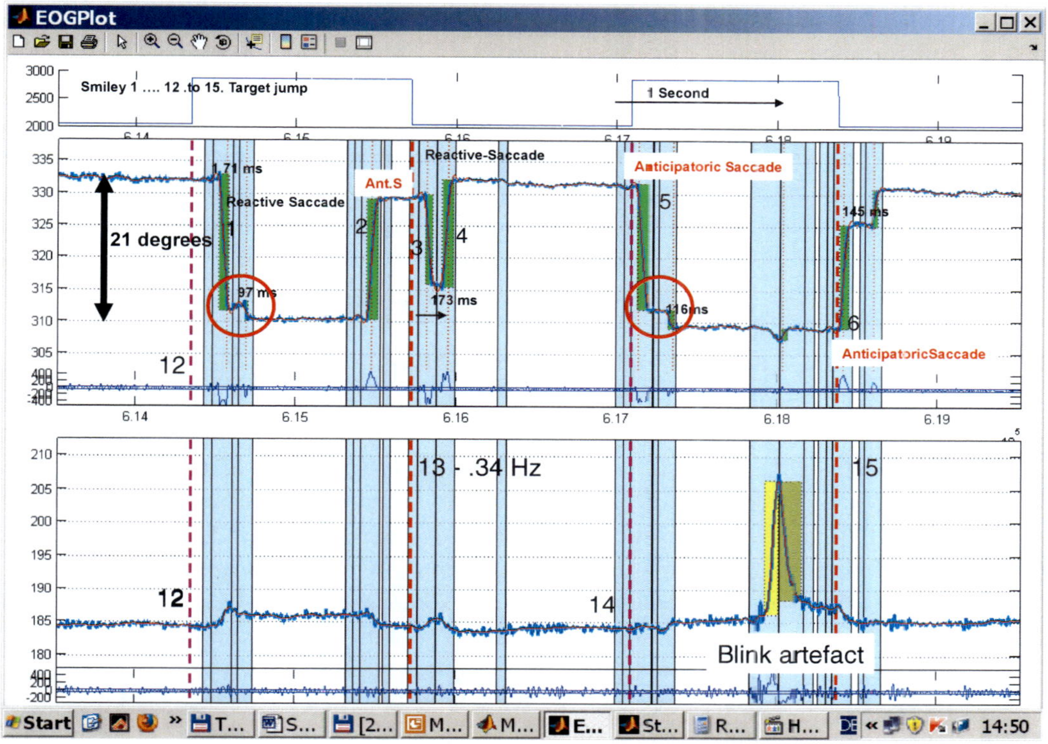

Figure 3. A screenshot of our computer program, EOGUI, which shows the horizontal EOG (first row) and the vertical EOG (second row) for a subject who followed a jumping target spot. The six large saccades that were identified are shown as green beams. They are gaze responses of the subject to target jumps number 12, 13, 14 and 15 in the sequence of 112 jumps with decreasing intervals. In the areas of the EOG that are circled in red, very small saccades can be detected, which were not identified by the program although the human inspector clearly traced these small steps as saccades.

In the task, *Jumping Point,* the subject had to follow a jumping target point on a screen with his gaze "as closely as possible". The target point jumped over a distance of 21 degrees (in this example) with continuously diminishing intervals. At the beginning, the frequency of the jumping was slow (0.2 Hz), but it sped up to 1.4 Hz, which is very demanding. Figure 3 is a detail of the horizontal (upper row) and vertical EOG channels (lower row) in which a blink artefact can be seen. Starting from jump number 12 the first response saccade (1) occurred 171 ms later. The next saccade (2) occurred approximately 250 ms before jump number 13 and is thus an anticipatory saccade. Very shortly after the jump a return saccade (3) can be seen. Very shortly afterwards another response saccade (4) occurred. Therefore, we had to decide if saccade 2 or 4 was the response saccade, because more than one response saccade for one target jump is not appropriate. We decided that the large saccade in the correct direction that came closest to the time of the target jump should be counted as the response saccade and all other saccades should not. In this case saccade 4 is the winner, because it is nearer to the time of the target jump than saccade 2.

A green beam overlaying the EOG signifies that our computer program EOGUI has identified a saccade at that time. Here is a URL where people can download our program: http://www.mathworks.com/matlabcentral/ fileexchange/ 32493.

The program is and has to be *conservative*: It is better for some very small saccades to be missed than for some noise to be identified as saccades. There are some consequences of using our machine to identify fixation durations. Every time a small saccade is missed, the fixation duration that is registered is too long. However, as one can see in figure 4, saccades aren't normally very small. If they were 2 degrees or larger, they were mostly well identified by the program. The percentage of saccades not identified by the program is 5 to 6 percent. By using the median of many fixations per subject and per task, the presence of some artificial, overly long fixations does not matter.

What Can the EOG (Not) Tell Us about Fixations and Eye Movements?

We have mentioned that noise in the electrooculogram can prevent saccades smaller than 1 to 2 degrees from being by identified by our computer program. However, there is another weakness of EOG: as you can see in Figure 1, the EOG is superimposed over signal drift. In concrete terms, the signal is not positionally stable over a long time period. It has a very slow inherent shift, which makes determining exact position information of the eyes impossible. Thus, the sometimes very important information some users hope to obtain from eye movement registration, namely, *where* the subject is looking, is not simply available from EOG. Therefore, in a comprehensive guide to methods and measures (Holmqvist, Nyström Andersson, Dewhurst, Jarodzka & Van de Weijer, 2011) for eye movement registration systems, EOG is only mentioned as a low-cost method that is not useful for research. This seems to be a too strict verdict, but it is worth asking what research *should not be conducted* with EOG:

- All research which needs exact information about the position of the gaze in relation to the target.
- All research on saccades of very small amplitude, which are called microsaccades. The question of how many microsaccades occur is relevant. Our computer program identified overly long fixation durations if a microsaccade was missed. However, fortunately microsaccades aren't very frequent (see below), and the few occurrences were made less important by using the median of the fixation duration.

There are at least three advantages of EOG over other systems of eye movement registration:

1) EOG and thus saccades, fixations and blink artefacts can be collected when *the eyes are closed*. The Eyes Closed Condition occurs not only during sleep and can serve as an interesting control condition for tasks with open eyes. Saccades are still present during very light sleep as well as during so-called REM sleep, which is *rapid eye movement* sleep while dreaming. The name REM was chosen by Aserinsky and Kleitman (1953), who were unaware that these rapid eye movements were saccades. However, rapid eye movements or saccades, as we now know, are absent in deep slow wave sleep, when the EEG is dominated by delta waves.
2) In the vertical EOG channel, there is an obvious *blink* artefact (see Figure 3), which enabled us to detect all blinks and to analyze the circumstances of their occurrence.

Blinks are short time interruptions of vision due to the covering of the pupil by the lid. A blink lasts for approximately 200 ms. Blink rates are very variable between people and signify attention or variations in vigilance as well as characteristics of the subject's arousal level.

3) As an electrical signal, EOG has good time resolution. Thus it is possible to obtain very exact fixation durations on a millisecond basis, which is crucial for our present topic.

How often Do Microsaccades Occur, and What Is the Function of These Very Small Saccades?

Because very small saccades, called microsaccades, are sometimes missed by computer identification one might wonder how often or how seldom these small saccades occur. In two comprehensive reports about microsaccades (Otero-Millan, Troncoso, Macknik, S.L., Serrano-Pedraza I. & Martinez-Conde , 2008; Rolfs, 2009) the authors wrote that microsaccades have a mean amplitude of half a degree and that their occurrence is a function of the task. Microsaccades become more frequent the longer a fixation duration lasts. However, they are rare during fixations shorter than 250 ms. Microsaccades occur unconsciously but can be inhibited by will. Rolfs (2009) listed seven functions for these very small saccades, of which the *reduction of perceptual fading, the continuity of perception* and the *control of fixation position* seem to be the most important ones.

In our *used standard tasks* histogram, curves of saccadic amplitudes show notable peaks at 2, 3 or 4 degrees and declines at smaller amplitudes (see Figure 4). The exceptions to this rule were the tasks *Eyes Closed* and *Interview,* during which small saccades, i.e., microsaccades, were frequent. However, during these tasks the subjects had no visual task. When the subjects performed *Picture Inspection* or followed a wandering sinusoidal point with their gaze (*Sinus*), solved the *Raven* task, or followed the *Jumping Point* they seldom showed very small saccades. Because we used the medians as the central tendency for fixation duration, the fact that the computer program overlooked some microsaccades had a negligible effect on fixation duration.

Saccade amplitudes differ in relation to the task, but amplitudes larger than 10 degrees are seldom seen with the exception of the J*umping Point* task, in which the task demands a specific amplitude saccade to be performed by the subject. Usually, the target point jumped 12 degrees. The value was 21 degrees in only a few studies, as seen in Figure 3. The responses to the target jumps are usually large amplitude saccades, but small saccades with short latencies do occur, for example when correcting the landing position of the gaze.

Correspondingly, the peak of the amplitudes in this task (see Figure 4) was at 11 degrees, mirroring the tendency of subjects to undershoot the target amplitude by 10 percent. The tendency to make small saccades to correct the undershoot is seen in the increase at 2 degrees for the curve of the jumping point shortly after the large response saccade. The function of other small saccades often remains obscure but may belong to the above-mentioned categories of microsaccades, to prevent the fading of the picture in central representation.

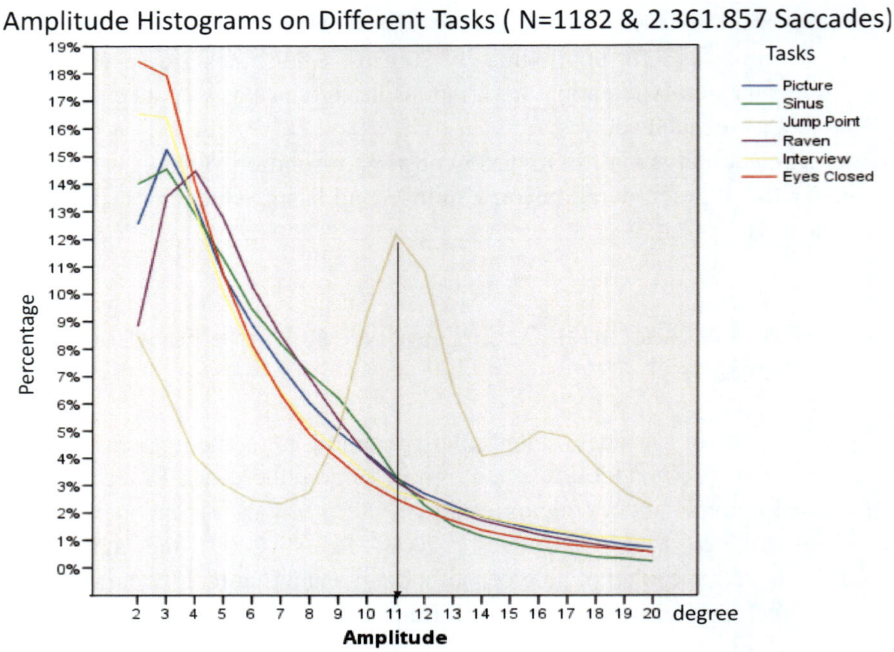

Figure 4. Distribution of histogram curves of saccadic amplitudes (in degrees) in our standard tasks: *Picture Inspection, Sinus, Jumping Point, Raven, Interview,* and *Eyes Closed.* In most tasks, amplitudes of 2,3 or 4 degrees dominate, with the exception of Jumping Point, in which most subjects [but not all (see Figure 3)] had to follow a 12 degree jump of the target.

Our Standard Battery of Tasks

In our research on eye movements with several populations (children, adults, very old people, but mostly students) we used some tasks consistently in different studies. Some of the results are published (Galley 1984; Galley 1987a; Galley, 1987b; Galley and Fritz 1987; Galley 1993; Galley 1998; Galley and Galley 1999; Galley 2001; Galley 2010), but here we report analyses of pooled data under the main aspect *which factors modulate the fixation duration*.

In the task *Picture Inspection,* subjects looked at an illustration by Ali Mitgutsch in which many events occur. Subjects are supposed to remember these events because they will be asked about them later. *Picture Inspection* was usually the first task in our standard battery of tasks. The next two were *Sinus* and *Jumping Point*. Tasks where a moving spot was accelerated from a very slow 0.2 Hz to a fast 1.2 Hz (for children) or to 1.6 Hz for adults over 12 or 20 degrees were strenuous. In the task *Sinus,* the horizontal sinusoid's target spot wanders back and forth, following the same frequency scale as in the task *Jumping Point*, but the *pursuit eye movement system* is prominently involved in this task (Thier & Ilg, 2005), while only the saccadic eye movement system is involved in *Jumping Point.* Subjects followed the *sinus* target with prominently smooth pursuit eye movements, nevertheless, many saccades can be seen. Thus the rests of the eyes on the moving target are overlaid by abrupt changes of position from time to time. Usually these saccades aren't large, thus, the target does not leave the zone around the fovea from which the pursuit system controls the eyes. Increasing the velocity of the sinusoidal movement of the target increases the incidence of bigger saccades.

In most of our own studies cited above, these tasks were followed by the *Raven* task in a children's form (see Figure 1) or a corresponding adult form. Here subjects had to decide which of the alternatives was the correct one to fill the gap in the top figure.

The last two tasks were the *Interview* and *Eyes Closed* tasks. In the *Eyes Closed* task subjects were asked which details of the viewed picture they remembered, while in the task, *Interview,* subjects were questioned about which tasks they judged most or least difficult, most interesting, and so on. In these last two tasks there was no visual presentation that could guide the gaze. During *Eyes Closed,* only the remembered events of the Ali-Mitgutsch-Picture could guide the path of the eyes, and in *Interview* the outside environment was present but irrelevant.

In several studies devoted to different themes, most of our subjects completed these six standard tasks, which lasted only two minutes or less, successively. Only the *Raven* task lasted for several minutes. In every task subjects made hundreds or more fixations. For each fixation the computer identification captured and parameterized the following values: the beginning and end of each saccade in milliseconds as well as in spatial coordinates and the maximal velocity of the saccade. Additionally all blinks, which sometimes mask the occurrence of a saccade, were identified by the algorithm and stored together with the values of the saccades on the hard disk. Pooling several studies for which our standard battery of tasks was used, we obtained a rather large number of subjects ranging from 4 to 90 years old and a huge amount of fixations.

Fixation As a Time Consuming Process Becomes Cognitive Controlled Not until after a while

We reported that sometimes fixation durations are very short, for example only 90 to 100 ms long. We wondered about these *express fixations:* How could visual information be processed so quickly by brain circuits? Visual information has to go through several stations in the retina, be transferred to the visual centers, and reach the oculomotor centers in the brainstem, and it must do all this in a few milliseconds. However, as one can see in Figure 5, a small fraction of fixation durations are *even shorter than 90 ms*. In this figure, the same data as in Figure 2 are analyzed and presented in a slightly different way.

We labelled the shortest range of fixations as *very short (1)* fixations, the next range as *express (2)* and the longer fixations as the *cognitive (3)* range. This is programmatic, and we will present evidence to justify these categorizations and the borderlines between these categories. In comparison with figure 2, we cut off the tail at *very long (4)* fixations in figure 5, but we shall go back to this category later on. The data in figure 5 were arranged into three curves, according to the IQs of the subjects. In figure 2, the three histograms show a slight trend for longer fixations when subjects *solved more difficult problems*, i.e., a shift to the right. In figure 5 the rightward shift is caused by the *lower competence of the subjects*. This corresponds nicely, because for people with lower intelligence the same problem seems to be more difficult. In other words, subjects with less competence *need more time for every fixation*. Thus, one factor that extends fixation duration seems to be the difficulty of the task or the lower competence of the subject.

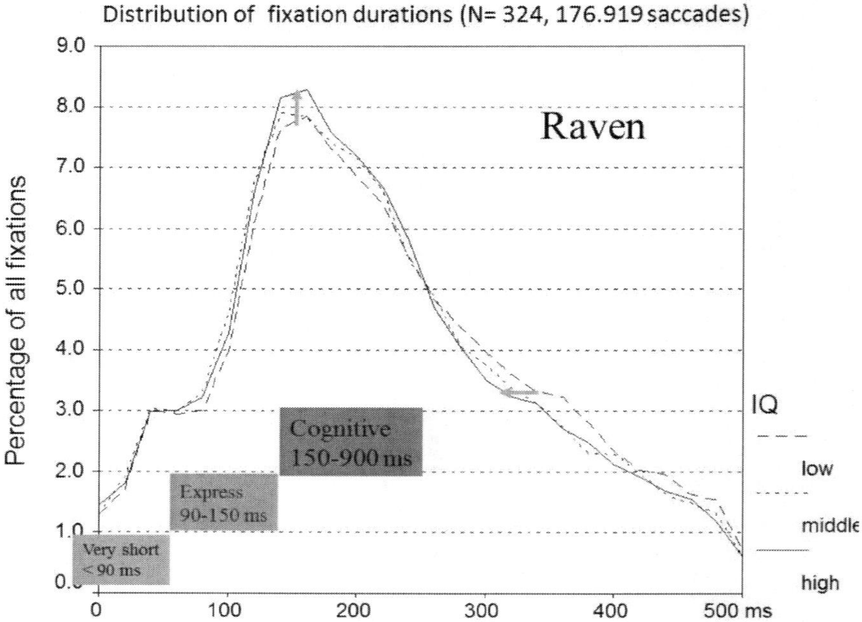

Figure 5. The same data are used here as in figure 2, but now the subject fixation durations during the Raven task are arranged in relation to three components of the subjects' IQ (**intelligence** scores). Additionally only fixation durations shorter than 500 ms were considered. Curves of the more intelligent subjects were shifted to the left, i.e., to shorter values.

The peculiarity of *express latencies* has attracted the attention of researchers due to the astonishingly very fast reaction of saccadic eye movements (less than 100 ms) in response to visual targets (Fischer & Weber, 1993). It has been proven that express reactions are truly visual *reactions* and not anticipatory behavior. However, there are to date open questions about what factors influence the time window of express reactions or express fixations. Thirty years ago, the typical way to obtain more or less express fixations in the laboratory was to have the subject fixate on a small spot, wait until a target appeared, and then look at the target. Usually the latency for the unexpected target is approximately 200 ms, which is double that of express reaction time. But when the fixation stimulus disappears 200 ms before the target appears – a so called *gap paradigm* – express latencies of approximately 100 ms latency often occur. Later on it was found that express fixations are often a rather small part of the normal reaction paradigm called the *overlap condition* and are seen in a multitude of normal visual tasks, such as reading (Radach, Heller & Inhoff, 1998) or searching (Sommer, 1994; McPeek, Skavenski & Nakayama, 2000).

In our task *Jumping Point* (see Figure 3 and 6) we learned about shortening response reaction time. At the beginning, subjects showed response saccade reaction times of approximately 200 ms. Later on subjects tended to shorten their reaction times (Figure 6: 180 ms, 10 ms, 90 ms) or began to anticipate the jump (- 120 ms) when the intervals between the jumps became shorter. *Response saccades* are those that were in the same direction as the target jump, more than half of the amplitude of the target jump and closest in time to the jump.

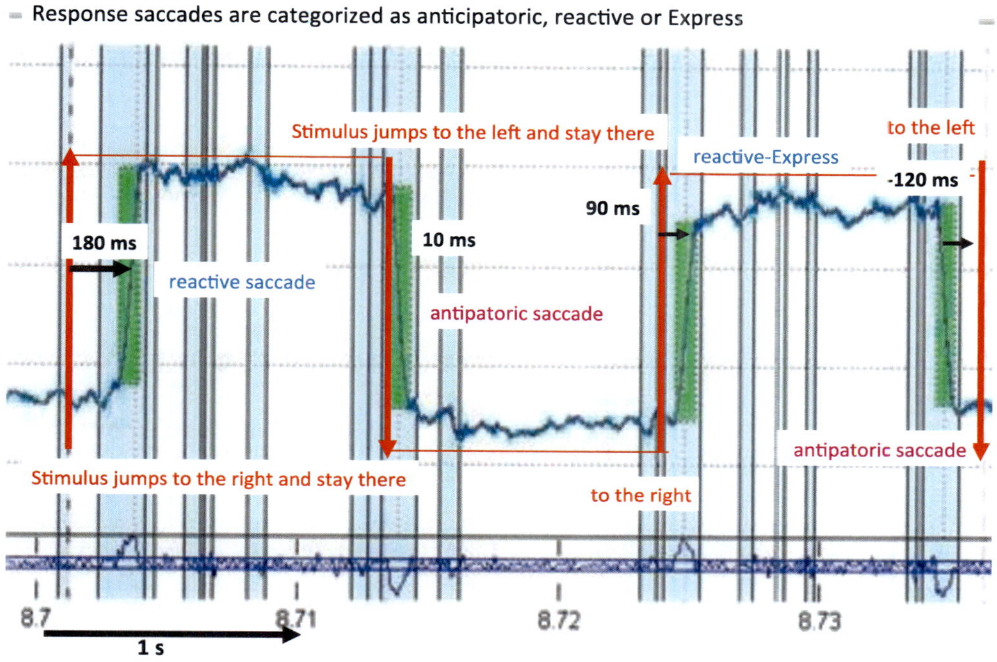

Figure 6. A section from the original registration of the horizontal EOG shows response saccades to target jumps as green beams. The subject's first response shown is a reaction with 180 ms latency after the jump. The next three are: an anticipatory response only 10 ms after the jump, which cannot be a reaction, an express reaction with 90 ms latency and then an anticipatory response, which occurs 120 ms before the target jumps.

The latencies of the responses do not indicate which times are reactive and which are anticipatory. A response 10 ms after the jump is obviously not a reaction but should be considered an anticipatory response. Responses 90 ms after the jump can be *express* reactions, and responses -120 ms before are in *anticipation*. A latency histogram of all response saccades from the large population of subjects who performed the task is shown in figure 7. It provides clues to help categorize the *anticipation*, *express* and *reaction* response modes.

One can see three sections or peaks in this histogram: a very broad peak for probable anticipatory responses and two small peaks at 122 ms and at 180 ms after the jump. These curves led us to *define the express range* as the time window between 90 to 150 ms on a rather small sample (Galley 1990). After we have collected data for a large population, we can now assess whether this decision was correct. Evidence for fundamental differences between *anticipatory*, *express* and *reactive* response saccades comes from the different velocities and amplitudes of these response categories (see Figures 8 and 9).

Computing the standardized mean velocity of the response saccades shows different velocities for the values (see Figure 8): anticipatory response saccades had lower velocities than express or reactive ones over the whole range of jumping frequencies.

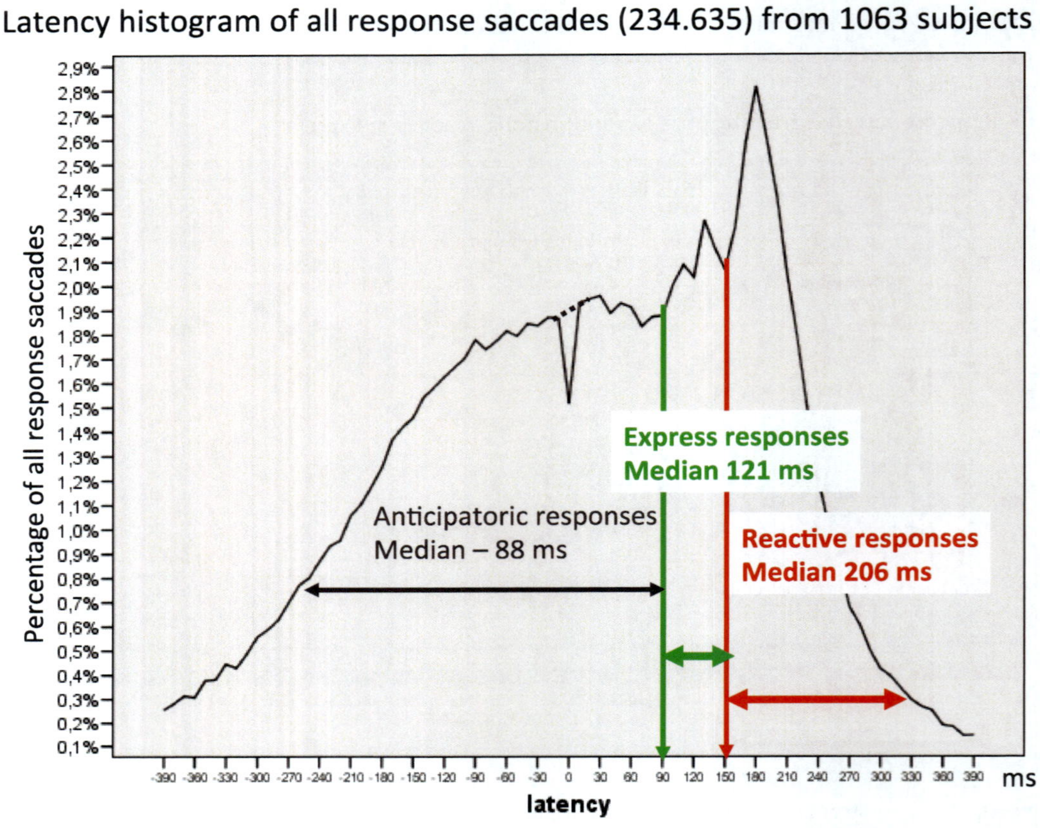

Figure 7. A latency histogram for all the response saccades from a large population ($N = 1063$) shows three sections or peaks. The first, labelled as *anticipatory,* ended approximately 90 ms after the target jump and had a median of – 88 ms ahead of the target jump. The second, labelled as *express,* ended at 150 ms and had a median of 121 ms. The third, called *reactive,* began at this time and had a median of 206 ms. The hollow at 0 ms is an artefact of the SPSS program that results from class construction around zero and is corrected by a dotted line.

Standardization of saccadic velocities is necessary because larger amplitude saccades have higher velocities, which is an undesirable effect.

Standardization computes the velocity of a specific saccade as the percentage of the value this velocity normally owes to this amplitude in a large population (Schleicher & Galley, 2005). For example if a specific saccade with an amplitude of 11 degrees had a velocity of 200 degrees/sec and the normal value was 220 degrees/sec, then the standardized velocity is 200*100/220 = 90.9 percent of the expected value. By this standardization, saccadic velocity becomes a value of the momentary activation, which varies as a function of fatigue, motivation, effort and so on (Galley, 1998).

Analyses of the amplitudes of response saccades in *Jumping Point* additionally show that anticipatory responses tend to have smaller amplitudes than reactive or express responses for the first periods up to 0.6 Hz (see Figure 9).

Response saccades differ in their velocities (N=1063 & 234.635 Saccades)

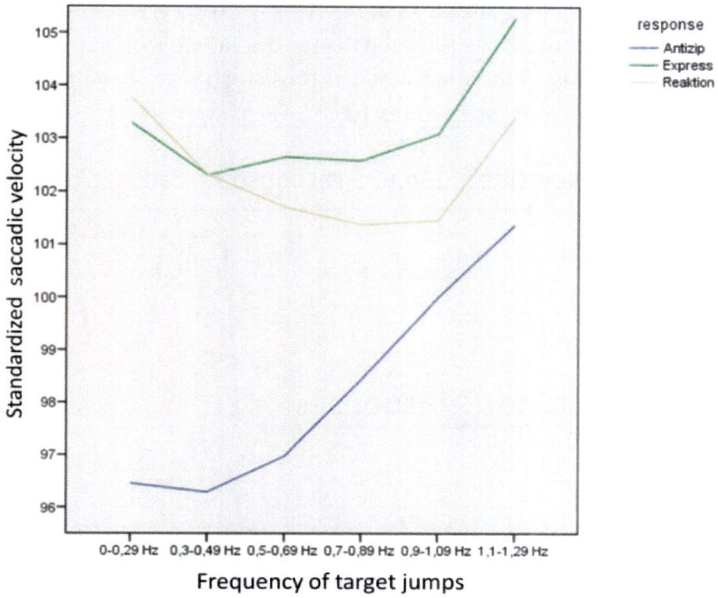

Figure 8. Standardized saccadic velocities in the three response categories (plotted as percentage of expected value) clearly differ. *Anticipatory* responses have lower velocities than *reactive* or *express* ones over the whole range of jumping frequencies.

Response saccades differ in their amplitudes (N=1063 & 234.635 Saccades)

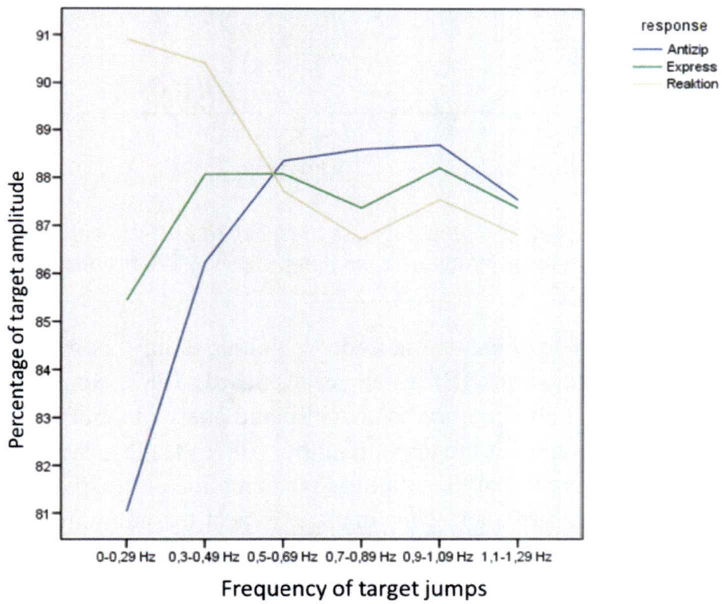

Figure 9. The amplitudes of response saccades with increasing target jump frequency in the different response categories are shown here. Anticipatory response amplitudes in the low frequency range from 0.2 and 0.4 Hz are clearly smaller than the express and reactive ones. Later on, when the jumping frequency increases, the amplitudes become more similar.

Using these different properties of anticipatory, express and reactive responses one can locate the borders of the categories (Galley, 1990) over the latency. Computing the standardized velocity of the response saccades over the latency of the response we found a characteristic increase roughly at the time when express responses began and a decrease when reactive responses began to occur (see Figure 10).

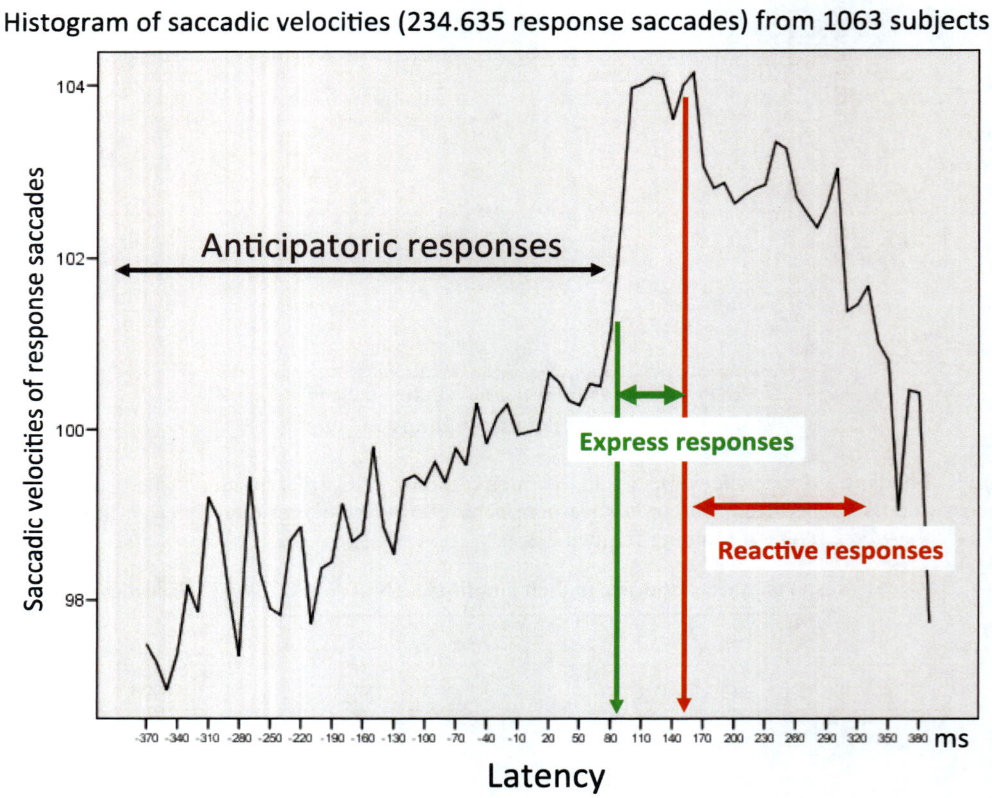

Figure 10. Response saccades show an abrupt increase in (standardized) velocity (plotted as percentage of expected value). Increase begins at 80 ms after the jump. Close to 170 ms one sees a downward trend.

The cause of the lower anticipatory saccade velocities is not known, but other research also confirms the lower velocities (Bronstein & Kennard, 1987; Smit & Van Gisbergen, 1989). Our guess is that that anticipatory behavior spared energy by not withholding the gaze while waiting for the appearance of the target (Galley, 1987b; Galley, 1989).

We have shown in Figure 9 that the amplitudes of anticipatory responses are smaller than reactive or express response saccades. Thus one can expect the amplitudes to show a profile over the latency of the response that reflects this behavior (see Figure 11).

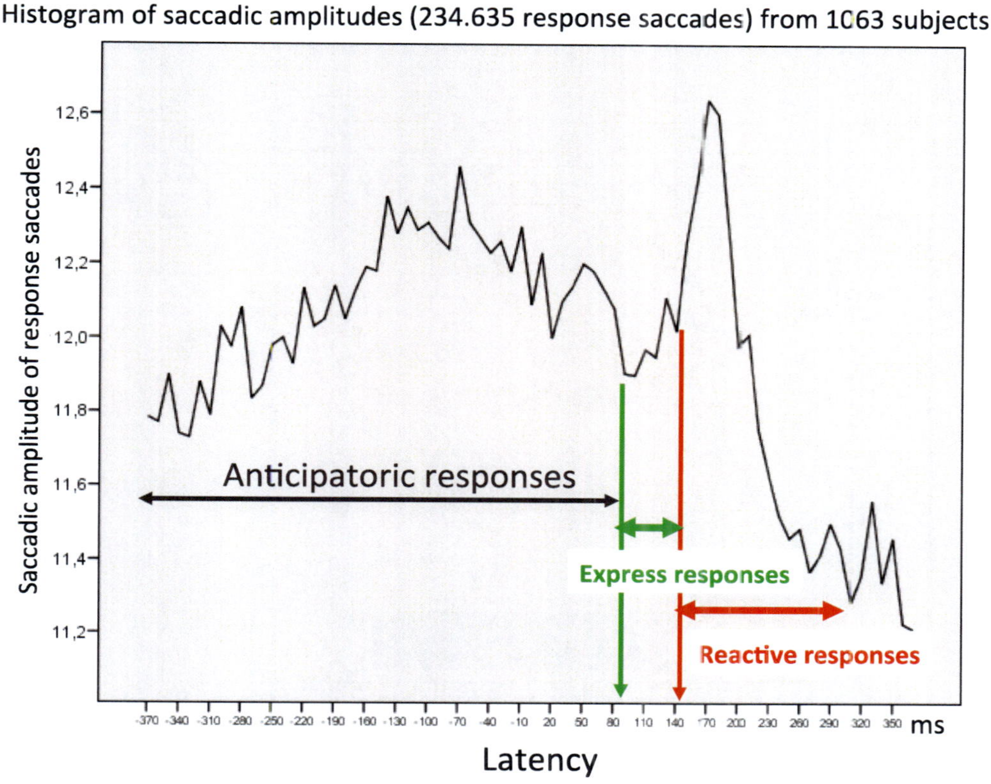

Figure 11. Response saccades show an abrupt increase in amplitude (in degrees) beginning roughly at 150 ms after the jump and a hole in the express range (90-150 ms).

Different saccade amplitudes and velocities permit us to separate express and anticipatory responses during the *Jumping Point* task. However, this is a very special task, and it is uncertain whether we can generalize the time windows for express saccades and the other proposed time ranges for fixation durations (see Figure 5) to other tasks. In Figure 12, the histograms of all fixation durations for our 6 standard tasks are shown.

While the *Raven* and *Picture Inspection* tasks have their peaks in the *cognitive* and *express* range, the tracking tasks, *Sinus* and *Jumping Point*, have their peaks at the target frequency and additionally at approximately 150 ms. In contrast, the *Interview* and the *Eyes Closed* tasks in the no-visual-task group show no peaks in the *cognitive* and *express* range but the highest values for short fixation durations followed by an exponential decay. It seems noteworthy that some tasks have low values in the *very short* range (<90 ms) while the *Interview* and the *Eyes Closed* tasks do not.

Sinus, *Picture Inspection*, *Raven* and *Jumping Point* – in this sequence – show decreasing values in the *very short* range. An obvious interpretation seems to be that more inhibition of gaze initiation is effective in these tasks and prevents irrelevant behavior. This is lacking in the tasks *Eyes Closed* and *Interview* and results in more early and short fixations.

Because amplitudes and velocities gave us hints as to the time window for express fixations in the *Jumping Point* task, we computed these parameters for our other standard tasks too (see Figures 13 and 15).

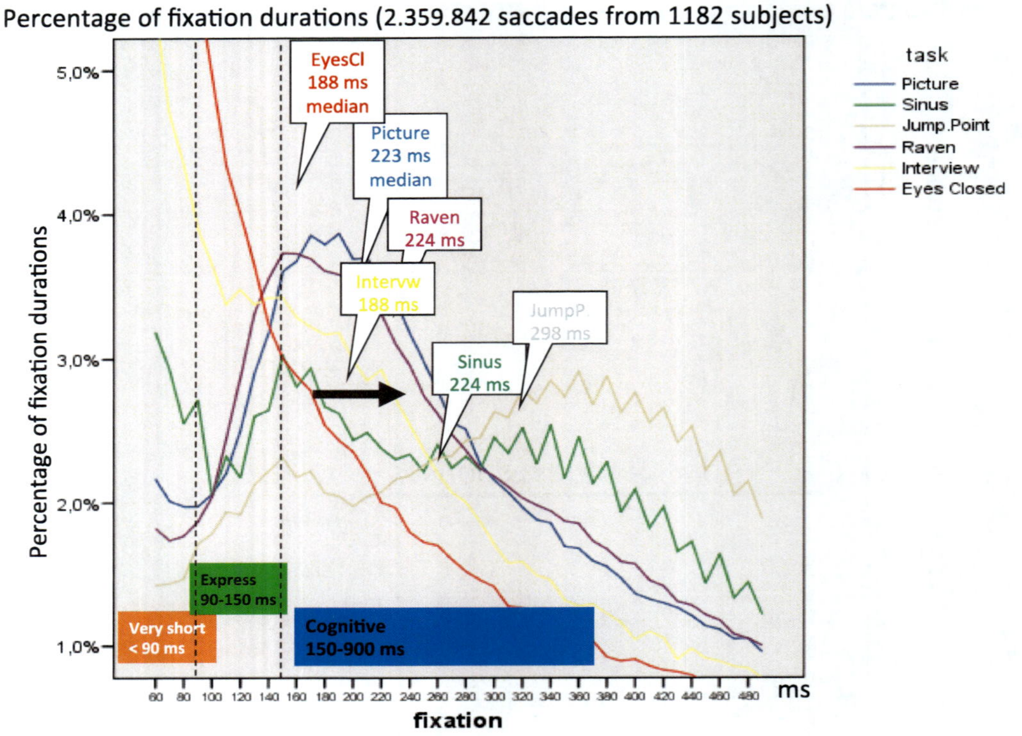

Figure 12. Fixation durations in our 6 standard tasks for all subjects. One can see three groups of curves: the *Raven* and the *Picture Inspection* task have their peaks at 130 to 220 ms, while the two tracking tasks, *Jumping Point* and *Sinus,* show double peaks from 300 to 400 ms and from 130 to 170 ms. The later peak at 300-400 ms is induced by the frequency of the target movement, which the subjects had to follow (see also figure 4). The third group of histogram curves stems from the interview tasks, *Interview* and *Eyes Closed*, during which subjects had no visual task to carry out. These curves show the highest values for short fixations, followed by an exponential decrease.

The amplitudes of the saccades were small in the *very short* range and increased in the *express* range, except in the *Jumping Point* task; here a dramatic increase began with the *cognitive* range at 150 ms. This seems to be a confirmation that at this point a new area begins. In the *express* range the amplitudes in this task were the lowest, which corresponds to the experience that small corrective saccades are often followed by undershooting response saccades. In the no visual task *Eyes Closed* the amplitudes remain nearly constant at 4 degrees. This may be a hint that the default condition for our inborn searching behavior that does not rest when we close our eyes is equipped with such an amplitude. This 3-fold range of our fovea may guarantee that new information in our nearby environment isn't overlooked but frees us from the strenuous looking for small details.

In Figure 14, a linear increase of fixation duration over saccadic amplitude in *Raven* and *Picture Inspection* is shown. When looking for the next object in the periphery, the visual systems needs an additional 11 ms per one degree of distance for evaluation. Other research has reported a slightly different value: 8 ms /degree for the shift of attention over the visual field (Tsal, 1983). The slopes for the *Picture Inspection* and *Raven* increases were separated by some 40 ms.

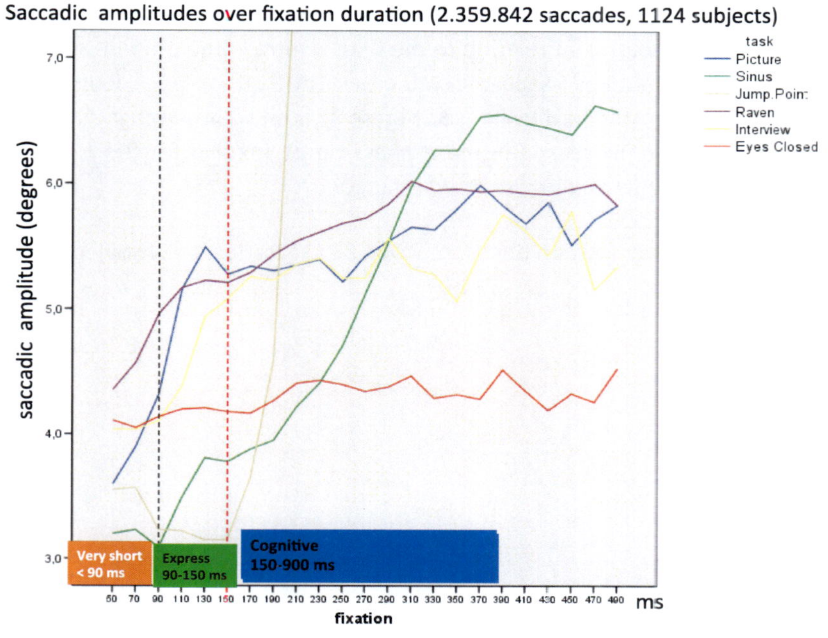

Figure 13. Amplitudes for all saccades (in degrees) over fixation duration (in ms) in our 6 standard tasks for all subjects. In all six tasks the median saccadic amplitudes are smaller in the *very short* range, increase in the *express* range (except in the Jumping Point task) and reach a plateau or increase further in the *cognitive* range. However, even in the *very short* range, amplitudes are larger than the microsaccade range (< 1 degree). The curve for *Jumping Point* shows a dramatic increase at the beginning of the *cognitive* range of fixations.

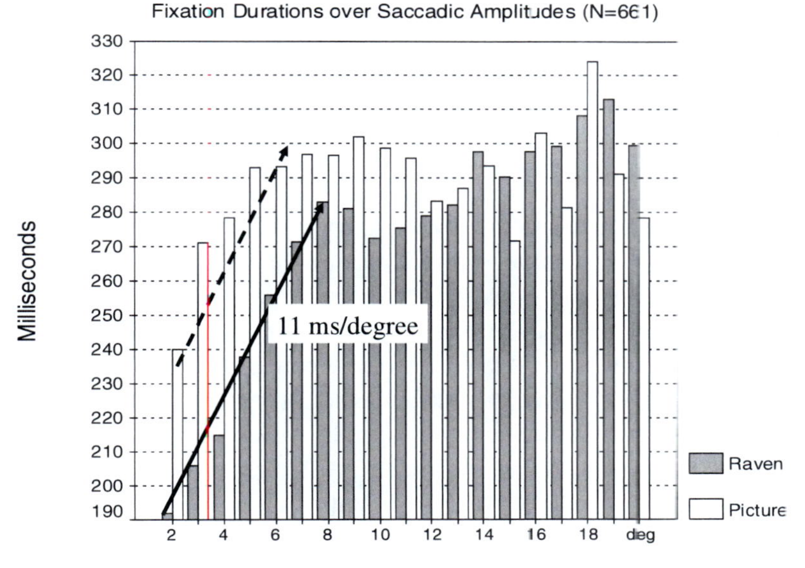

Figure 14. Fixation durations increase over saccadic amplitude with approximately 11 ms per degree distance until a plateau is reached, which occurs at 6 degrees in *Picture Inspection* and 8 degrees in *Raven*.

The fixation durations for *Picture Inspection* were greater, which seems to be caused by the lower contrast of the pictures in relation to the high-contrast line drawings in the *Raven*.

Looking at the (standardized) saccadic velocities (in degrees per second) over fixation duration (in ms) during our standard tasks (see Figure 15), one can see that the velocities were low in the *very short* range, increased in the *express* range (except for the *Eyes Closed* task) and showed different tendencies in the *cognitive* range.

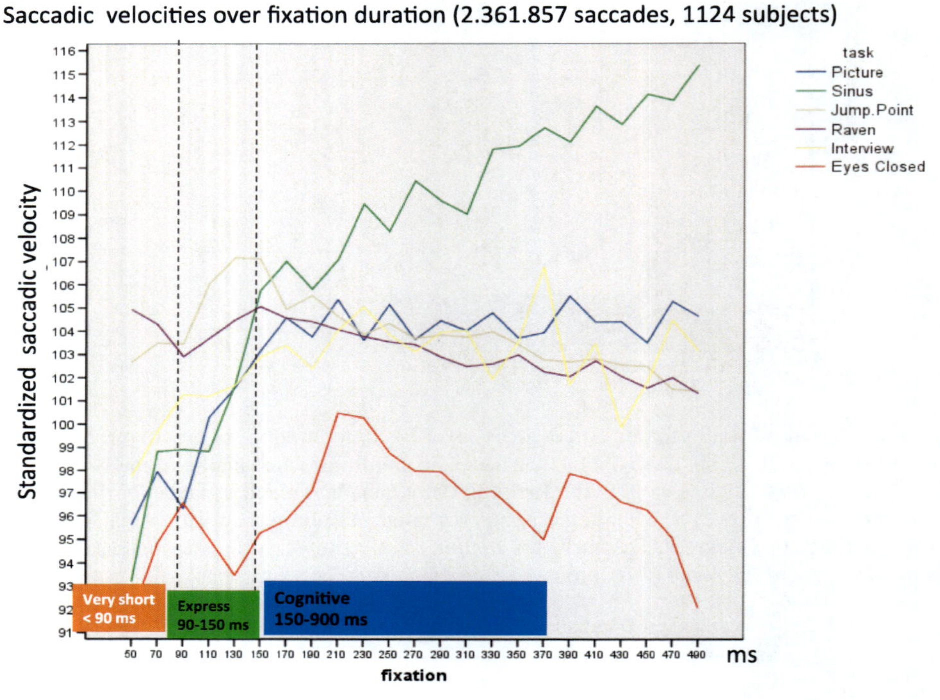

Figure 15. The (standardized) velocities for all saccades over fixation duration (in ms) in our 6 tasks were lowest in the *very short* range, increased in the *express* range (except for the *Eyes Closed* task) and showed different tendencies in the *cognitive* range.

The lowest velocity in the *Eyes Closed* task is partly caused by the braking effect of the closed lid on the eyeball. The tasks showed the lowest values in the *very short* range, increases in the *express* range and showed differences in the *cognitive* range. Here the *Sinus* task showed the highest values and further increases. This corresponds to the fact that subjects judged the continuous tracking of an accelerated moving point to be the most strenuous task, while *Jumping Point* was judged as less strenuous, although it had the same frequency. However, the task allowed rests between the jumps and did not need uninterrupted attention to the target. At exactly the beginning point of the *cognitive* range (150 ms) a plateau is reached by the velocity curves. This confirms the borderlines between the time windows. Thus we have presented evidence that separation of fixation duration into three ranges - *very short*, *express*, and *cognitive* - is supported by different parameters of gaze behavior: the peaks in the distribution curves, the behavior of saccadic velocities and saccadic amplitudes. We learned that the difficulty of the task as well as the IQ of the subjects had a small effect on fixation duration. As we can see in Figures 16 and 17, the age of the probands had a greater impact on fixation.

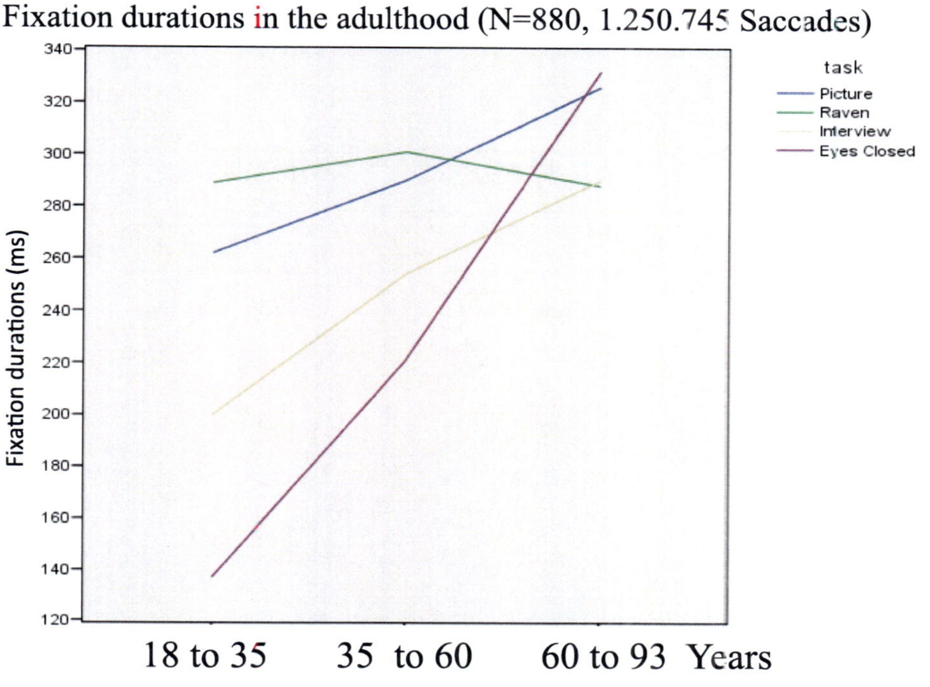

Figure 16. Median fixation duration in adulthood increases with the age of the subject. With the exception of the *Raven* task, fixation durations increased continuously over age.

Increasing age increased fixation duration in most tasks. The effect is dramatic: elderly subjects needed 60 ms more during *Picture Inspection* than middle-aged persons and 200 ms longer during *Eyes Closed*. It seems that mental processes take longer with age. That is exactly what the mental speed theory had described (Salthouse, 1996). Therefore, the reverse should also be found for youth. Becoming mature, i.e. an adult, speeds up mental processes, as seen in Figure 17.

Fixation duration in youth decreased when age increased: young children (3-4 years old) looked for 440 ms at a detail in the *Picture* before moving to the next one, while 14-year-old needed only 360 ms. Only the *Eyes Closed* task did not show such a systematic trend of increasing speed. However, in this task there is no picture for the visual system to process.

Until this point we haven't examined the long and the *very long* fixations, our fourth category of fixation durations. All the fixation duration medians we have shown are in the *cognitive* range. But, this is a characteristic of medians: extremes are left out.

In a study of 129 drivers during a prolonged trip in a driving simulator we found that tired drivers showed more short fixations < 150 ms, less cognitive fixations (150 to 900 ms) and more very long fixations, i.e., longer than 900 ms (Schleicher, Galley, Briest & Galley, 2008). From these data we concluded that there must be a fourth category of very long fixations outside the *cognitive* window. Very long fixation durations are usually very rare, so there is not enough data for an undeniable functional interpretation. However, the non-cognitive connotation seems justified by the increase in very long fixations in the Falling Asleep Condition as well as their more frequent occurrence in very old people (our own unpublished data).

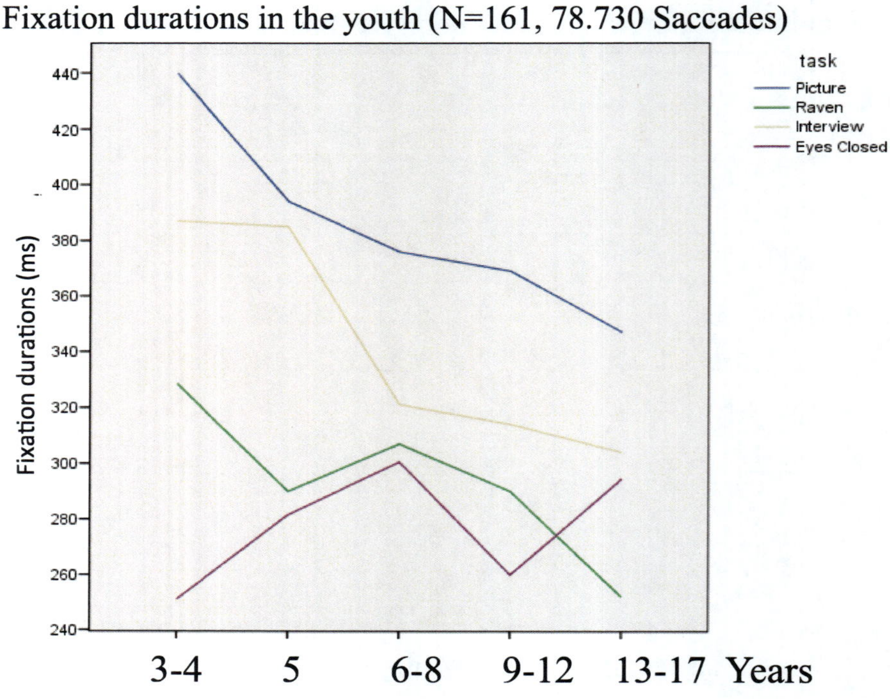

Figure 17. Median fixation duration in youth decreases with the age of the subject. The exception is the Eyes Closed task, in which the increasing speed of fixation durations did not occur.

Discussion and Conclusion

We have attempted to provide an explanation for the apparently high variability of fixation durations by looking at the distribution curves of fixations during different tasks (Figures 2, 4, 5, and 12). This led us to believe that fixation is a process in time that has four ranges: (1) *very short fixations*, (2) *express fixations*, (3) *cognitive* and (4) *very long fixations*. We found evidence for the first three ranges in the histograms of the latencies, velocities, and amplitudes of the response saccades in the *Jumping Point* task (Figures 7, 10, 11). In Figures 13 and 15, the behavior of saccadic amplitudes and velocities from the other tasks over the fixation duration provided evidence that these ranges are valid for other tasks, too. Obviously, the task had an enormous influence on the distribution curves of fixation duration, much more than the value of the central tendency reveals (Figure 12). For example, the tasks *Raven* and *Sinus* show the same 224 ms median fixation duration but have very different distribution curves.

It has often been suggested that the phenomenon of fixation has to be understood as the interplay of two systems: the visual and oculomotor system on one side and the cognitive system on the other side. This is in accord with our results. We often found that lengthening the fixation duration was accompanied by signs of inhibition, for example fewer very short fixations (see Figure 12 and the related text), which signify attention and cognitive control. The task *Jumping Point* tolerates fewer irrelevant, very small gazes than *Sinus* and *Raven*, but during *Interview* small saccades do not disrupt the task and are disinhibited or allowed. Thus signs of inhibition can be absent in other tasks, and the oculomotor system can work in its default mode as a searching system with a high frequency of movements, for example in the *Eyes Closed* task. A closer look at Figure 12 shows that the curve of *Interview* is shifted to the right for approximately 60 ms in relation to *Eyes Closed*. In other words, having an image (*Interview*) lengthened fixation compared with not having an image (*Eyes Closed*).

In a comprehensive study about the factors that guide the eyes while searching Pomplun (1998) reported a small difference in two nearly identical pictures. Pomplun suggested a model "which should generate fixations and saccades on the basis of assumed mental processes and their parameters (strategies, visual acuity, attention, working memory etc." (p. 185). The inputs for the model generator were a) overall reaction time for finding the target, b) fixation durations, c) saccadic amplitudes, d) the probability of missing the target and some derived measures. He stated that basic research has found that fixation can be ambiguous in the sense that one gaze can eventually process two items if their distance is small enough that both items fall in the area covered per fixation. He reported that fixation duration increased with item intensity and in the last verification phase compared with the beginning exploration phase. Unfortunately Pomplun used the mean of fixation duration as a measure of the central tendency. This is an inappropriate descriptor for the measurement of the central tendency; thus his reported values of most values over 200 ms seem to be overtaxed by some very long fixation durations (see his Figure 3.3. on p. 56, where all fixations <100 ms have been excluded. This is another sign that most researcher are not interested in very short fixations). Interestingly, he proposed a category called 'long fixations', as we also did, but he used 500 ms (p. 56) as the critical value, while we used 900 ms as the critical value. Pomplun did not report if these values were excluded from the 'mean' computation. Thus Pomplun could not use the probabilities of different time ranges to draw conclusions about inhibition processes as we did.

What are the functional implications of dividing fixation duration into four ranges?

Firstly, very short fixations could not be controlled by cognitive, for example conscious mental processes. They are therefore often excluded from further analysis; but the proportion of fixations in this range can signify the inhibitory influence of the cognitive system. For example, it is minimal in *Eyes Closed* and maximal in *Jumping Point*.

Secondly, the *express* range seems to reflect simple cognitive processes, for example, "this is not the intended position - I must go further in this direction". This is often the case in corrective saccades, but they can hardly be detected in most tasks with the exception of *Jumping Point*. Other examples of reduced costs of cognitive control are *express* range response saccades, which can be seen in decreased latencies when the jumps were expected in *Jumping Point*. However, these express reactions are not anticipatory saccades, which are characterized by smaller amplitudes and lower velocities, as we have seen. Often, *express* fixations seem to reflect simply the tendency of the vigilant oculomotor system to function as a high frequency search system and the absence of cognitive inhibition.

Thirdly, in the *cognitive* range, there is enough time for cognitive operations to detect matches or mismatches between the object seen and the expected object. If time is insufficient, the cognitive system allows a microsaccade, which does not remove the object from the fixation area. If the cognitive operation on the object is concluded, a new object outside the fixation area is grasped. However, this takes time, which we had calculated as 11 ms per degree (Figure 14).

Fourthly, although the consideration of fixation frequencies in the categories *express* range and *very short* range gives hints that the cognitive systems has inhibited the saccadic system, it contains no simple indications as to what the cognitive system is working on. For many years, researchers believed that scan path analysis could help, because it seems obvious that the sequence of different areas of fixation mirrors different mental content. However, the problem lies in the uncertainty as to whether a microsaccade was voluntarily controlled or happened automatically, for example to prevent the fading out of visual perception. Another ambiguity arises because longer fixation durations can suggest more difficult identification or detection processes or the incidence of two neighboring items being processed by one fixation. Thus the mental processes behind a sequence of fixations are complicated and cannot simply be deduced by oculomotor parameters (Schütz, Braun & Gegenfurtner, 2011).

References

Aserinsky, E. & Kleitman, N. (1953). Regularly Occurring Periods of Eye Motility, and Concomitant Phenomena, during Sleep. *Science*, *118* (3062), 273-274. doi: 10.1126/science.118.3062.273

Bronstein, A. M. & Kennard, C. (1987). Predictive eye saccades are different from visually triggered saccades. *Vision Research*, *27*(4), 517-520. doi: 10.1016/0042-6989(87)90037-X

Fischer, B. & Weber, H. (1993). Express saccades and visual attention. *Behavioral and Brain Sciences*, *16*(3), 553-567. doi: 10.1017/ S0140525X00031575

Galley, N. (1984). An activation paradigm using saccadic movements. In A. G. Gale & F. Johnson (Eds.), *Theoretical and applied aspects of eye movement research*, (511-521). Amsterdam: Elsevier.

Galley, N. (1987a). Saccadic velocity is regulated by the command mode of the subject and not by the stimulus parameters per se. In G. Lueer & U. Lass (Eds.), *Fourth European Conference on Eye Movements*, (127-129). Toronto: Hogrefe.

Galley, N. (1987b). Saccadic velocity varies as a function of 'activation'. In J. K O'Regan & A. Lévy-Schoen (Eds.), *Eye movements - from physiology to cognition*, (154-155). Amsterdam: Elsevier.

Galley, N. (1989). Saccadic eye movement velocity as an indicator of (de)activation. A review and some speculations. *Journal of Psychophysiology*, *3*, 229-244.

Galley, N. (1990). *Von Augen-blick zu Augen-blick. Eine experimentelle Psychologie der sakkadischen Augenbewegungen.* Habilitationsschrift. Philosophische Fakultät der Universität zu Köln, Deutschland.

Galley, N. (1993). Augenbewegungen, Antizipation und Leistung. Auf dem Wege zu einem neuropsychologischen Modell der Konzentration. In J. Beckmann, H. Strang & E. Hahn (Eds.), *Aufmerksamkeit und Energetisierung. Facetten von Konzentration und Leistung*, (229-246). Göttingen: Hogrefe.

Galley, N. (1998). An enquiry into the relationship between activation and performance using saccadic eye movement parameters. *Ergonomics*, *41*(5), 698-720. doi: 10.1080/ 001401398186865

Galley, N. (2001). Physiologische Grundlagen, Meßmethoden und Indikatorfunktion der okulomotorischen Aktivität. In F. Rösler (Ed.), *Enzyklopädie der Psychologie. Grundlagen und Methoden der Psychophysiologie. Biologische Psychologie*, (Vol. *4*, 237-316). Göttingen: Hogrefe.

Galley, N. (2010). Cognitive Development over the Life Span as Indicated by Eye Movements. In R. Zukauskiene (Ed.), *XIV European Conference on Developmental Psychology*, (33-41). Vilnius, Lithuania: Medimond.

Galley, N. & Fritz, A. (1987). Augenbewegungen von Kindern mit unterschiedlich diagnostizierten Hirnfunktionsstörungen. *Zeitschrift für Kinder- und Jugendpsychiatrie*, *15*, 342-354.

Galley, N. & Galley, L. (1999). Saccadic latency and fixation durations as indicators of mental speed. In I. Mervielde, I. Deary, F. De Fruyt & F. Ostendorf (Eds.), *Personality Psychology in Europe*, (Vol. *7*, 221-234). Tilburg: Tilburg University Press.

Holmqvist, K., Nyström M., Andersson, R., Dewhurst, R., Jarodzka, H. & Van de Weijer, J. (Eds.) (2011). *Eye Tracking. A comprehensive guide to methods and measures*. Oxford, Oxford University Press.

McPeek, R. M., Skavenski, A. A. & Nakayama, K. (2000). Concurrent processing of saccades in visual search. *Vision Research*, *40* (18), 2499-2516. doi:10.1016/S0042-6989(00)00102-4.

Otero-Millan, J., Troncoso, X. G., Macknik, S. L., Serrano-Pedraza, I. & Martinez-Conde, S. (2008). Saccades and microsaccades during visual fixation, exploration, and search: Foundations for a common saccadic generator. *Journal of Vision*, *8*(14), 21, 1-18. doi: 10.1167/8.14.21

Pomplun, M. (1998). *Analysis and models of eye movements in comparative visual search*. Göttingen: Cuvillier.

Radach, R., Heller, D. & Inhoff, A. (1999). Occurence and function of very short fixation durations in reading. In W. Becker, H. Deubel & T. Mergner (Eds.), *Current Oculomotor Research: Physiological and Psychological Aspects*, (321-332). New York, N.Y.: Plenum Press. doi: 10.1007/978-1-4757-3054-8_46

Raven, J. C., Court, J. & Raven, J. (1978). Coloured Progressive Matrices. CPM. *Raven-Matrizen-Test.* Weinheim: Beltz Test.

Rolfs, M. (2009). Microsaccades: Small steps on a long way. *Vision Research*, *49*, 2415–2441. doi: 10.1016/j.visres.2009.08.010

Salthouse, T. A. (1996). The processing-speed theory of adult age differences in cognition. *Psychological Review*, *103*(3), 403-428. doi: 10.1037/0033-295X.103.3.403

Schleicher, R. & Galley, N. (2005). Saccadic velocity and duration as psychological variables I. Standardization procedure. *13th European Conference on Eye Movements*. Bern: University of Bern.

Schleicher, R., Galley, N., Briest, S. & Galley, L. (2008). Looking tired? Blinks and saccades as indicators of fatigue in sleepiness warners. *Ergonomics*, *51*(7), 982-1010. doi: 10.1080/00140130701817062

Schütz, A. C., Braun, D. I. & Gegenfurtner, K. R. (2011). Eye movements and perception: A selective review. *Journal of Vision*, *11*(5), 9, 1-30. doi: 10.1167/11.5.9

Schweigert, M. (2003). *Fahrerblickverhalten und Nebenaufgaben*. Dissertationsschrift. Fakultät für Maschinenwesen, Technische Universität München, Deutschland.

Smit, A. C. & Van Gisbergen, J. A. M. (1989). A short-latency transition in saccadic dynamics during square-wave tracking and its significance for the differentiation of visually-guided and predictive saccades. *Experimental Brain Research, 20*, 64-74.

Sommer, M. A. (1994). Express saccades elicited during visual scan in the monkey. *Vision Research, 34* (15), 2023-2038. doi: 10.1016/0042-6989(94)90030-2

Thier, P. & Ilg, U. J. (2005). The neural basis of smooth-pursuit eye movements. *Current Opinion in Neurobiology, 15*, 645-652. doi: 10.1016/ j.conb.2005.10.013

Tsal, Y. (1983). Movements of attention across the visual field. *Journal of Experimental Psychology: Human Perception and Performance*, *9*(4), 523-530.

In: Advances in Visual Perception Research
Editor: Thomas Heinen
ISBN: 978-1-63482-455-2
© 2015 Nova Science Publishers, Inc.

Chapter 6

Attention Deficit Hyperactivity Disorder: Precise Time Reproduction, but Accelerated Saccadic Peak Velocity of Voluntary Eye Movements after MPH-Medication

Kristian Folta-Schoofs[1,*], Carina Hilke[1], Hans-Jörg Bethge[2] and Dieter Felbel[2]
[1]Educational Neurocience Lab, Institute of Psychology, University of Hildesheim, Germany.
[2]AMEOS Clinic, Child and Youth Psychiatry and Psychotherapy, Hildesheim, Germany

Abstract

Attention deficit hyperactivity disorder (ADHD) is a prevalent developmental disorder, which is characterized by symptoms of impulsiveness, hyperactivity, and/or inattention. Here, we investigated ADHD-dependent modulations in time perception and distractibility, as well as changes in the velocity profile of saccadic eye movements. We tested independent groups of children including I) healthy children, II) ADHD children tested OFF-medication, and III) ADHD children tested ON-medication. A subsample of the latter group was tested ON- and OFF-medication, successively. All children participated in a temporal distractor paradigm requiring the precise reproduction of a target-interval in the seconds-range, while saccades to eccentric visual distractors either have to be suppressed, or voluntarily initiated. Our results showed comparable abilities with regards to precise time reproduction for all groups and conditions. Additionally, a comparable number, latency, amplitude, and duration of erroneously and voluntarily

* Corresponding author: Institute of Psychology, University of Hildesheim, Universitätsplatz 1, D-31141 Hildesheim, Germany. Tel.: +49 5121 883 109 10. Email: foltak@uni-hildesheim.de.

executed saccades had been observed. Most importantly, children tested both ON- and OFF-medication revealed accelerated peak velocities for voluntarily executed saccades, when tested ON-medication. This acceleration indicates a pharmacologically induced increase in brainstem excitation.

Keywords: ADHD, Time perception, Interval timing, Distraction, Interference control, Executive control, Eye-tracking

Introduction

Attention deficit hyperactivity disorder (ADHD) is a prevalent developmental disorder (Graham, 2010; Lloyd, Stead & Cohen, 2006). Its prevalence was demonstrated to be independent of socio-economic, national and cultural influences (Barkley, 1997; Biederman, Newcorn & Sprich, 1991). Children diagnosed with ADHD show an age-inappropriate high level of impulsiveness, hyperactivity, and/or inattention. These cardinal symptoms occur in at least two different spheres of life (e.g., in school and family), and remarkably impair children's psychosocial and subjective wellbeing. On the cognitive level, deficits in precise timing, a lack of inhibitory behavioral control, and deficits in executive functions such as working memory, attention, interference control, task-switching, or self-regulation had been reported (Imhof, 2004; Kempton et al., 1999; Pennington & Ozonoff, 1996; Petermann & Toussaint, 2009; Tannock, 1998). According to the *DSM IV* or *DSM V* (American Psychiatric Association, 1994, 2013), ADHD affects 3% to 10% of all children (Lehmkuhl et al., 1998; Polanczyk, de Lima, Horta, Biederman & Rohde, 2007; Tannock, 1998) and can persist even into adolescence and adulthood (Barkley, 1997; Biederman et al., 1991).

At present, the etiology and neurobiological foundations of ADHD remain poorly defined. Existing studies suggest disruptions to the child's behavioral inhibition system to sufficiently explain several of the behavioral and cognitive deficits characterizing ADHD (Cairney et al., 2001). This inhibition system depends on the integrity of the frontostriatal circuitry connecting the frontal cortex (FC), the thalamus, and the basal ganglia (BG; Giedd, Blumenthal, Molloy & Castellanos, 2001; Munoz, Armstrong, Hampton & Moore, 2003; Thier, 2006; Ullsperger & von Cramon, 2006). Structural and functional brain imaging studies demonstrated anatomical alterations of the FC and the BG, as well as reductions of the dopamine-dependent transmission of neural signals within the frontostriatal circuitry as one of the likely causes for the observed frontocortical hypoexcitation in ADHD-diagnosed children (Banaschewski, Roessner, Uebel & Rothenberger, 2004; Castellanos et al., 1994, 1996, 2001, 2002; Giedd et al., 1994; Pliszka, 2005; Rubia et al., 1999). In addition, regional blood flow and glucose metabolic studies revealed an increased density and sensitivity of dopamine transporter molecules in the FC, and substantial changes in the expression and sensitivity of dopamine receptors in regions of the BG of ADHD patients (Lou, Henriksen & Bruhn, 1984, 1989; Zametkin et al., 1990). Methylphenidate (MPH), the main pharmacotherapy for ADHD treatment, proved to be effective in reducing ADHD symptoms by blocking the frontocortical dopamine reuptake and thereby compensating for the deficit of excitation within the FC. Accordingly, after MPH-medication significant increases in regional cerebral blood flow were observed in in the FC, the thalamus, and the BG (Kim, Lee, Cho & Lee, 2001; Kim, Lee, Shin, Cho & Lee, 2002; Lee et al., 2005).

Despite its involvement in the pathophysiology of ADHD, the frontostriatal circuitry is considered to be of major importance for the precise estimation, anticipation, and (re)production of short temporal durations (Barkley, 1997; Castellanos et al., 2002; Durston et al., 2004; Giedd et al., 2001; Kim et al., 2002). It is thus conceivable to expect remarkable timing deficits in non-medicated ADHD patients. Indeed, some studies on ADHD (see for review: Toplak, Dockstader & Tannock, 2006) were able to observe significant timing deficits in tasks requiring duration discrimination (Rubia, Norloos, Smith, Grunning & Sergeant, 2003), duration production (Van Meel, Oosterlaan, Heslenfeld & Sergeant, 2005), time reproduction (Barkley, Edwards, Laneri, Fletcher & Metevia, 2001a; Barkley, Murphy & Bush, 2001b; Kerns, McInerney & Wilde, 2001; Meaux & Chelonis, 2003; Mullins, Bellgrove, Gill & Robertson, 2005; Sonuga-Barke, Saxton & Hall, 1998; Toplak, Rucklidge, Hetherington, John & Tannock, 2003; West et al., 2000), and finger tapping (Ben-Pazi, Gross-Tsur, Bergman & Shaley, 2003; Rubia et al., 1999, 2003). However, other studies completely or at least partly failed to reveal temporal processing deficits in tasks requiring duration discrimination (Radonovich & Mostofsky, 2004), temporal judgement (Brown & Vickers, 2004), time reproduction (Bauermeister et al., 2005; Folta & Mähler, 2011; Smith, Taylor, Warner, Newman & Rubia, 2002), and finger tapping (Tiffin-Richards, Hasselhorn, Richards, Banaschewski & Rothenberger, 2004). Similarly to deficits in time perception, an increased distractibility is often assigned to the typical characteristics of ADHD, even though there is little empirical evidence that ADHD children are indeed more distractible than their healthy peers (see for review: Douglas & Peters, 1979; Gumenyuk et al., 2005; Huang-Pollock, Nigg & Carr, 2005; Mason, Humphreys & Kent, 2003; van der Meere & Sergeant, 1988). The high number of contradictory results suggests that timing is not always disrupted, and distraction is not always distracting in children and adults diagnosed with ADHD. One probable explanation for the obvious discrepancy of results might be, that most studies on timing or distraction cannot be considered as ecologically valid measures of timing and distraction in daily life situations. In daily life, timing becomes regularly distracted by environmental stimuli, which appear outside the current task, but nevertheless compete for attention and for a limited amount of information processing resources. Therefore, deficits in the frontostriatal circuitry might primarily be expected to influence the acuity and precision in timing tasks, which require an allocation of information processing resources away from the timing task, and towards environmental stimuli or events. Similarly, distractibility in ADHD children might critically depend on the characteristics and number of concurrent tasks or environmental stimuli. In line with this argument, children diagnosed with ADHD were shown to perform worse in tasks with incorporated distractor stimuli that interfered with the primary task, thus requiring interference control, and a (re-)allocation of information processing resources (Imhof, 2004; Nigg, 2001; Pearson, Lane & Swanson, 1991; van Mourik, Osterlaan, Heslenfeld, Konig & Sergeant, 2007; van Mourik, Osterlaan & Sergeant, 2005; Wood, Maruff, Levy, Farrow & Hay, 1999).

Besides from timing and distraction, recent studies indicated ADHD-correlated changes in the frontostriatal circuitry to influence the characteristic of fast ballistic eye movements (saccades), which move the high acuity of the retinal fovea to visual stimuli in more peripheral parts of the visual field. Saccades are characterized by their latency, duration, amplitude, and peak velocity, and are always followed by fixations, which are relatively stable rest phases of the eye (Huey, 1900). The latency of a saccade is a good indicator of cognitive decision processes (Groner & Groner, 1989), and corresponds to the time between the presentation of a target stimulus and the initiation of a saccade to this target. The amplitude of the saccade reflects the spatial distance between two fixations, and is usually measured in degree (°) of visual angle. The duration of a saccade corresponds to the time, needed to move the eye from one point of fixation to another. Finally, the peak velocity reflects the maximum speed of a saccade (measured in degree per second, °/s), and becomes affected by subjects' mental workload and attentional state during ecologically valid tasks (DiStasi et al., 2010).

Until today, an overwhelming amount of studies have provided a detailed outline of anatomical structures and neural connections (Figure 1), which are involved in the control of saccades and fixations (Kömpf & Heide, 1998; Leigh & Zee, 1999; Matsuda et al., 2004; Pierrot-Deseilligny, Milea & Müri, 2004; Sparks, 2002). This allows for designing eye-tracking experiments probing the functionality of neural structures and pathways of the frontostriatal circuitry (Everling & Fischer, 1998; Folta & Mähler, 2011; Heinrichs & Reinhold, 2010; Kemner, van der Geest, Verbaten & van Engeland, 2004; Munoz et al., 2003; Ramus, 2003; Ross, Harris, Olincy & Radant, 2000; Sweeney, Takarae, Macmillan, Luna & Minshew, 2004; Trillenberg, Lencer & Heide, 2004).

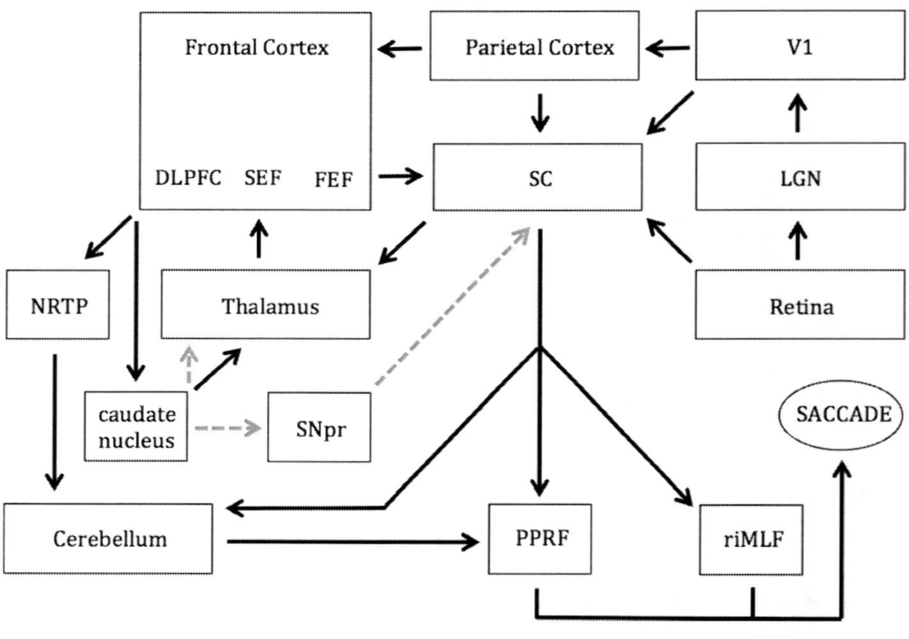

Figure 1. Saccade system. Depicted are several subsystems processing different aspects of visual stimuli, and producing saccades with different saccadic reaction times and temporal velocity profiles. Solid black arrows represent excitatory connections, and dashed gray arrows indicate inhibitory projections. Of special importance for the control of saccadic peak velocity are the rostral interstitial nucleus of the medial longitudinal fasciculus (riMLF) and the paramedian pontine reticular formation (PPRF), which receive most of their excitatory input from the superior colliculus (SC). The SC receives its input from the retina and from occipital, parietal, and frontal cortical areas (including the frontal eye field, FEF). Saccade-inhibition depends on structures of the frontal cortex and the striatum (e.g., caudate nucleus). Further abbreviations: DLPFC, dorsolateral prefrontal cortex; LGN, lateral geniculate nucleus; NRTP, nucleus reticularis tegmenti pontis; SEF, supplementary eye field; SNpr, substantia nigra, pars reticulata; V1, primary visual cortex.

Because of the apparent overlap of structures and pathways underlying time processing, executive control (particularly in the presence of distractors), and saccade execution (Kustov & Robinson, 1996), eye-tracking methods were successfully applied to a number of studies on developmental and psychiatric disorders, such as OCD (Rosenberg, Dick, O'Hearn & Sweeney, 1997), autism (Kemner et al., 2004; Takarae, Minshew, Luna, Krisky & Sweeney, 2004a; Takarae, Minshew, Luna & Sweeney, 2004b), dyslexia (Ramus, 2003), and ADHD (Folta & Mähler, 2011; Munoz et al., 2003; Ross et al., 2000). As it was hypothesized from neurobiological models, eye movement studies on ADHD children revealed remarkable deficits in saccadic suppression and an altered characteristic of saccades (Cairney et al., 2001; Gould, Bastain, Israel, Hommer & Castellanos, 2001; Hanisch, Radach, Holtkamp, Hepertz-Dahlmann & Konrad, 2006; Klein, Raschke & Brandenbusch, 2003). When tested OFF-medication, ADHD children (compared to healthy children) produced an increased number of reflexive (i.e., involuntary and stimulus-driven) saccades, although fixation was required (Cairney et al., 2001; Gould et al., 2001; Hanisch et al., 2006; Klein et al., 2003). Several studies reported voluntary (i.e., consciously driven) prosaccades (pro = in the direction of a target stimulus) in non-medicated ADHD children to be characterized by longer latencies (Klein et al., 2003; Mostofsky, Lasker, Cutting, Denckia & Zee, 2001; Munoz et al., 2003), but other authors failed to confirm such a difference (Hanisch et al., 2006; Ross et al., 2000).

Besides from latency differences, Munoz et al. (2003) reported a deceleration of peak velocities for voluntarily initiated prosaccades in non-medicated children with a diagnosis of ADHD. On the other hand, Folta & Mähler (2011) observed accelerated peak velocities for voluntarily initiated prosaccades, when comparing medicated ADHD children with their age- and IQ-matched healthy peers. Considering the ADHD-correlated alterations in neuronal excitation within the frontostriatal circuitry, such differences in peak velocity might best be explained by a passive flow of neuronal excitation from the FC - via the superior colliculus (SC) of the midbrain tectum - to burst neurons in the paramedian zone of the paramedian pontine reticular formation (PPRF), and the rostral interstitial nucleus of the medial longitudinal fasciculus (riMLF), coding for the peak velocity of horizontal and vertical saccades (Figure 1; Sparks, 2002), respectively. Burst neurons in the PPRF and the riMLF 'translate' excitation from the SC into an acceleration of the eye. One subdivision of the FC, the frontal eye field (FEF, see Figure 1), might primarily be involved in the passive flow of frontocortical excitation to the midbrain SC. If these assumptions can considered to be correct, ADHD-dependent accelerations or decelerations of saccadic peak velocities (i.e., MPH-dependent acceleration in saccadic peak velocity vs. deceleration in non-medicated ADHD children) might best be explained by the magnitude of frontocortical excitation within the FEF, which is decreased in ADHD children, and might become increased as an compensatory effect of medication. In this study, we further tested this notion using an experimental paradigm, which allowed for the registration of voluntarily and erroneously executed saccades, and additionally provided ecologically valid measures of children's abilities of precise timing and interference control (as indicators of intact executive functions). Previous timing studies successfully investigated distractor-induced (re)allocations of information processing resources using an experimental paradigm that required time reproductions of a previously trained target interval in the presence and absence of visual distractors (Folta & Mähler, 2011; Folta-Schoofs, Wolf, Treue & Schoofs, 2014; Fortin & Massé, 2000). We adapted a modified version of this paradigm to the peculiarities of combined psychophysical testing and eye movement registration in children. All children were required to reproduce a previously trained time interval, while prosaccades to eccentric visual distractors either have to be suppressed (saccade-inhibition condition), or voluntarily executed (cued prosaccade condition). Between-subjects comparisons of the characteristics of time response functions and saccades were conducted in independent groups of I) healthy control children, II) ADHD children tested OFF-MPH-medication, and III) ADHD children tested ON-MPH-medication. Additionally, a subsample of the latter group was tested ON-MPH- and OFF-MPH-medication, successively, and thus allowed for within-subjects comparisons. Within- and between-subjects comparisons of time reproduction and eye movement data were considered to allow for proving the functionality of the frontostriatal circuitry on both the cognitive and oculomotor level.

Method

Participants

A total of $N = 33$ children (21 boys, 12 girls) aged between 7;11 (years;months) and 11;0 (years;months) participated in this study. Only children with a general IQ > 85 were included (IQ-range: 91 to 136; *HAWIK IV*; Petermann & Petermann, 2008). All children had normal or corrected-to-normal vision, and were assigned to one of three experimental groups containing I) healthy control children ($N = 12$), II) ADHD children being ON-MPH-medication ($N = 12$), and III) ADHD children being OFF-MPH-medication ($N = 10$). All groups were comparable in age (*Kruskal-Wallis-test*: $\chi^2(2) = 1.439$; $p > .05$), and intelligence (*Kruskal-Wallis-test*: $\chi^2(2) = 5.013$; $p > .05$). In addition, all groups demonstrated comparable arithmetic abilities (*DEMAT*; Gölitz, Roick & Hasselhorn, 2006; Krajewski, Liehm & Schneider, 2004; Roick, Gölitz & Hasselhorn, 2004; *Kruskal-Wallis-test*: $\chi^2(2) = 2.29$; $p > .05$), and produced comparable reaction times in an alertness task (*TAP 2.0*; Zimmermann & Fimm, 2002; *Kruskal-Wallis-test*: $\chi^2(2) = 1.247$; $p > .05$). However, the three groups significantly differed in children's ability of reading (*WLLP*; Küspert & Schneider, 1998; *Kruskal-Wallis-test*: $\chi^2(2) = 10.749$; $p < .01$) and writing (*WRT*; Birkel, 2007; *Kruskal-Wallis-test*: $\chi^2(2) = 12.827$; $p < .01$), and showed significant performance differences in an attentional Go-/Nogo-task (*TAP 2.0*; Zimmermann & Fimm, 2002; *Kruskal-Wallis-test*: $\chi^2(2) = 7.564$; $p < .05$). Detailed subject characteristics are summarized in Table 1. Prior to the study, written informed consent was obtained from the children's parents. All children had to agree by writing down their name on the permission form. Parents received EUR 15,00 as a monetary compensation for travel costs. In addition, all children were rewarded for their participation with a gift. The study was approved by the Medical Ethical Committee of the Goettingen University Hospital, and was conducted in accordance with the Declaration of Helsinki.

Healthy control children (5 boys, 7 girls; mean age: 9;5, see Table 1) were recruited from three local primary schools. Based on reports by parents and teachers, none of the children in the control group had any history of neurological, sensorimotor or psychiatric problems. All children in this group demonstrated age-appropriate abilities in reading (*WLLP*: $T \geq 40$; range of T-values: 43 to 68), writing (*WRT*: $T \geq 40$; range of T-values: 40 to 67), and arithmetic (*DEMAT*: $T \geq 40$; range of T-values: 40 to 69). To completely exclude the occurrence of

ADHD symptoms in control children, parents and teachers completed the German teachers' and parental report on ADHD symptoms (*FBB-ADHS* from the *DISYPS-II*; Döpfner, Götz-Dorten & Lehmkuhl, 2008). The *FBB*-rating comprises an inattention scale, a hyperactivity scale, and an impulsivity scale. Relative *FBB*-scores ranging from 0 to .49 are considered as inconspicuous, scores ranging from .5 to .99 are considered as somewhat conspicuous, and scores above 1.00 are considered as conspicuous or very conspicuous (relative scores > 1.49). None of the control children obtained relative *FBB*-scores above 1.00 on one or more of the three scales. Additionally, parents completed the *Child Behavioral Checklist* (*CBCL/4-18*; Aschenbach, 1991a), whereas teachers completed the corresponding *Teachers' Report Form* (*TRF*; Aschenbach, 1991b). Children were excluded from the control group, when *CBCL-/TRF*-scores exceeded cut-off values for at least one of eight behavioral scales (social withdrawal, somatic complaints, phobic/depressive behavior, social problems, schizoid/compulsive behavior, attention deficits, dissocial behavior, and aggressive behavior).

Table 1. Demographic data (mean age, sex) and results from psychological tests (IQ, Writing, Arithmetic, Reading, Alertness) of healthy control children, and ADHD children tested with and without methylphenidate (MPH)-medication (ADHD ON-MPH-medication vs. ADHD OFF-MPH-medication group). Children in the ADHD ON-/OFF-MPH-medication group constitute a subgroup of the ADHD ON-MPH-medication group, and were tested with and without MPH-medication, successively (to allow for within-subjects comparisons). Cognitive performance measures are indicated with mean *T*-values (*M*) and standard errors (*S.E.*)

	ADHD (ON MPH-medication)	*ADHD (OFF MPH-medication)*	*ADHD ON/OFF MPH*	*Healthy Control*
Mean Age (years, months)	9;5	9;2	9;3	9;5
Sex (male, female)	9m, 3f	7m, 2f	5m, 2f	5m, 7f
	M ± S.E.	*M ± S.E.*	*M ± S.E.*	*M ± S.E.*
IQ (HAWIK-IV)	106 ± 3.3	102 ± 2.3	110 ± 4.1	113 ± 3.5
Writing (WRT)	44 ± 2.8	44 ± 2.3	48 ± 2.2	56 ± 2.0
Calculating (DEMAT)	49 ± 4.1	47 ± 3.6	53 ± 4.4	55 ± 2.6
Reading (WLLP)	43 ± 3.3	44 ± 2.7	44 ± 3.7	57 ± 2.4
Alertness (TAP 2.0)				
Alertness RT	51 ± .5	52 ± .9	52 ± .7	50 ± .8
Go-Nogo RT	57 ± 1.2	53 ± 3.4	58 ± 1.7	51 ± 1.1

Abbreviations: DEMAT: Deutscher Mathematiktest (Gölitz et al., 2006; Krajewski et al., 2004; Roick et al., 2004); HAWIK-IV: Hamburg-Wechsler-Intelligenztest für Kinder (Petermann & Petermann, 2008); MPH: methylphenidate; RT: reaction time; TAP 2.0: Test battery of Attentional Performance 2.0 (Zimmermann & Fimm, 2002); WRT: Weingartner Rechtschreibtest (Birkel, 2007); WLLP: Würzburger Leise Leseprobe (Küspert & Schneider, 1998). .

Children with approved ADHD symptoms were recruited from a local psychiatric hospital. Before participation in this study, all children underwent pediatric examination, child psychiatric diagnostics, and psychological testing. Inclusion to one of the two independent ADHD groups (ON-MPH-medication group vs. OFF-MPH-medication group) required a formal diagnosis of ADHD according to *DSM-IV* (American Psychiatric Association, 1994) or *ICD-10* (World Health Organization, 1992). Furthermore, inclusion required relative *FBB*-scores of above 1.00 (as indicated by parents or teachers; *FBB-ADHS* from the *DISYPS-II*; Döpfner et al., 2008) on the inattention, hyperactivity, and/or impulsivity scale, and/or reports of attentional deficits on either the *Child Behavioral Checklist* (*CBCL/4-18*; Aschenbach, 1991a), or the *Teachers' Report Form* (*TRF*; Aschenbach, 1991b). ON-MPH- and OFF-MPH-medication groups demonstrated comparable abilities in reading and writing (*WLLP* & *WRT*; *Mann-Whitney-U-tests*: $p > .05$), but were significantly worse than in the control group (*Mann-Whitney-U-tests*: $p < .01$; see Table 1). In addition, mean reaction time in the attentional Go-/Nogo-task was significantly higher for the ON-MPH-medication group than for the control group (*Mann-Whitney-U-tests*: $p < .01$).

ADHD children in the ON-MPH-medication group (9 boys, 3 girls; mean age: 9;5, see Table 1) belonged to the ADHD mixed type ($N = 7$) or the pure attentional type ($N = 5$), and were at least 2 months under regular MPH-medication (Medikinet, 10 to 30mg). On the day of the experiment, intake of MPH-medication was ensured at least 1.5 hours before testing. This procedure guaranteed the effectiveness of MPH-medication for the complete period of testing.

A total of $N = 7$ children from the ON-MPH-medication group (5 boys, 2 girls; mean age: 9;3, see Table 1) participated in a follow-up measurement conducted without MPH-medication, to allow for within-subjects comparisons. Children of this subgroup were of the mixed type ($N = 4$) or the pure attentional type ($N = 3$), and the follow-up measurement was conducted between 1 and 8 months (mean = 5 months; S.E. = 1.01) after being tested ON-MPH-medication. When tested OFF-MPH-medication, children stopped their medication at least 12 h before testing, allowing for a complete washout of the active ingredient (Pelham et al., 2005, 1999; Rapport & Denney, 1997).

ADHD children in the OFF-MPH-medication group (7 boys, 2 girls; mean age: 9;2, see Table 1) were of the mixed type ($N = 1$) or the pure attentional type ($N = 8$). They had never received psychoactive medication ($N = 4$) before, or had been OFF-MPH-medication for at least 12 h before testing ($N = 5$).

Apparatus and Stimuli

The experiment was conducted in an acoustically shielded chamber (2 x 4 x 2.5m). The diffuse illumination of the chamber was adapted to the luminance of the screen (50cd/m^2). Children were seated in front of a monitor on a height-adjustable chair, and used a height-adjustable chin-rest, and a forehead support to ensure stable fixation on the screen. Viewing distance was 100cm. Visual stimuli comprised a central fixation stimulus (white square, 2° x 2°), a marker stimulus (black square, 2° x 2°), and white or green squares (2° x 2°) as visual distractors. All stimuli were displayed on a Quato Intelli Proof 240 24 inch TFT-monitor (1920 x 1200pixel, 60Hz, 12ms S/W). The background of the monitor was set to gray. Distractors (white or green squares) were presented at a distance of 5° from the center of the screen, and were randomly placed in one of four peripheral screen positions (upper left, lower left, upper right or lower right position). The experiment was controlled by MATLAB 7.8.0 (R2009a, TheMathworks, Inc., Natick, MA, USA) running on an iMac 24 inch (Intel Core 2 Duo Processor, 1066 MHz; system software: Mac OS X, Version 10.5.7). Participants responded by pressing or releasing the 'ENTER'-key on a standard numerical keyboard, and were instructed to respond with the middle or index finger of their dominant hand.

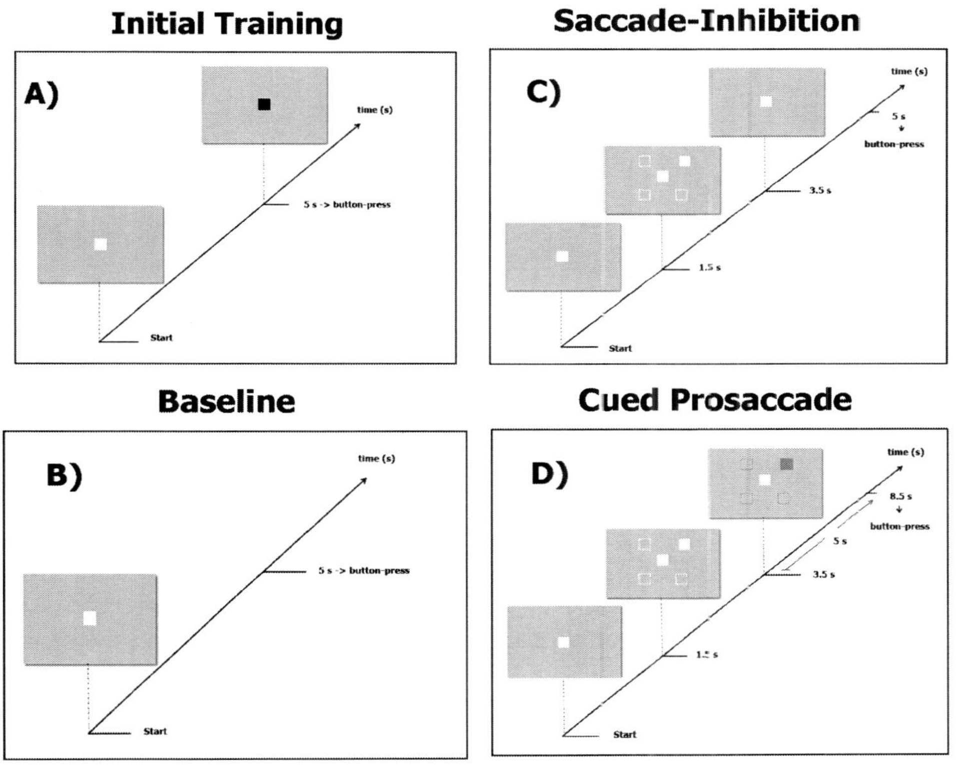

Figure 2. A) Initial Training: Each session started with a block of 20 training trials. Subjects had to fixate a centrally presented white square, and to press the response key after appearance of a central black square (appearing always after 5s). B) Baseline: In 60 baseline trials, subjects had to fixate a central white square, and to press the response key when they expected appearance of a black square (which actually never appeared in these trials). Baseline trials measured children's ability of precise time reproduction (as a critical test of executive functioning). C) Saccade-Inhibition: In 60 saccade-inhibition trials, children had to fixate a centrally presented white square, and to reproduce the previously trained target duration. During time reproduction (and always 1.5s after initiation of each trial) visual distractor stimuli (white squares) were presented in one of 4 peripheral positions (presentation-duration: 2s). Children were required to ignore the distractor, and to press the response key when they expected the end of the trained target duration. D) Cued Prosaccade: In 60 cued prosaccade trials, children had to fixate the central white square until the peripheral white distractor changed its color to green (always 3.5s after initiation of the trial). In the moment of the color-switch, children had to quickly move their eyes from central fixation to the peripheral green stimulus, and to restart the reproduction of the trained target duration, while fixating the peripheral green square.

In parallel to the psychophysical time reproduction task, eye movements were recorded for the left monocular eye using an infrared high-speed eye-tracking system (iView X Hi-Speed 1250Hz System, SensoMotoric Instruments, Teltow, Germany) at a sampling rate of 1250Hz. Recording of eye movements was controlled by a PC (Intel Core 2 Duo Processor, 2.66 GHz; system software: Windows XP, Version 2002), and by the recording software iViewX (Version 2.0.23b, SensoMotoric Instruments, Teltow, Germany). A network connection allowed for the exchange of stimulus-trigger between the stimulus computer and the recording system. In the beginning of the experiment, a calibration of the eye-tracking system was conducted using a nine-point calibration matrix.

Distraction Paradigm

All children participated in a psychophysical double-task, requiring precise time reproduction of a 5s-interval in combination with an oculomotor task. Previous timing studies in humans successfully investigated attention-dependent effects of distraction using a time reproduction paradigm with visual distractors (Folta & Mähler, 2011; Folta-Schoofs et al., 2014; Fortin & Massé, 2000). In this study, we adapted a modified version of this paradigm to the peculiarities of combined psychophysical testing and eye movement registration in children with and without ADHD. Our experiment contained an initial training (N = 60 trials), and a subsequent experimental session (N = 180 trials).

Training of the Critical Target Duration

In the beginning of the experiment, all children were initially trained to mentally represent a fixed target duration of 5s (Figure 2A). Importantly, all children were unaware of the explicit time period they were trained to. All children were not allowed to use any form of explicit or implicit counting strategies (e.g., rhythmic head movements, foot-, or finger-tapping). The whole training contained a total of N = 60 trials. Children initiated each trial by pressing and releasing the response key. Immediately after key press, a fixation stimulus (white square) was presented centrally on the gray screen for a total duration of 5s. Thereafter, a central marker stimulus (black square) appeared for a total duration of 1s, before the white square reappeared. Children were required to again press the response key immediately after the occurrence of the color switch from white to black, and to memorize the critical target interval comprising the time interval between the first and second press of the response key. No feedback about correct performance was provided throughout the session. After the second press of the response key, children were prompted to initiate the next trial (i.e., children initiated each trial at their own pace). In the case of no response, training trials were terminated after a maximum trial duration of 30s. At the end of the training, all children were asked if they were able to successfully memorize the critical target duration. Afterwards, they paused for 2 to 3min before they continued with the experimental session.

Experimental Session

The experimental session contained a total of N = 180 time reproduction trials, and served to test for the accuracy and precision of time reproduction of the memorized target duration (5s) in the presence (distractor trials) and absence of visual distractors (baseline trials). No feedback about timing performance was provided throughout the experimental session. Comparable to the training session, children were not allowed to use any form of explicit or implicit counting strategies (e.g., rhythmic head movements, foot-, or finger-tapping), and were instructed not to count the length of distractors as part of the to-be-reproduced duration. Children initiated each trial at their own pace. In the case of no response, all trials were terminated after a maximum trial duration of 30s.

A total of N = 60 baseline trials (Figure 2B) were conducted to measure children's ability of precise time reproduction (as a critical test of executive functioning and interference control) in the absence of visual distraction, and were characterized by presentation of a central white square that continued for the further duration of the trial. Children were instructed to reproduce the memorized criterion time, and to press the response key when they felt that the critical target interval had passed by. Baseline trials were randomly intermingled with a total of N = 120 distractor trials that were divided in N = 60 trials requiring saccade-inhibition and N = 60 trials requiring the execution of cued prosaccades. Trials requiring saccade-inhibition (Figure 2C) contained an initial time period of 1.5s of a centrally presented white square, followed by an additional 2s distractor presentation of a white square in one of four randomly chosen peripheral screen positions (i.e., 15 distractor presentations per screen position). Children were instructed to fixate the centrally presented white square and to continue their time reproduction in the face of a peripherally presented second white square, so that the time between the first and second press of the response key approximately corresponded to the trained target duration. Previous studies revealed an effect of distractor location on human time reproduction with small temporal distortions induced by distracting signals presented in the beginning, and relatively higher distortions induced by distracting signals presented near the end of the to-be-timed interval (Fortin & Massé, 2000; Fortin, Bédard & Champagne, 2005; Tremblay & Fortin, 2003). This location-effect was suggested to depend on the expectancy of the distracting signal producing different amounts of time- or resource-sharing (Fortin, 2003; Fortin & Massé, 2000). To ensure a comparable amount of time- or resource-sharing, we presented all distractors always 1.5s after the initiation of the trial, and defined a fixed distractor duration of 2s (comparable to Folta-Schoofs et al., 2014). In cued prosaccade trials (Figure 2D), children were instructed to fixate the central white square, and to continue fixation for the duration of the peripheral white distractor, which appeared randomly in one of four peripheral screen positions (i.e., 15 distractor presentations per screen position appearing always 1.5s after the initiation of the trial). Thereafter, always 3.5s after the initiation of the trial, the peripheral square changed its color to green. In the moment of the color-switch, children had to quickly move their eyes from central fixation to the peripheral stimulus, and to restart the reproduction of the trained time interval, while fixation on the peripheral green square had to be maintained.

Data Analysis and Statistics

Analysis of Time Reproduction Data

Fitted time response functions were applied to time reproduction data using MATLAB 7.8.0 (R2009a, The Mathworks, Inc., Natick, MA, USA). Time response functions provide an ideal illustration of the accuracy and precision of time reproductions in baseline and distractor trials (see Figure 2), and were regularly reported in studies investigating timing in the seconds-to-minute range (interval timing). Comparable to existing interval timing studies (e.g., Buhusi, 2012; Buhusi & Meck, 2000, 2006a, b; Folta & Mähler, 2011; Olton, Wenk, Church & Meck, 1988; Roberts, 1981), time response functions were calculated by first dividing the maximum trial length (30s) into subintervals (bins) of 1s duration. Then, for each experimental condition (baseline, saccade-inhibition condition, cued prosaccade condition) the response-frequency (responses/min) was determined by summating all timing responses for each subject and bin, and then dividing the resulting bin-count by the absolute number of trials for the corresponding experimental condition. Using the MATLAB curve fitting toolbox, Gaussian-fits (equation: a × exp (– ((x – b) / c) ^ 2)) were obtained from response-frequency data using the nonlinear least square method with further refinement by minimizing least absolute residuals. Individual fits were approved with Goodness-of-fit-tests, which on average revealed a very good quality of the fits (adjusted $r^2 > .94$). Parameters (*a, b, c*) corresponding to the accuracy of time reproduction (peak time, *b*), maximum response rate at peak time (peak amplitude, *a*), and precision of timing (width, *c*) were extracted from individual fits, and were subjected to further statistical analysis.

Saccade Analysis

Saccade analysis was conducted using the SMI BeGaze analysis software (Sensomotric Instruments, Teltow, Germany). Firstly, blink artifacts were removed from the recorded data, and latency, speed, duration and amplitude of saccade-like events (SLE) were determined. Saccades were defined as SLE, when peak velocity exceeded a threshold of 150°/s in a time window comprising 20 to 80% of the duration of a SLE. Additionally, saccades were required to point to the direction of the peripheral target stimulus, to show a latency between 80 to 1000ms, an amplitude between 2.5° and 15°, and a fixation duration of at least 100ms.

Statistics

Statistical analyses were conducted using IBM SPSS Statistics 22.0.0 (IBM Corp., 1989-2013, USA). Non-parametric tests were used to verify statistical significance ($p < .05$, *two-sided*) of effects. Independent factors were tested using *Kruscal-Wallis-tests* and *Mann-Whitney-U-tests*. Dependent factors were tested using *Wilcoxon-tests*.

Results

Time Reproduction of the Trained Target Duration in Baseline Trials without Distraction

Children's characteristic of mean time response functions during baseline trials (without presentation of peripheral distractors) is summarized in Table 2. Descriptive analysis revealed a mean peak time of 5.7s (S.E. = .37s) for children in the control group, a mean peak time of 5.5s (S.E. = .38s) for children in the ADHD ON-MPH-medication group, and a mean peak time of 5.7s (S.E. = .4s) for children in the ADHD OFF-MPH-medication group (see Table 2 for further characteristics of mean time response functions, i.e. peak amplitude, width, and r^2-values indicating the quality of fits). Non-parametric statistical comparisons between the three independent experimental groups (ADHD children tested ON-MPH-medication vs. ADHD children tested OFF-MPH-medication vs. healthy control children) revealed no significant differences in peak time (*Kruskal-Wallis-test*: $\chi^2(2) = .384$; $p > .05$), peak amplitude (*Kruskal-Wallis-test*: $\chi^2(2) = .409$; $p > .05$), and width (*Kruskal-Wallis-test*: $\chi^2(2) = .305$; $p > .05$) of time response functions in baseline trials without any distraction. These results were in line with children's reports of having been able to successfully memorize the critical target duration (5s) during training.

Table 2. Subjective time reproduction in baseline trials (without presentation of visual distractors) for children in the ADHD ON-MPH-medication group, ADHD OFF-MPH-medication group, and the control group. For the three independent experimental groups, parameters of peak time, peak amplitude, and width of mean time response functions (Mean ± standard error, S.E.) are depicted. Goodness-of-fit-values (r-square) indicate the quality of fits for the different time response functions (1 = perfect fit)

Baseline-Trials	ADHD (ON MPH-medication)	ADHD (OFF MPH-medication)	Healthy controls (no medication)
Peak Time	5.5s ± .38 (S.E.)	5.7s ± .40 (S.E.)	5.7s ± .37 (S.E.)
Peak Amplitude	7.5 resp./bin ± .67 (S.E.)	7.3 resp./bin ± .95 (S.E.)	6.9 resp./bin ± .77 (S.E.)
Width	1.5s ± .16 (S.E.)	1.90s ± .42 (S.E.)	1.5s ± .21 (S.E.)
r-square	.97 ± .01 (S.E.)	.98 ± .01 (S.E.)	.94 ± .02 (S.E.)

In addition to between-subjects comparisons, within-subjects comparisons were conducted on time reproduction data for one group of ADHD children that was tested ON-MPH- and OFF-MPH-medication, successively. The descriptive analysis of baseline trials for this group revealed a mean peak time of 5.8s (S.E. = .53s; see Table 4), mean peak amplitude of 6.7 responses/bin (S.E. = .8 resp./bin), and a mean width of 1.6s (S.E. = .25s) when tested ON-MPH-medication, and a mean peak time of 5.1s (S.E. = .55s), a mean peak amplitude of 7.6 responses/bin (S.E. = .89 resp./bin), and a mean width of 1.5s (S.E. = .18s) when tested OFF-MPH-medication. Comparable to what was observed from between-subjects comparisons, within-subjects comparisons revealed no significant differences in mean peak time (*Wilcoxon-test*: $U = 1.521$; $p > .05$), peak amplitude (*Wilcoxon-test*: $U = .507$; $p > .05$), and width (*Wilcoxon-test*; $U = .507$; $p > .05$) of time response functions extracted from baseline trials without visual distraction.

Time Response Functions from Trials with Visual Distraction

Children's characteristic of mean time response functions for distractor trials (saccade-inhibition vs. cued prosaccade trials) is summarized in Table 3. Descriptive analysis of trials requiring saccade-inhibition to peripheral visual distractors revealed a mean peak time of 5.4s (S.E. = .20s) for children in the control group, a mean peak time of 5.1s (S.E. = .19s) for children in the ADHD ON-MPH-medication group, and a mean peak time of 5.6s (S.E. =

.47s) for children in the ADHD OFF-MPH-medication group (see Table 3 for further characteristics of mean time response functions, i.e. peak amplitude, width, and r^2-values indicating the quality of fits). Non-parametric statistical comparisons between the three independent experimental groups (ADHD children tested ON-MPH-medication vs. ADHD children tested OFF-MPH-medication vs. healthy control children) revealed no significant differences in peak time (*Kruskal-Wallis-test*: $\chi^2(2) = .829$; $p > .05$), and peak amplitude (*Kruskal-Wallis-test*: $\chi^2(2) = 3.130$; $p > .05$), but demonstrated a significant small difference in the width (*Kruskal-Wallis-test*: $\chi^2(2) = 6.368$; $p < .05$) of time response functions. Pairwise comparisons revealed this significance to be due to a slightly smaller width in the ON-MPH-medication group (Mean width = .9s, S.E. = .07s) compared to the control group (Mean width = 1.2s, S.E. = .06s; *Mann-Whitney-U-tests*: $U = 2.483$; $p < .05$). However, pairwise comparisons revealed no significant differences in mean width between the control group and OFF-MPH-medication group, or between ON- and OFF-MPH-medication groups (*Mann-Whitney-U-tests*: $p > .05$). Therefore (and because of limitations resulting from the binning- and fitting-procedure), the observed differences in width of time response functions are practically of no major importance.

Descriptive analysis of trials requiring the voluntary execution of a saccade to a peripherally presented visual distractor (cued prosaccade trials) revealed a mean peak time of 4.5s (S.E. = .45s) for children in the control group, a mean peak time of 3.7s (S.E. = .65s) for children in the ADHD ON-MPH-medication group, and a mean peak time of 3.9s (S.E. = .38s) for children in the ADHD OFF-MPH-medication group (see Table 3 for further characteristics of mean time response functions, i.e. peak amplitude, width, and r^2-values indicating the quality of fits). Non-parametric statistical comparisons between the three independent experimental groups (ADHD children tested ON-MPH-medication vs. ADHD children tested OFF-MPH-medication vs. healthy control children) revealed no significant differences in peak time (*Kruskal-Wallis-test*: $\chi^2(2) = 2.369$; $p > .05$), peak amplitude (*Kruskal-Wallis-test*: $\chi^2(2) = 2.704$; $p > .05$), and width (*Kruskal-Wallis-test*: $\chi^2(2) = 1.567$; $p > .05$) of time response functions.

Across groups, pairwise comparisons between experimental conditions were conducted. Statistical comparisons of time response functions for baseline and cued prosaccade trials revealed comparable amplitudes (*Wilcoxon-test*: $U = 1.653$; $p > .05$) and widths (*Wilcoxon-test*: $U = 1.331$; $p > .05$). However, mean peak time was demonstrated to be significantly shorter in cued prosaccade trials (Mean peak time = 4.1s, S.E. = .3s) compared to baseline trials (Mean peak time = 5.6s, S.E. = .21s; *Wilcoxon-test*: $U = 4.226$; $p < .001$) or saccade-inhibition trials (Mean peak time = 5.4s, S.E. = .16s; *Wilcoxon-test*: $U = 3.672$; $p < .001$). Time response functions in saccade-inhibition trials clearly differed from those observed in baseline trials and cued prosaccade trials with respect to peak amplitude and width of time response functions (*Wilcoxon-tests*: $p < .001$). Saccade-inhibition trials showed a slightly increased peak amplitude (Mean peak amplitude = 10.3 responses/bin, S.E. = .59 resp./bin), and a slightly reduced width of time response functions (Mean width = 1.1s, S.E. = .05s) compared to baseline trials (Mean peak amplitude = 7.2 responses/bin, S.E. = .44 resp./bin; Mean width = 1.6s, S.E. = .15s) or cued prosaccade trials (Mean peak amplitude = 7.8 responses/bin, S.E. = .36 resp./bin; Mean width = 1.4s, S.E. = .09s).

Table 3. Characteristics of time reproductions (peak time, amplitude, width, and r-square-values), and saccade characteristics (number, latency, duration, peak amplitude, and peak velocity of saccades) calculated for the saccade-inhibition and cued prosaccade condition. Data (Mean ± standard error) are depicted for independent groups containing ADHD children tested ON-MPH-medication, ADHD children tested OFF-MPH-medication, and healthy control children (tested without any medication). Across groups, children showed significant differences (*p* < .05) in number, latency, amplitude, and peak velocity of voluntary saccades (cued prosaccade condition) compared to erroneously executed saccades (saccade-inhibition condition)

	Saccade-Inhibition:			*Cued Prosaccade:*		
	ADHD (ON-MPH-medication)	*ADHD (OFF-MPH-medication)*	*Healthy Control*	*ADHD (ON-MPH-medication)*	*ADHD (OFF-MPH-medication)*	*Healthy Control*
Time reproduction						
Peak time (s)	5.1 ± .19	5.6 ± .47	5.4 ± .20	3.7 ± .65	3.9 ± .38	4.5 ± .45
Amplitude (resp./bin)	11.8 ± 1.05	9.4 ± 1.03	9.4 ± .89	8.6 ± .59	7.5 ± .77	7.2 ± .51
Width (s)	.9 ± .07	1.2 ± .13	1.2 ± .06	1.3 ± .11	1.7 ± .26	1.4 ± .11
r-square	.99 ± .004	.97 ± .01	.97 ± .01	.97 ± .01	.97 ± .01	.95 ± .01
Saccades						
Number (%)	25.7 ± 5.2	28.2 ± 6.5	19.5 ± 3.8	47.5 ± 6.6	49.3 ± 6.8	54.7 ± 4.9
Latency (ms)	523 ± 34	525 ± 45	541 ± 26	650 ± 27	663 ± 25	613 ± 20
Duration (ms)	43 ± 1.0	43 ± 1.7	38 ± 1.3	44 ± 1.2	44 ± 1.6	42 ± 1.3
Amplitude (°)	4.9 ± .22	4.8 ± .25	4.6 ± .13	5.3 ± .15	5.1 ± .2	5.4 ± .2
Peak Velocity (°/s)	251 ± 12.5	220 ± 9.0	238 ± 8.2	261 ± 10.8	237 ± 13.7	265 ± 12.5

Finally, within-subjects comparisons were conducted on time reproduction data for a group of ADHD children that was tested ON-MPH- and OFF-MPH-medication, successively. For saccade-inhibition trials, the analysis revealed a mean peak time of 5.1s (S.E. = .17s; see Table 4), mean peak amplitude of 11.8 responses/bin (S.E. = 1.7 resp./bin), and a mean width of .9s (S.E. = .11s) when tested ON-MPH-medication, and a mean peak time of 4.9s (S.E. = .15s), a mean peak amplitude of 12.3 responses/bin (S.E. = 1.56 resp./bin), and a mean width of .9s (S.E. = .11s) when tested OFF-MPH-medication. Non-parametric statistical comparisons between both measures revealed no significant differences in mean peak time (*Wilcoxon-test*: $U = 1.183$; $p > .05$), peak amplitude (*Wilcoxon-test*: $U = .507$; $p > .05$), and width (*Wilcoxon-test*: $U = .169$; $p > .05$) of time response functions.

Table 4. Peak times and saccade characteristics (number, latency, duration, peak amplitude, and peak velocity of saccades) for baseline trials (only peak time), saccade-inhibition trials, and cued prosaccade trials. Data (Mean ± standard error, S.E.) are depicted for dependent groups of ADHD children tested both ON-MPH-medication and OFF-MPH-medication, successively. Within-subjects comparisons revealed a significant acceleration ($p < .05$) in peak velocity for the cued prosaccade condition, but no significant changes in peak velocity for the saccade-inhibition condition. Similarly, number, duration and amplitude of saccades were not significantly different between both experimental conditions ($p > .05$)

	ADHD ON-MPH	S.E.	ADHD OFF-MPH	S.E.
Peak time (s)				
Baseline	5.8	.53	5.1	.55
Saccade Inhibition	5.1	.17	4.9	.15
Cued Prosaccade	3.9	.84	5.1	.51
Number (%)				
Saccade Inhibition	18.2	5.2	9.6	2.7
Cued Prosaccade	52.0	9.5	50.2	8.8
Latency (ms)				
Saccade Inhibition	527	57	559	27
Cued Prosaccade	620	31	621	37
Duration (ms)				
Saccade Inhibition	44	1.3	43	1.6
Cued Prosaccade	44	1.2	44	1.9
Amplitude (°)				
Saccade Inhibition	4.7	.20	4.9	.15
Cued Prosaccade	5.2	.14	5.0	.20
Peak-Velocity (°/s)				
Saccade Inhibition	247	16.3	238	9.8
Cued Prosaccade	261	8.4	243	12.1

Cued prosaccade trials were analyzed using within-subjects comparisons between ADHD children tested ON-MPH- and OFF-MPH-medication, successively. The analysis revealed a mean peak time of 3.9s (S.E. = .84s; see Table 4), mean peak amplitude of 8.5 responses/bin (S.E. = .91 resp./bin), and mean width of 1.3s (S.E. = .16s) when tested ON-MPH-medication, and a mean peak time of 5.1s (S.E. = .51s), a mean peak amplitude of 9.4 responses/bin (S.E. = 1.28 resp./bin), and a mean width of 1.1s (S.E. = .09s) when tested OFF-MPH-medication. Non-parametric statistical comparisons between both dependent measures revealed a significant difference in mean peak time (*Wilcoxon-test*: $U = 2.028$; $p < .05$), but no significant differences in peak amplitude (*Wilcoxon-test*: $U = 1.014$; $p > .05$), and width (*Wilcoxon-test*: $U = 1.521$; $p > .05$) of time response functions. Thus, the accuracy of time reproduction was significantly reduced under MPH-medication, when voluntarily executed prosaccades to visual distractors were required. Interestingly, this effect has not been observed in baseline and saccade-inhibition trials, where time reproductions perfectly matched to the trained target duration.

Saccades to Peripheral Distractors: Between-Subjects Comparisons

Saccade characteristics for the saccade-inhibition and cued prosaccade condition are summarized in Table 3 for the three independent groups of children (ADHD ON-MPH-medication group, ADHD OFF-MPH-medication group, and healthy control group). All experimental groups showed a comparable number, latency, amplitude, and peak velocity of saccades for the saccade-inhibition (*Kruskal-Wallis-test*: $p > .05$) and the cued prosaccade condition (*Kruskal-Wallis-test*: $p > .05$). Statistical comparisons of saccade duration revealed a significant difference for the saccade-inhibition task (*Kruskal-Wallis-test*: $\chi^2(2) = 7.172$; $p < .05$), but not for the cued prosaccade task (*Kruskal-Wallis-test*: $\chi^2(2) = 1.1$; $p > .05$). Additional group-comparisons revealed this significant difference in saccade duration (see Table 3) to be due to a small duration difference of 5ms for the ADHD ON-MPH-medication group (Mean duration = 43ms, S.E. = 1.0ms) compared to the control group (Mean duration = 38ms, S.E. = 1.3ms; *Wilcoxon-test*: $U = 2.656$; $p < .01$). Since all groups showed comparable saccade amplitudes, this small difference in duration can practically be neglected.

Across the three experimental groups, dependent nonparametric *Wilcoxon-tests* were conducted to test for differences in saccade characteristics between erroneously executed saccades in saccade-inhibition trials, and voluntarily executed saccades in trials requiring cued prosaccades. The analysis revealed significant differences between the two experimental conditions for the number of executed saccades (Mean percentage of saccades in saccade-inhibition trials = 24%, S.E. = 2.9%; Mean percentage of saccades in cued prosaccade trials = 51%, S.E. = 3.5%; *Wilcoxon-test*: $U = 3.694$; $p < .001$), as well as the latency (Mean latency of saccades in saccade-inhibition trials = 530ms, S.E. = 19ms; Mean latency of saccades in cued prosaccade trials = 640ms, S.E. = 14ms; *Wilcoxon-test*: $U = 3.851$; $p < .001$), amplitude (Mean amplitude of saccades in saccade-inhibition trials = 4.7°, S.E. = .11°; Mean amplitude of saccades in cued prosaccade trials = 5.3°, S.E. = .1°; *Wilcoxon-test*: $U = 3.654$; $p < .001$), and peak velocity (Mean peak velocity of saccades in saccade-inhibition trials = 238°/s, S.E. = 6.2°/s; Mean peak velocity of saccades in prosaccade trials = 256°/s, S.E. = 7.2°/s; *Wilcoxon-test*; $U = 2.796$; $p < .01$) of saccades. Only for the parameter ‘saccade duration’, no significant difference was observed (Mean duration of saccades in saccade-inhibition trials = 41ms, S.E. = .82ms; Mean duration of saccades in prosaccade trials = 43ms, S.E. = .75ms;

Wilcoxon-test: $U = 1.474$; $p > .05$). These results clearly indicate substantial differences in the characteristics of voluntarily and erroneously executed saccades.

Saccades to Peripheral Visual Distractors: Within-Subjects Comparisons

In addition to between-subjects comparisons, within-subjects comparisons were conducted on eye movement data for a group of ADHD children that was tested ON-MPH- and OFF-MPH-medication, successively. Saccade characteristics for the saccade-inhibition and cued prosaccade condition for this group (ADHD ON-/OFF-MPH-medication group) are summarized in Table 4. For both distractor conditions (saccade inhibition vs. cued prosaccade condition), ADHD children produced a comparable number, latency, amplitude, and duration of saccades, irrespectively of the fact that MPH-medication was taken or not (*Wilcoxon-tests*: $p > .05$). However, non-parametric pairwise comparisons revealed a significant difference in saccadic peak velocity for the cued prosaccade task (*Wilcoxon-test*: $U = 2.197$; $p < .05$), but not for the saccade-inhibition task (*Wilcoxon-test*: $U = .676$; $p > .05$). In cued prosaccade trials, ADHD children showed a higher peak velocity of voluntarily executed saccades (Mean peak velocity = 261°/s, S.E. = 8.4°/s) when tested ON-MPH-medication, compared to peak velocity of cued prosaccades executed without MPH-medication (Mean peak velocity = 243°/s, S.E. = 12.1°/s; see Table 4 and Figure 3).

Non-parametric statistical comparisons between individual saccade characteristics for the saccade-inhibition and cued prosaccade condition were separately conducted for children tested in the ON- and OFF-MPH-medication condition. For the ON-MPH-medication condition, no significant differences between erroneously and voluntarily executed saccades were observed for the latency (*Wilcoxon-test*: $U = 1.352$; $p > .05$), duration (*Wilcoxon-test*: $U = .507$; $p > .05$), and peak velocity (*Wilcoxon-test*: $U = .845$; $p > .05$) of saccades. On the other hand, significant differences were observed for the number (*Wilcoxon-test*: $U = 1.997$; $p < .05$), and amplitude (*Wilcoxon-test*: $U = 2.366$; $p < .05$) of erroneously and voluntarily executed saccades. The descriptive analysis revealed a higher number of voluntarily executed saccades (Mean percentage of saccades in saccade-inhibition trials = 18.2%, S.E. = 5.2%; Mean percentage of saccades in prosaccade trials = 52%, S.E. = 9.5%; see Table 4), and a higher amplitude of voluntarily executed saccades (Mean amplitude of saccades in saccade-inhibition trials = 4.7°, S.E. = .2°; Mean amplitude of saccades in prosaccade trials = 5.2°, S.E. = .14°; see Table 4). For the OFF-MPH-medication condition, non-parametric analysis revealed no significant differences in duration (*Wilcoxon-test*: $U = .676$; $p > .05$), amplitude (*Wilcoxon-test*: $U = .845$; $p > .05$), and peak velocity (*Wilcoxon-test*: $U = .338$; $p > .05$) of erroneously and voluntarily executed saccades. On the other hand, significant differences were observed for the number (*Wilcoxon-test*: $U = 2.366$; $p < .05$), and latency (*Wilcoxon-test*: $U = 2.028$; $p < .05$) of erroneously and voluntarily executed saccades. The descriptive analysis revealed a higher number of voluntarily executed saccades (Mean percentage of saccades in saccade-inhibition trials = 9.6%, S.E. = 2.7%; Mean percentage of saccades in prosaccade trials = 50.2%, S.E. = 8.8%; see Table 4), and a longer latency of voluntarily executed saccades (Mean latency of saccades in saccade-inhibition trials = 559ms, S.E. = 27ms; Mean latency of saccades in prosaccade trials = 621ms, S.E. = 37ms; see Table 4). As expected, in both MPH-medication conditions (ON-MPH- vs. OFF-MPH-medication) a higher number of saccades were generated, when a voluntary execution of saccades were required. Comparable to results from between-subjects comparisons (see previous section), within-subjects comparisons confirmed a tendency to longer latencies and slightly increased amplitudes of voluntarily executed saccades in the cued prosaccade condition.

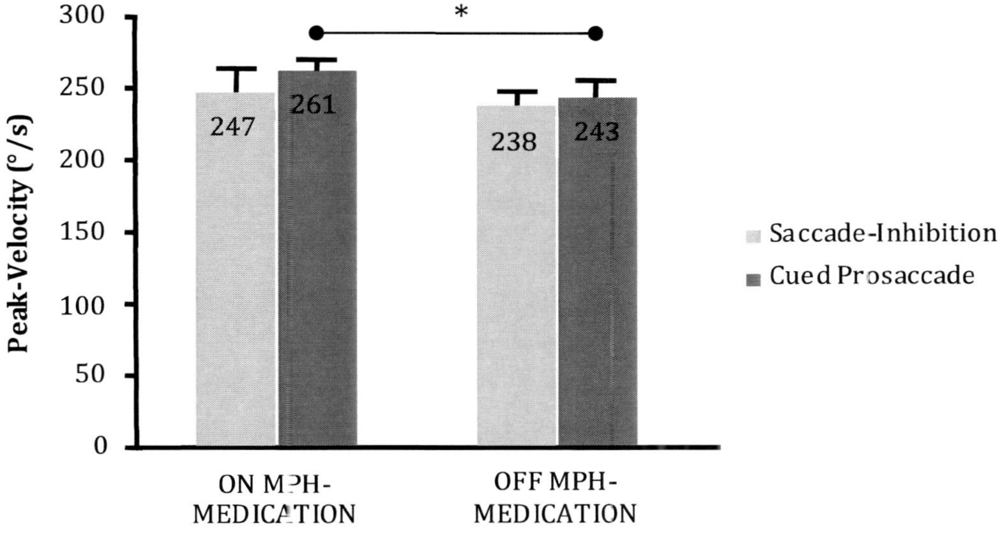

Figure 3. Saccadic peak velocity of ADHD children tested both ON-MPH- and OFF-MPH-medication, successively. Data are shown for both experimental conditions (saccade-inhibition vs. cued prosaccade task). Error-bars denote standard error (S.E.).

Peak Velocity of Saccades in the ON/OFF-MPH-Medication Group vs. the Control Group

Voluntarily executed prosaccades showed a significant increase in peak velocity when children were tested ON-MPH-medication compared to testing in the OFF-MPH-medication condition (Table 4; see previous section). However, this increase in peak velocity failed to reach significance level for between-subjects comparisons of independent groups of ADHD children tested with and without MPH-medication (Table 3), although a trend in the right direction was observable also in these data. We conducted additional independent non-parametric statistics to compare peak velocities of prosaccades in the ADHD ON-/OFF-MPH medication group (N = 7) and in the independent group of healthy control children (N = 12). This analysis revealed no significant differences between both experimental groups (*Mann-Whitney-U-tests*: $p > .05$). Most importantly, peak velocity of cued prosaccades was not significantly different for control children (Mean peak velocity = 265°/s, S.E. = 12.5°/s), and ADHD-children tested both ON-MPH-medication (Mean peak velocity = 261°/s, S.E. = 8.4°/s; *Mann-Whitney-U-tests*: U = .085; $p > .05$) and OFF-MPH-medication (Mean peak velocity = 243°/s, S.E. = 12.1°/s; *Mann-Whitney-U-tests*: U = 1.268; $p > .05$), successively. Thus, when contrasted to healthy control children, between-subjects comparisons were not successful in demonstrating significant changes in peak velocity, although a non-significant trend to decelerated peak velocities was observed also in non-medicated ADHD children.

Discussion and Conclusion

In daily life, perception of time becomes regularly distracted by environmental stimuli, which compete for attention and information processing resources (Imhof, 2004; Nigg, 2001; Pearson et al., 1991; van Mourik et al., 2005, 2007; Wood et al., 1999). To allow for ecologically valid measures of timing and distraction, we employed a temporal distractor paradigm requiring the precise reproduction of a previously trained target interval, while saccades to eccentric visual distractors either have to be suppressed (saccade-inhibition condition) or voluntarily initiated (cued prosaccade condition). This paradigm was considered to allow for proving deficits (or the integrity) of the child's behavioral inhibition system (Cairney et al., 2001; Kerns et al., 2001; McInerney & Kerns, 2003; Meaux & Chelonis, 2003; Mullins et al., 2005). Accurate and precise time reproductions of memorized time intervals, as well as successful saccade-inhibition in the presence of distracting visual stimuli were considered to effectively prove the integrity of the frontostriatal circuitry, which constitutes an important neural correlate of the behavioral inhibition system in humans (Giedd et al., 2001; Munoz et al., 2003; Thier, 2006; Ullsperger & von Cramon, 2006). Deficits in the frontostriatal circuitry were expected to result in distractor-induced changes of the characteristic of time response functions or specific modulations of saccade characteristics in time reproduction trials with and without visual distraction.

Characteristic of Time Response Functions

The current study revealed time reproductions that were characterized by time response functions demonstrating a smoothly increasing response density to a peak near criterion time (5s), followed by a smooth and symmetrical decrease of the response rate to near zero levels of responding. This general response pattern confirmed the effectiveness of our training procedure, and was in line with children's reports of having been able to successfully memorize the critical target interval. In addition, the observed pattern of time response functions is in perfect correspondence to time reproduction data as they were previously reported for rodents and birds (Cheng & Westwood, 1993; Church, Meck & Gibbon, 1994; Gibbon, 1977; Gibbon & Church, 1990), and also for human subjects (Folta-Schoofs et al., 2014; Hinton & Meck, 2004; Lustig & Meck, 2005; Rakitin et al., 1998; Wearden & McShane, 1988). Unlike previous studies (i.e., Rubia et al., 1999), which reported a higher variability of timing responses (i.e., loss of temporal precision) in ADHD children, our study showed (apart from small variations in amplitude and width of time response functions, which can easily be attributed to limitations of the binning and fitting procedure) no meaningful differences in peak amplitude, and width of time response functions produced by healthy children and ADHD children tested OFF-MPH- and ON-MPH-medication. Similarly, no changes in peak time were observed between the different experimental groups. However, across groups, pairwise comparisons revealed a significantly shorter mean peak time for cued prosaccade trials compared to baseline or saccade-inhibition trials. Moreover, within-subjects comparisons between ADHD children successively tested ON-MPH- and OFF-MPH-medication revealed a significantly reduced mean peak time of 3.9s for cued prosaccade trials when tested ON-MPH-medication. Thus, the accuracy of time reproduction was significantly reduced for the ON-MPH-medication condition, where voluntary execution of prosaccades to visual distractors was required. Interestingly, this effect was not observed for baseline and saccade-inhibition trials, where time reproductions perfectly matched to the trained target duration. Further studies are necessary to investigate the precise neural mechanisms underlying this apparent (and probably pharmacologically induced) reduction in acuity of time reproductions.

We expected deficits in the frontostriatal circuitry to influence the acuity and precision in timing tasks, which require an allocation of information processing resources away from the timing task, and towards environmental stimuli or events. For this reason, we employed an ecologically valid measure of timing and distraction by incorporating perceptual simple distractor stimuli that interfered with the primary timing task. In rodents and birds, time reproduction studies with gaps or distractors revealed underestimations (or overproductions) of critical target durations (Buhusi, 2012; Buhusi & Meck, 2000, 2006 a,b; Cabeza de Vaca, Brown & Hemmes, 1994; Roberts, 1981; Roberts, Cheng & Cohen, 1989), which were not observed in the current study. One might argue, that – at least in human subjects – less salient distractors require less information processing, so that most processing resources can still be concentrated on the timing task, when meaningless distractors (e.g., white squares) are presented. Thus, the functionality of interference control and the involvement of a supervisory attentional system might critically depend on the number and characteristics of externally presented distractor stimuli. Indeed, salience- and stimulus-dependent effects on timing performance have been demonstrated for human subjects (van Wassenhove, Buonomano, Shimojo & Shams, 2008; Wittmann, van Wassenhove, Craig & Paulus, 2010). Recently, Folta-Schoofs et al. (2014) investigated the effect of distractor characteristics on human time reproductions in the several seconds-range, and demonstrated temporal overproductions to occur after presentation of perceptual complex but not perceptually simple visual distractors. Comparable to what was observed in the current study, presentation of simple geometric figures (i.e., white rectangles) produced no significant shifts of peak time in adult and healthy participants (Folta-Schoofs et al., 2014). Thus comparable to adult participants, children in the current study might have learned to automatically ignore perceptual simple distractor stimuli, and required – if at all – only limited amounts of interference control to successfully solve the timing task. In situations where temporal accuracy has to be maintained despite ‘noisy’ and distracting natural environments, complexity-dependent changes of timing performance constitute an efficient and economic strategy for children and adults to ensure precise timing even in the presence of distracting stimuli. Further studies should employ more salient distractors to further investigate the functionality of the behavioral inhibition system in healthy and developmentally disturbed children.

Characteristic of Erroneously and Voluntarily Executed Saccades

Analyses of eye movement data revealed remarkable differences between saccade-characteristics of erroneously and voluntarily executed saccades. Compared to the cued prosaccade condition, a lower number, shorter latency, and slightly lower amplitude of saccades was observed for the saccade-inhibition condition. The latter might be attributable to group-differences in orienting gaze predominantly in the direction of the upper or lower border of the distractor stimulus. The relatively high percentage of erroneously executed saccades (10 to 30%) matched to findings from a previous study, employing a comparable experimental timing and saccade paradigm in medicated ADHD children and healthy controls (Folta & Mähler, 2011). The high number of erroneously executed saccades supports the notion of a general problem in active suppression of prosaccades in children younger than ten years of age (Paus, 1989; Paus, Babenko & Radil, 1990). For example, Paus (1989) presented peripheral distractor stimuli and asked healthy children between 8 and 12 years of age to actively suppress the execution of prosaccades. Ten years old children produced erroneously executed saccades in only 1.5% of all trials, whereas eight years old children executed such saccades in 26% of all trials (Paus, 1989). This high number perfectly matched to the percentages of erroneously executed saccades as they were observed for the current study. In contrast to studies that reported a significant increase in the number of erroneously executed saccades for ADHD children compared to healthy children (Cairney et al., 2001; Gould et al., 2001), the current study was not able to confirm such a difference. Despite from differences in the number of saccades, we observed longer latencies for the cued prosaccade condition. Previous studies on human adults reported latencies of about 200ms for prosaccades when gaze was reoriented from central fixation to a peripheral target stimulus. In the current study, saccadic latencies of between 520 and 560ms were observed for the saccade-inhibition condition, and even longer latencies of between 610 and 660ms were reported for the cued prosaccade condition. These long latencies confirm a general problem related to the suppression of an ongoing active saccade-inhibition in children younger than ten years of age (Paus, 1989; Paus et al., 1990). Indeed, Ross & Ross (1983) reported increased latencies for prosaccades in children aged between 8 and 11 years, and Ross, Young, Hommer & Radant (1994) found these latencies to decrease until age 14 or 15, where latencies approximated to that of adult participants. In addition, several studies reported changes in prosaccade-latency in ADHD children compared to healthy controls (Klein et al., 2003; Mostofsky et al., 2001; Munoz et al., 2003). However, similar to other authors (e.g., Hanisch et al., 2006; Ross et al., 2000), we failed to confirm such a difference. The controversy of results might best be explained by difficulties in correctly identifying ADHD-subtypes, which might differ in their saccade characteristics (Folta & Mähler, 2011).

Between experimental groups, statistical comparisons of number, latency, duration, amplitude, and peak velocity of correctly and erroneously executed saccades only revealed a non-significant trend of reduced peak velocities in the ADHD OFF-MPH-medication group (237°/s), compared to the ADHD ON-MPH-medication group (261°/s), and the healthy control group (265°/s). Generally, these results confirm intact executive functions and saccadic control in ADHD children and healthy control children. However, within-subjects comparisons revealed significantly increased peak velocities for correctly executed prosaccades in ADHD children tested ON-MPH-medication (261°/s), compared to peak velocities as they were observed in the OFF-MPH-medication condition (243°/s). Additionally, mean peak velocity of cued prosaccades was not significantly different in the ON-MPH-medication group and the healthy control group (261°/s vs. 265°/s). In summary, data of the current study suggest saccadic peak velocity to increase in ADHD children from about 240°/s before MPH-medication to about 260°/s after MPH-medication. This pattern of result confirms existing studies demonstrating the effectiveness of oral medication for successful compensation of behavioral deficits in children diagnosed with ADHD (e.g., Folta & Mähler, 2011; Klein, Fischer Jr., Fischer & Hartnegg, 2002; Munoz, Hampton, Moore & Goldring, 1999).

Modulations of saccadic peak velocities were previously observed in stutterers (Doslak, Healey & Rise, 1986), and in healthy subjects after intake of psychopharmacological agents (Aschoff, 1968; Bittencourt, Wade, Smith & Richens, 1981; Kahn, Taylor & Jones, 2000). In addition, there is evidence of variations in peak velocity depending on the mental workload required to perform different tasks (App & Debus, 1998; DiStasi et al., 2010; Galley, 1998). Khan et al. (2000) demonstrated the peak velocity of saccades to increase with increasing alertness. Munoz et al. (2003) reported a significant deceleration in peak velocity in non-medicated ADHD children that was not accompanied by changes in saccade amplitude. Compared to non-medicated healthy children, Folta & Mähler (2011) observed an accelerated peak velocity in medicated ADHD children that was not accompanied by significant modulations of saccade duration or amplitude. Interestingly, also in the current study, an increase in peak velocity was observed that was not accompanied by changes in the duration and amplitude of the saccade. Traditionally, the relationship between the amplitude, duration and velocity of a saccade has been called the 'main sequence', to indicate that peak velocity and saccadic duration increase systematically with the amplitude of the saccade (Becker, 1989; DiStasi et al., 2010). However, it is important to consider that the peak velocity is independent of the saccadic duration since it is not linked to it, a priori, by mathematical definition (Becker, 1989, DiStasi et al., 2010). Additionally, our observation, that changes in peak velocity were not accompanied by changes in amplitude or saccade duration, was also reported in previous studies (e.g., Folta & Mähler, 2011; DiStasi et al., 2010; Munoz et al., 2003), and suggest the relationship between peak velocity, amplitude, and duration probably to be more complex than has previously been assumed (Schmidt, Abel, Dell'Osso & Aroff, 1979).

Considering the ADHD-correlated alterations in neuronal excitation within the frontostriatal circuitry, the observed differences in peak velocity might best be explained by a passive flow of neuronal excitation from the FC - via the SC of the midbrain tectum - to burst neurons in the PPRF, and the riMLF, coding for the peak velocity of horizontal and vertical saccades, respectively (Figure 1; Leigh & Kennard, 2004; Sparks, 2002; Sparks, Barton, Gandhi & Nelson, 2002). One subdivision of the FC, the FEF, might primarily be involved in the passive flow of frontocortical excitation to the midbrain SC (Hanes & Wurtz, 2001; Hutton, 2008; Pierrot-Deseilligny, Rivaud, Gaymard & Agid, 1994; Schiller, True & Conway, 1980). We suggest ADHD-dependent accelerations or decelerations of saccadic peak velocities (i.e., MPH-dependent acceleration in saccadic peak velocity vs. deceleration of peak velocity in non-medicated ADHD children) to depend on the magnitude of frontocortical excitation within the FEF, which is decreased in non-medicated ADHD children (due to frontocortical hypoexcitation), and might become increased as a compensatory effect of MPH-medication. Alternatively, ADHD symptoms might be accompanied by anatomical and/or physiological changes in brainstem regions (Lahat et al., 1995; Sohmer & Student, 1978), which are responsible for generating the velocity profile of rapid eye movements.

Excitatory burst neurons (EBNs) in the brainstem PPRF and riMLF ‚translate' excitation from the SC into an acceleration of the eye. Duration, amplitude, and peak velocity of saccades are functions of the burst duration, number of spikes generated, and peak firing rate of EBNs, respectively (King & Fuchs, 1979). Activity in the PPRF is specifically related to the velocity profile of horizontal saccades and the horizontal component of oblique saccades. Omnipause neurons (OPNs) discharge at a relatively constant rate, and allow for fixation of the eyes. When saccade execution is required, the SC sends a trigger signal to inhibit the OPNs for the duration of the saccade. Simultaneously, neurons in SC excite long-lead burst neurons (LLBNs) and EBNs both generating high-frequency bursts of activity for the execution of saccades. EBNs are tightly coupled to saccade onset and make excitatory, monosynaptic connections (Strassman, Highstein & McCrea, 1986) with motor neurons in the ipsilateral abducens. Microstimulation of neurons in the PPRF was shown to produce horizontal eye movements (Cohen & Komatsuzaki, 1972). In addition, the peak velocity of saccades to horizontal targets was demonstrated to largely decrease after reversible lidocaine inactivation of neurons in the rostral PPRF, whereas the peak velocity of vertical saccades was not significantly affected (Sparks et al., 2002). Interestingly, a lidocaine-induced reduction in saccadic peak velocity was accompanied by an increase in saccade duration, indicating a compensation for velocity changes, as would be expected if the activity of EBNs is under feedback control (Sparks et al., 2002; Zee, Optican, Cook, Robinson & Engel, 1976). In contrast to activity in the PPRF, activity in the riMLF is specifically related to the velocity profile of vertical saccades and the vertical component of oblique saccades. For saccade initiation, neurons in the riMLF generate high-frequency bursts and convey these signals monosynaptically to the motor neurons that are responsible for moving the eye (Buttner, Buttner-Ennever & Henn, 1977; Dalezios, Scudder, Highstein & Moschovakis, 1998; King & Fuchs, 1979; Kokkoroyannis, Scudder, Highstein, Balaban & Moschovakis, 1996). Oblique saccades have both horizontal and vertical components, which onsets become synchronized in order to establish a relatively straight trajectory, and to avoid markedly curved oblique saccades (Sparks, 2002).

To summarize, presentations of visual distractors, as well as an execution of prosaccades within the to-be-reproduced time interval were not sufficient to distract ADHD children from accurate (i.e., peak times near criterion time) and precise time reproduction (i.e., narrow width of time response functions). These results suggest an intact ability of time reproduction and interference control in both healthy children and children with a diagnosis of ADHD. This observation is in accordance with results from previous studies demonstrating intact temporal abilities and interference control in ADHD children (Douglas & Peters, 1979; Folta & Mähler, 2011; Gumenyuk et al., 2005; Huang-Pollock et al., 2005; Mason et al., 2003; Tiffin-Richards et al., 2004; van der Meere & Sergeant, 1988; West et al., 2000). However, our results are in contrast to studies on ADHD children reporting severe deficits in accurate and precise timing (see for review: Toplak et al., 2006) or interference control (see for review: Douglas & Peters, 1979).

Further studies are necessary to clarify a potential role of distracter saliency for the involvement of mechanisms of interference control in healthy and developmentally disturbed children. In addition, further studies are necessary to clarify the neural basis of the observed ADHD- and MPH-dependent changes in saccade characteristics of voluntarily executed prosaccades.

Probably in the future, the peak velocity of saccades might be proved a useful indicator of frontocortical excitation, and might be used to improve the diagnosis and medical treatment of ADHD.

Acknowledgments

We thank all the children and their parents for support of this study. Additionally, we thank Larissa Bonin, Stephan Polowinski, and Rauni Rüter for their invaluable assistance in recruiting and testing participants, and Katharina Klabunde for her help in post-processing of eye movement data.

References

American Psychiatric Association. (2013). *Diagnostic and statistical manual of mental Disorders – DSM-V* (5th ed.). Arlington, VA: American Psychiatric Press.

American Psychiatric Association. (1994). *Diagnostic and statistical manual of mental disorders – DSM-IV* (4th ed.). Washington, DC: American Psychiatric Press.

App, E. & Debus, G. (1998). Saccadic velocity and activation: development of a diagnostic tool for assessing energy regulation. *Ergonomics*, *41*, 689-697.

Aschenbach, T. M. (1991a). *CBCL. Child Behaviour Checklist 4-18.* Burlington, VT: Department of Psychiatry, University of Vermont.

Aschenbach, T. M. (1991b). *TRF. Teacher Report Form.* Burlington, VT: Department of Psychiatry, University of Vermont.

Aschoff, C. J. (1968). Veränderungen rascher Blickbewegungen (Saccaden) beim Menschen unter Diazepam (Valium). *Archiv für Psychiatrie und Nervenkrankheiten*, *211*, 325-332.

Banaschewski, T., Roessner, V., Uebel, H. & Rothenberger, A. (2004). Neurobiologie der Aufmerksamkeitsdefizit- / Hyperaktivitätsstörung (ADHS). *Kindheit und Entwicklung*, *13*, 180-189.

Barkley, R. A. (1997). Behavioral inhibition, sustained attention, and executive functions: constructing a unifying theory of ADHD. *Psychological Bulletin*, *121*, 65-94.

Barkley, R. A., Edwards, G., Laneri, M., Fletcher, K. & Metevia, L. (2001a). Executive functioning, temporal discounting, and sense of time in adolescents with attention deficit hyperactivity disorder (ADHD) and oppositional defiant disorder (ODD). *Journal of Abnormal Child Psychology*, *29*, 541-556.

Barkley, R. A., Murphy, K. R. & Bush, T. (2001b). Time perception and reproduction in young adults with attention deficit hyperactivity disorder. *Neuropsychology*, *15*, 351-360.

Bauermeister, J. J., Barkley, R. A., Martinez, J. V., Cumba, E., Ramirez, R. R., Reina, G., et al. (2005). Time estimation and performance on reproduction tasks in subtypes of children with attention deficit hyperactivity disorder. *Journal of Clinical Child and Adolescence Psychology*, *34*, 151-162.

Becker, W. (1989). Saccadic eye movements as a control system: Metrics. In R.H. Wurtz, & M.E. Goldberg (Eds.), *Reviews of ocuolomotor research (Vol. 3): The neurobiology of saccadic eye movements*, (13-67). Hillsdale: Elsevier.

Ben-Pazi, H., Gross-Tsur, V., Bergman, H. & Shalev, R. S. (2003). Abnormal rhythmic motor response in children with attention-deficit-hyperactivity disorder. *Developmental Medicine and Child Neurology*, *45*, 743-750.

Biederman, J., Newcorn, J. & Sprich, S. (1991). Comorbidity of attention deficit hyperactivity disorder with conduct, depressive, anxiety and other disorders. *American Journal of Psychiatry*, *148*, 564-577.

Birkel, P. (2007). *Weingartener Grundwortschatz Rechtschreib-Test*. Göttingen: Hogrefe.

Bittencourt, P. R. M., Wade, P., Smith, A. T. & Richens, A. (1981). The relationship between peak velocity of saccadic eye movements and serum benzodiazepine concentration. *British Journal of Clinical Pharmacology*, *12*, 523-533.

Brown, L. N. & Vickers, J. N. (2004). Temporal judgments, hemispheric equivalence, and interhemispheric transfer in adolescents with attention deficit hyperactivity disorder. *Experimental Brain Research*, *154*, 76-84.

Buhusi, C. V. (2012). Time-sharing in rats: Effect of distracter intensity and discriminability. *Journal of Experimental Psychology: Animal Behavior Processes*, *38*, 30-39.

Buhusi, C. V. & Meck, W. H. (2006a). Interval timing with gaps and distracters: Evaluation of the ambiguity, switch, and time-sharing hypotheses. *Journal of Experimental Psychology: Animal Behavior Processes*, *32*, 329-338.

Buhusi, C. V. & Meck, W. H. (2006b). Time sharing in rats: A peak-interval procedure with gaps and distracters. *Behavioral Processes*, *71*, 107-115.

Buhusi, C. V. & Meck, W. H. (2000). Timing for the absence of a stimulus: The gap paradigm reversed. *Journal of Experimental Psychology: Animal Behavior Processes*, *26*, 305-322.

Buttner, U., Buttner-Ennever, J. A. & Henn, V. (1977). Vertical eye movement related unit activity in the rostral mesencephalic reticular formation of the alert monkey. *Brain Research*, *130*, 239-252.

Cabeza de Vaca, S., Brown, B. L. & Hemmes, N. S. (1994). Internal clock and memory processes in animal timing. *Journal of Experimental Psychology: Animal Behavior Processes*, *20*, 184-198.

Cairney, S., Maruff, P., Vance, A., Barnett, R., Luk, E. & Currie, J. (2001). Contextual abnormalities of saccadic inhibition in children with attention deficit hyperactivity disorder. *Experimental Brain Research*, *141*, 507-518.

Castellanos, F. X., Giedd, J. N., Eckburg, P., Marsh, W. L., Vaituzis, A. C., Kaysen, D., Hamburger, S. D. & Rappoport, J. L. (1994). Quantitative morphology of the caudate nucleus in attention deficit hyperactivity disorder. *American Journal of Psychiatry*, *151*, 1791-1796.

Castellanos, F. X., Giedd, J. N., Marsh, W. L., Hamburger, S. D., Vaituzis, A. C., Dickstein, D. P. et al. (1996). Quantitative brain magnetic resonance imaging in attention-deficit hyperactivity disorder. *Archives of General Psychiatry*, *53*, 607-616.

Castellanos, F. X., Giedd, J. N., Berquin, P. C., Walter, J. M., Sharp, W., Tran, T. et al. (2001). Quantitative brain magnetic resonance imaging in girls with attention-deficit hyperactivity disorder. *Archives of General Psychiatry*, *58*, 289-295.

Castellanos, F. X., Lee, P. P., Sharp, W., Jeffries, N. O., Greenstein, D. K., Clasen, L. S. et al. (2002). Developmental trajectories of brain volume abnormalities in children and adolescents with attention-deficit hyperactivity disorder. *JAMA*, *288*, 1740-1748.

Cheng, K. & Westwood, R. (1993). Analysis of single trials in pigeons' timing performance. *Journal of Experimental Psychology: Animal Behavior Processes*, *19*, 56-67.

Church, R. M., Meck, W. H. & Gibbon, J. (1994). Applications of scalar timing theory to individual trials. *Journal of Experimental Psychology: Animal Behavior Processes*, *20*, 135-155.

Cohen, B. & Komatsuzaki, A. (1972). Eye movements induced by stimulation of the pontine reticular formation: evidence for integration in oculomotor pathways. *Experimental Neurology*, *36*, 101-117.

Dalezios, Y., Scudder, C. A., Highstein, S. M. & Moschovakis, A. K. (1998). Anatomy and physiology of the primate interstitial nucleus of Cajal. II. Discharge pattern of single efferent fibers. *Journal of Neurophysiology*, *80*, 3100-3111.

DiStasi, L. L., Renner, R., Staehr, P., Helmert, J. R., Velichkovsky, B. M., Canas, J. J., Catena, A. & Pannasch, S. (2010). Saccadic peak velocity sensitivity to variations in mental workload. *Aviation, Space, and Environmental Medicine*, *81*, 413-417.

Doslak, M. J., Healey, E. C. & Riese, K. (1986). Eye movements of stutterers. *Investigative Ophthalmololgy Visual Science*, *27*, 1410-1414.

Döpfner, M., Götz-Dorten, A. & Lehmkuhl, G. (2008). *DISYPS-II. Diagnostik-System für psychische Störungen nach ICD-10 und DSM-IV für Kinder und Jugendliche – II*. Verlag Hans Huber: Bern.

Douglas, V. I. & Peters, K. G. (1979). Toward a clearer definition of the attentional deficit of hyperactive children. In: Hale, G. A., Lewis, M. (Eds.). *Attention and the development of cognitive skills*, (173-246). New York: Plenum Press,

Durston, S., Hulshoff-Pol, H. E., Schnack, H. G., Buitelaar, J. K., Steenhuis, M. P., Minderaa, R. B. et al. (2004). Magnetic resonance imaging of boys with attention deficit/hyperactivity disorder and their unaffected siblings. *Journal of the American Academy of Child and Adolescent Psychiatry*, *43*, 332-340.

Everling, S. & Fischer, B. (1998). The antisaccade: a review of basic research and clinical studies. *Neuropsychologia*, *36*, 885-899.

Folta, K. & Mähler, C. (2011). Schnelle Augenbewegungen und visuelle Fixation bei Kindern mit ADHS. *Kindheit und Entwicklung*, *20*, 21-30.

Folta-Schoofs, K., Wolf, O. T., Treue, S. & Schoofs, D. (2014). Perceptual complexity, rather than valence or arousal accounts for distracter-induced overproductions of temporal durations. *Acta Psychologica*, *147*, 51-59.

Fortin C. (2003). Attentional time-sharing in interval timing. In W. H. Meck (Ed.), *Functional and neural mechanisms of interval timing*, (235-260). Boca Raton, FL: CRC Press.

Fortin, C. & Massé, N. (2000). Expecting a break in time estimation: Attentional time-sharing without concurrent processing. *Journal of Experimental Psychology: Human Perception and Performance*, *26*, 1788-1796.

Fortin, C., Bédard, M. C. & Champagne, J. (2005). Timing during interruptions in timing. *Journal of Experimental Psychology: Human Perception and Performance*, *31*, 276-288.

Galley, N. (1998). An enquiry into the relationship between activation and performance using saccadic eye movement parameters. *Ergonomics*, *41*, 698-720.

Gibbon, J. (1977). Scalar expectancy theory and Weber's law in animal timing. *Psychological Review*, *84*, 279-325.

Gibbon, J. & Church, R. M. (1990). Representation of time. *Cognition*, *37*, 23-34.

Giedd, J. N., Blumenthal, J., Molloy, E. & Castellanos, F. X. (2001). Brain imaging of attention deficit hyperactivity disorder. *Annals of the New York Academy of Sciences, 931*, 33-49.

Giedd, J. N., Castellanos, F. X., Casey, B. J., Kozucg, P., King, A. C., Hamburger, S. D. & Rapoport, J. L. (1994). Quantitative morphology of the corpus callosum in attention deficit hyperactivity disorder. *American Journal of Psychiatry, 151*, 665-669.

Gölitz, D., Roick, T. & Hasselhorn, M. (2006). *DEMAT 4. Deutscher Mathematiktest für vierte Klassen*. Göttingen: Beltz.

Gould, T. D., Bastain, T. M., Israel, M. E., Hommer, D. W. & Castellanos, F. X. (2001). Altered Performance on an Ocular Fixation Task in Attention Deficit/Hyperactivity Disorder. *Biological Psychiatry, 50*, 633-635.

Gumenyuk, V., Korzyukov, O., Escera, C., Hämäläinen, M., Huotilainen, M., Häyrinen, T. et al. (2005). Electrophysiological evidence of enhanced distractibility in ADHD children. *Neuroscience Letters, 374*, 212-217.

Graham, L. J. (2010). *(De)Constructing ADHD: A critical guide for teachers and Teacher educators*. New York: Peter Lang Publishing.

Groner, R. & Groner, M. T. (1989). Attention and eye movement control: an overview. *European Archives of Psychiatry and Clinical Neuroscience, 239*, 9-16.

Hanes, D. P. & Wurtz, R. H. (2001). Interaction of the frontal eye field and superior colliculus for saccade generation. *Journal of Neurophysiology, 85*, 804-815.

Hanisch, C., Radach, R., Holtkamp, K., Herpertz-Dahlmann, B. & Konrad, K. (2006). Oculomotor inhibition in children with and without attention-deficit hyperactivity disorder (ADHD). *Journal of Neural Transmission, 113*, 671-684.

Heinrichs, N. & Reinhold, N. (2010). Experimentelle Augenbewegungsmessung bei Kindern und Jugendlichen: Relevanz für psychopathologische Prozesse am Beispiel der sozialen Angst. *Kindheit und Entwicklung, 19*, 12-20.

Hinton, S. C. & Meck, W. H. (2004). Frontal-striatal circuitry activated by human peak-interval timing in the supra-seconds range. *Cognitive Brain Research, 21*, 171-182.

Huang-Pollock, C. L., Nigg, J. T. & Carr, T. H. (2005). Deficient attention is hard to find: applying the perceptual load model of selective attention to attention deficit hyperactivity disorder subtypes. *Journal of Child Psychology and Psychiatry, 46*, 1211-1218.

Huey, E. B. (1900). On the psychology and physiology of reading. I. *American Journal of Psychology, 11*, 283-302.

Hutton, S. B. (2008). Cognitive control of saccadic eye movements. *Brain and Cognition, 68*, 327-340.

Imhof, M. (2004). Diagnostik von Konzentration und Aufmerksamkeit in der Schule. In G. Büttner, & L. Schmidt-Atzert (Eds.), *Diagnostik von Konzentration und Aufmerksamkeit* (Tests & Trends, N. F. Bd. 3, 232- 247). Göttingen: Hogrefe.

Kemner, C., van der Geest, J. N., Verbaten, M. N. & van Engeland, H. (2004). In search of neurophysiological markers of pervasive developmental disorders: smooth pursuit eye movements? *Journal of Neural Transmission, 111*, 1617-1626.

Kempton, S., Vance, A., Maruff, P., Luk, E., Costin, J. & Pantelis, C. (1999). Executive function and attention deficit hyperactivity disorder: stimulant medication and better executive function performance in children. *Psychological Medicine, 29*, 527-538.

Kerns, K., McInerney, R. & Wilde, N. (2001). Time reproduction, working memory, and behavioral inhibition in children with ADHD. *Child Neuropsychology, 7*, 21-31.

Khan, O. A., Taylor, S. R. & Jones, J. G. (2000). Anaesthesia and saccadic eye movements. *Anaesthesia*, *55*, 877-882.

Kim, B. N., Lee, J. S., Shin, M. S., Cho, S. C. & Lee, D. S. (2002). Regional cerebral perfusion abnormalities in attention deficit/hyperactivity disorder. Statistical parametric mapping analysis. *European Archives of Psychiatry and Clinical Neuroscience*, *252*, 219-225.

Kim, B. N., Lee, J. S., Cho, S. C. & Lee, D. S. (2001). Methylphenidate increased regional cerebral blood flow in subjects with attention deficit/hyperactivity disorder. *Yonsei Medical Journal*, *42*, 19-29.

King, W. M. & Fuchs, A. F. (1979). Reticular control of vertical saccadic eye movements by mesencephalic burst neurons. *Journal of Neurophysiology*, *42*, 861-876.

Klein, C. H., Raschke, A. & Brandenbusch, A. (2003). Development of pro- and antisaccades in children with attention deficit hyperactivity disorder (ADHD) and healthy controls. *Psychophysiology*, *40*, 17-28.

Klein, C., Fischer Jr. B., Fischer, B. & Hartnegg, K. (2002). Effects of methylphenidate on saccadic responses in patients with ADHD. *Experimental Brain Research*, *145*, 121-125.

Kokkoroyannis, R., Scudder, C. A., Highstein, S. M., Balaban, C. & Moschovakis, A. K. (1996). The anatomy and physiology of the primate interstitial nucleus of Cajal. I. Efferent projections. *Journal of Neurophysiology*, *75*, 725-739.

Kömpf, D. & Heide, W. (1998). Zentralnervöse Strukturen - two goals, two modes, six systems. Eine Einführung. In A. Huber, & D. Kömpf (Eds.), *Klinische Neuroophthalmologie* (48-57). Stuttgart: Georg Thieme Verlag.

Krajewski, K., Liehm, S. & Schneider, W. (2004). *DEMAT 2+. Deutscher Mathematiktest für zweite Klassen*. Göttingen: Beltz.

Küspert, P. & Schneider, W. (1998). WLLP. Würzburger Leise Leseprobe. Göttingen: Hogrefe.

Kustov, A. A. & Robinson, D. L. (1996). Shared neural control of attentional shifts and eye movements. *Nature*, *384*, 74-77.

Lahat, E., Avital, E., Barr, J., Berkovitch, M., Arlazoroff, A. & Aladjem, M. (1995). BAEP studies in children with attention deficit disorder. *Developmental Medicine and Child Neurology*, *37*, 119-123.

Lee, J. S., Kim, B. N., Kang, E., Lee, D. S., Kim, Y. K, Chung, J. K., et al. (2005). Regional cerebral blood flow in children with attention deficit hyperactivity disorder: Comparison before and after methylphenidate treatment. *Human Brain Mapping*, *24*, 157-164.

Lehmkuhl, G., Döpfner, M., Plück, J., Berner, W., Fegert, J., Huss, M., et al. (1998). Häufigkeit psychischer Auffälligkeiten und somatischer Beschwerden bei vier- bis zehnjährigen Kindern in Deutschland im Urteil der Eltern – ein Vergleich normorientierter und kriterienorientierter Modelle. *Zeitschrift für Kinder- und Jugendpsychiatrie und Psychotherapie*, *26*, 83-96.

Leigh, J. R. & Kennard, C. (2004). Using saccades as a research tool in clinical neurosciences. *Brain*, *127*, 460-477.

Leigh, J. R. & Zee, D. S. (1999). *The Neurology of Eye Movements* (3rd ed.). Philadelphia: F. A. Davis Company.

Lloyd, G., Stead, J. & Cohen, D. (2006). *Critical New Perspectives on ADHD*. London: Routledge.

Lustig, C. & Meck, W. H. (2005). Chronic treatment with haloperidol induces deficits in working memory and feedback effects of interval timing. *Brain and Cognition*, *58*, 9-16.

Lou, H. C., Henriksen, L. & Bruhn, P. (1984). Focal cerebral hyperfusion in children with dysphasia and/or attention deficit disorder. *Archives of Neurology*, *41*, 825-829.

Lou, H. C., Henriksen, L. & Bruhn, P. (1989). Striatal dysfunction in attention deficit and hyperkinetic disorder. *Archives of Neurology*, *46*, 48-52.

Mason, D. J., Humphreys, G. W. & Kent, L. S. (2003). Exploring selective attention in ADHD: visual search through space and time. *Journal of Child Psychology and Psychiatry*, *44*, 1-20.

Matsuda, T., Matsuura, M., Ohkubo, T., Ohkubo, H., Matsushima, E., Inoue, K., Taira, M. & Kojima, T. (2004). Functional MRI mapping of brain activation during visually guided saccades and antisaccades: cortical and subcortical networks. *Psychiatry Research*, *131*, 147-155.

McInerney, R. & Kerns, K. (2003). Time reproduction in children with ADHD: motivation matters. *Child Neuropsychology*, *9*, 91-108.

Meaux, J. & Chelonis, J. (2003). Time perception differences in children with and without ADHD. *Journal of Pediatric Health Care*, *17*, 64-71.

Mostofsky, S. H., Lasker, A. G., Cutting, L. E., Denckia, M. D. & Zee, D. S. (2001). Oculomotor abnormalities in attention deficit hyperactivity disorder: a preliminary study. *Neurology*, *57*, 423-430.

Mullins, C., Bellgrove, M., Gill, M. & Robertson, I. (2005). Variability in time reproduction: differences in ADHD combined and inattentive subtypes. *Journal of the American Academy of Child and Adolescent Psychiatry*, *44*, 169-176.

Munoz, D. P., Armstrong, I. T., Hampton, K. A. & Moore, K. D. (2003). Altered control of visual fixation and saccadic eye movements in attention-deficit hyperactivity disorder. *Journal of Neurophysiology*, *90*, 503-514.

Munoz, D. P., Hampton, K. A., Moore, K. D. & Goldring, J. E. (1999). Control of purposive saccadic eye movements and visual fixation in children with attention deficit hyperactivity disorder. In W. Becker, & H. Deubel (Eds.), *Current oculomotor research. Physiological and psychological aspects*, (415–423). New York, NY: Plenum Press.

Nigg, J. T. (2001). Is ADHD a disinhibitory disorder? *Psychological Bulletin*, *127*, 571-598.

Olton, D. S., Wenk, G. L., Church, R. M. & Meck, W. H. (1988). Attention and the frontal cortex as examined by simultaneous temporal processing. *Neuropsychologia*, *26*, 307-318.

Paus, T. (1989). The development of sustained attention in children might be related to the maturation of frontal cortical functions. *Acta Neurobiologiae Experimentalis (Warsaw)*, *49*.

Paus, T., Babenko, V. & Radil, T. (1990). Development of an ability to maintain verbally instructed central gaze fixation studied in 8- to 10-year-old children. *International Journal of Psychophysiology*, *10*, 53-61.

Pearson, D. A., Lane, D. M. & Swanson, J. M. (1991). Auditory attention switching in hyperactive children. *Journal of Abnormal Child Psychology*, *19*, 479-492.

Pelham, W. E., Burrows-MacLean, L., Gnagy, E. M., Fabiano, G. A., Coles, E. K., Tresco, K. E., et al. (2005). Transdermal methylphenidate, behavioral, and combined treatment for children with ADHD. *Experimental and Clinical Psychopharmacology*, *13*, 111-126.

Pelham, W. E., Gnagy, E. M., Chronis, A. M., Burrows-MacLean, L., Fabiano, G. A., Onyango, A. N. et al. (1999). A comparison of morning-only and morning/late afternoon Adderall to morning-only, twice-daily, and three times-daily methylphenidate in children with attention-deficit/ hyperactivity disorder. *Pediatrics*, *104*, 1300-1311.

Pennington, B. F. & Ozonoff, S. (1996). Executive functions and developmental psychology. *Journal of Child Psychology and Psychiatry*, *37*, 51-87.

Petermann, F. & Petermann, U. (2008). *HAWIK-IV. Hamburg-Wechsel-Intelligenztest für Kinder – IV*. Bern: Verlag Hans Huber.

Petermann, F. & Toussaint, A. (2009). Neuropsychologische Diagnostik bei Kindern mit ADHS. *Kindheit und Entwicklung*, *18*, 83-94.

Polanczyk, G., de Lima, M., Horta, B., Biederman, J. & Rohde, L. (2007). The worldwide prevalence of ADHD: a systematic review and metaregression analysis. *American Journal of Psychiatry*, *164*, 942-948.

Pierrot-Deseilligny, C., Milea, D. & Müri, R. M. (2004). Eye movement control by the cerebral cortex. *Current Opinion in Neurology*, *17*, 17-25.

Pierrot-Deseilligny, C., Rivaud, S., Gaymard, B. & Agid, Y. (1994). Cortical control of reflexive visually-guided saccades. *Brain*, *114*, 1473-1485.

Pliszka, S. R. (2005). The neuropsychopharmacology of attention-deficit/ hyperactivity disorder. *Biological Psychiatry*, *57*, 1385-1390.

Polanczyk, G., de Lima, M., Horta, B., Biederman, J. & Rohde, L. (2007). The worldwide prevalence of ADHD: A systematic review and metaregression analysis. *American Journal of Psychiatry*, *164*, 942-948.

Radonovich, K. J. & Mostofsky, S. H. (2004). Duration judgments in children with ADHD suggest deficient utilization of temporal information rather than general impairment in timing. *Child Neuropsychology*, *10*, 162-172.

Rakitin, B. C., Gibbon, J., Penney, T. B., Malapani, C., Hinton, S. C. & Meck, W. H. (1998). Scalar expectancy theory and peak-interval timing in humans. *Journal of Experimental Psychology: Animal Behavior Processes*, *24*, 15-33.

Ramus, E. (2003). Developmental dyslexia: specific phonological deficit or general sensorimotor dysfunction? *Current Opinion in Neurobiology*, *13*, 212-218.

Rapport, M. D. & Denney, C. (1997). Titrating methylphenidate in children with attention deficit/hyperactivity disorder: Is body mass predictive of clinical response. *Journal of Attention Disorders*, *36*, 523-530.

Roberts, S. (1981). Isolation of an internal clock. *Journal of Experimental Psychology: Animal Behavior Processes*, *7*, 242-268.

Roberts, W. A., Cheng, K. & Cohen, J. S. (1989). Timing light and tone signals in pigeons. *Journal of Experimental Psychology: Animal Behavior Processes*, *15*, 23-35.

Roick, T., Gölitz, D. & Hasselhorn, M. (2004). *DEMAT 3+. Deutscher Mathematiktest für dritte Klassen*. Göttingen: Beltz.

Rosenberg, D. R., Dick, E. L., O'Hearn, K. M. & Sweeney, J. A. (1997). Response-inhibition deficits in obsessive-compulsive disorder: an indicator of dysfunction in frontostriatal circuits. *Journal of Psychiatry and Neuroscience*, *22*, 29-38.

Ross, S. M. & Ross, L. E. (1983). The effects of onset and offset warning and post-target stimuli on the saccade latency of children and adults. *Journal of Experimental Child Psychology*, *36*, 340-355.

Ross, R. G., Harris, J. G., Olincy, A. & Radant, A. (2000). Eye movement task measures inhibition and spatial working memory in adults with schizophrenia, ADHD, and a normal comparison group. *Psychiatry Research*, *95*, 35-42.

Ross, R. G., Young, D. A., Hommer, D. W. & Radant, A. (1994). Saccadic eye movements in normal children from 8 to 15 years of age: a developmental study of visuospatial attention. *Journal of Autism and Developmental Disorders*, *24*, 413-431.

Rubia, K., Norloos, J., Smith, A., Gunning, B. & Sergeant, J. (2003). Motor timing deficits in community and clinical boys with hyperactive behavior: the effect of methylphenidate on motor timing. *Journal of Abnormal Child Psychology*, *31*, 301-313.

Rubia, K., Overmeyer, S., Taylor, E., Brammar, M., Williams, S. C. R., Simmons, A. et al. (1999). Hypofrontality in attention deficit hyperactivity disorder during high-order motion control: a study with functional MRI. *American Journal of Psychiatry*, *156*, 891-896.

Schiller, P. H., True, S. D. & Conway, J. L. (1980). Deficits in eye movements following frontal eye-field and superior colliculus ablations. *Journal of Neurophysiology*, *44*, 1175-1189.

Schmidt, D., Abel, L. A., Dell'Osso, F. & Aroff, R. B. (1979). Saccadic velocity characteristics: intrinsic variability and fatigue. *Aviation, Space, and Environmental Medicine*, *50*, 393-395.

Smith, A., Taylor, E., Warner, R. J., Newman, S. & Rubia, K. (2002). Evidence for a pure time perception deficit in children with ADHD. *Journal of Child Psychology and Psychiatry*, *43*, 529-542.

Sohmer, H. & Student, M. (1978). Auditory nerve and brainstem evoked responses in normal, autistic, minimal brain dysfunction and psychomotor retarded children. *Electroencephalography and Clinical Neurophysiology*, *44*, 380-388.

Sonuga-Barke, E. J. S., Saxton, T. & Hall, M. (1998). The role of interval underestimation in hyperactive children's failure to suppress responses over time. *Behavioral Brain Research*, *94*, 45-50.

Sparks, D. L. (2002). The brainstem control of saccadic eye movements. *Nature Reviews Neuroscience*, *3*, 952-964.

Sparks, D. L., Barton, E. J., Gandhi, N. J. & Nelson, J. (2002). Studies of the role of the paramedian pontine reticular formation (PPRF) in the control of head-restrained and head-unrestrained gaze shifts. *Annual New York Academic Science*, *956*, 85-98.

Strassman, A., Highstein, S. M. & McCrea, R. A. (1986). Anatomy and physiology of saccadic burst neurons in the alert squirrel monkey. I. Excitatory burst neurons. *Journal of Comparative Neurology*, *249*, 337-357.

Sweeney, J. A., Takarae, Y., Macmillan, C., Luna, B. & Minshew, N. J. (2004). Eye movements in neurodevelopmental disorders. *Current Opinion in Neurology*, *17*, 37-42.

Tannock, R. (1998). Attention deficit hyperactivity disorder: advancers in cognitive, neurobiological, and genetic research. *Journal of Child Psychology and Psychiatry*, *39*, 65-69.

Takarae, Y., Minshew, N. J., Luna, B., Krisky, C. M. & Sweeney, J. A. (2004a). Pursuit eye movement deficits in autism. *Brain*, *127*, 2584-2594.

Takarae, Y., Minshew, N. J., Luna, B. & Sweeney, J. A. (2004b). Oculomotor abnormalities parallel cerebellar histopathology in autism. *Journal of Neurology, Neurosurgery and Psychiatry*, *75*, 1359-1361.

Thier, P. (2006). Die funktionelle Architektur des präfrontalen Kortex. In H. -O. Karnath, & P. Thier (Eds.), *Neuropsychologie* (2nd ed., 471-478). Heidelberg: Springer Medizin Verlag.

Tiffin-Richards, M. C., Hasselhorn, M., Richards, M. L., Banaschewski, T. & Rothenberger, A. (2004). Time reproduction in finger tapping tasks by children with attention-deficit hyperactivity disorder and/or dyslexia. *Dyslexia*, *10*, 299-315.

Toplak, M. E., Dockstader, C. & Tannock, R. (2006). Temporal information processing in ADHD: Findings to date and new methods. *Journal of Neuroscience Methods*, *151*, 15-29.

Toplak, M. E., Rucklidge, J. J., Hetherington, R., John, S. C. F. & Tannock, R. (2003). Time perception deficits in attention-deficit/hyperactivity disorder and comorbid reading difficulties in child and adolescent samples. *Journal of Child Psychology and Psychiatry*, *44*, 1-16.

Tremblay, S. & Fortin, C. (2003). Break expectancy in duration discrimination. *Journal of Experimental Psychology: Human Perception and Performance*, *29*, 823-831.

Trillenberg, P., Lencer, R. & Heide, W. (2004). Eye movements and psychiatric disease. *Current Opinion in Neurology*, *17*, 43-47.

Ullsperger, M. & von Cramon, D. Y. (2006). Funktionen frontaler Strukturen. In H. -O. Karnath, & P. Thier (Eds.), *Neuropsychologie* (2nd ed., 479-488). Heidelberg: Springer Medizin Verlag.

Van der Meere, J. & Sergeant, J. A. (1988). Focused attention in pervasively hyperactive children. *Journal of Abnormal Child Psychology*, *16*, 627-639.

Van Meel, C. S., Oosterlaan, J., Heslenfeld, D. J. & Sergeant, J. A. (2005). Motivational effects on motor timing in attention-deficit/hyperactivity disorder. *Journal of the American Academy of Child and Adolescent Psychiatry*, *44*, 451-460.

Van Mourik, R., Osterlaan, J. & Sergeant, J. A. (2005). The stroop revisited: a meta-analysis of interference control in AD/HD. *Journal of Child Psychology and Psychiatry*, *46*, 150-165.

Van Mourik, R., Osterlaan, J., Heslenfeld, D. J., Konig, C. E. & Sergeant, J. A. (2007). When distraction is not distracting: A behavioral and ERP study on distraction in ADHD. *Clinical Neurophysiology*, *118*, 1855-1865.

Van Wassenhove, V., Buonomano, D. V., Shimojo, S. & Shams, L. (2008). Distortions of subjective time perception within and across senses. *PLoSONE*, *1*, e1437, 1-13.

West, J., Douglas, G, Houghton, S., Lawrence, V., Whiting, K. & Glasgow, K. (2000). Time perception in boys with attention-deficit/hyperactivity disorder according to time duration, distraction, and mode of presentation. *Child Neuropsychology*, *6*, 241-250.

Wearden, J. H. & McShane, B. (1988). Interval production as an analogue of the peak procedure: Evidence for similarity of human and animal timing processes. *Quarterly Journal of Experimental Psychology*, *40*, 363-375.

Wittmann, M., van Wassenhove, V., Craig, A. D. & Paulus, M. P. (2010). The neural substrates of subjective time dilation. *Frontiers in Human Neuroscience*, *4*, 1-9.

Wood, C. Maruff, P., Levy, F., Farrow, M. & Hay, D. (1999). Covert orienting of visual spatial attention in attention deficit hyperactivity disorder: does comorbidity make a difference? *Arch. Clinical Neuropsych.*, *14*, 179-189.

World Health Organization. (1992). *International classification of diseases* (10th ed.). Geneva, Switzerland: Author.

Zametkin, A. J., Nordahl, T. E., Gross, M., King, C., Semple, W. E., Rumset, J., Hamburger, S. & Cohen, R. M. (1990). Cerebral glucose metabolism in adults with hyperactivity of childhood onset. *New England Journal of Medicine*, *323*, 1361-1366.

Zee, D. S., Optican, L. M., Cook, J. D., Robinson, D. A. & Engel, W. K. (1976). Slow saccades in spinocerebellar degeneration. *Archives of Neurology*, *33*, 243-251.

Zimmermann, P. & Fimm, B. (2002). A test battery of attentional performance. In M. Leclercq, & P. Zimmermann (Eds.), *Applied Neuropsychology of Attention: Theory, Diagnosis and Rehabilitation* (110-151). Psychology Press.

In: Advances in Visual Perception Research
Editor: Thomas Heinen
ISBN: 978-1-63482-455-2
© 2015 Nova Science Publishers, Inc.

Chapter 7

Why What Comes Down Must First Look Like It's Going up: A Perceptual-Cognitive Regularity Dominates Online Perception

Dennis M. Shaffer*, Andrew B. Maynor, Benjamin K. Madden, April L. Utt and Ciara N. Adamrovich
The Ohio State University, Mansfield, OH, US

Abstract

Here we document a new perceptual-cognitive regularity -that people mentally represent thrown or launched objects to rise and fall in a parabolic motion irrespective of where the observer is relative to the trajectory. We then show that this representation persists in spite of obvious contradictory information presented to observers. Finally, we demonstrate that simply referring to a dot moving downward as that of a football causes observers to represent what they saw as the entire up-down parabolic motion a thrown football physically makes. This extends previous reports by showing the extent to which dynamical perceptual representations may dominate online perception of the motion of objects.

Keywords: Vision, motion perception, American football

Introduction

The perceptual system is attuned to invariant properties in the ambient array of light, which provides information about the layout of the surfaces in the environment (Gibson,

* The Ohio State University-Mansfield, 1760 University Drive, Mansfield, OH 44906. Email: shaffer.247@osu.edu

1979). These invariant properties are those in the environment that remain constant irrespective of our movement through it. These invariants include but are not limited to strategies that geometrically guarantee collision with airborne (Chapman, 1968; McBeath, Shaffer, & Kaiser, 1995) and ground-based targets (Fajen & Warren, 2007). Consistent with this, there have been many closely related perceptual-cognitive mechanisms documented, which Dolgov, McBeath, and Sugar (2009) term "perceptual regularities, or mental attunements to natural or physical regularities" (p. 399). These include the internalization of a spatially three-dimensional world (Shepard, 2001), embodied cognition -particularly that words may invoke dynamic perceptual representations (Zwaan, Madden, Yaxley, & Aveyard, 2004), and the axis-aligned motion bias -the tendency of an observer to perceive alignment between an object's motion direction and axial orientation (Dolgov et al., 2009). The first goal of the present work is to document a new perceptual-cognitive regularity -that people mentally represent thrown or launched objects to rise and fall in a parabolic motion irrespective of where the observer is relative to the trajectory or how much of the trajectory is visible to the thrower. This work then investigates the causes of people's unwavering reliance on their mental representation of the ball's physical up-down motion.

We first determined what exactly the optical flight path of a football looks like from the perspective of someone throwing it (i.e., the path of the ball relative to where the thrower is looking at each point in time). When approaching an airborne target, observers maintain their gaze in a monotonically increasing straight line (e.g., McBeath et al., 1995). For a receding airborne target like a thrown football, we expected that the flight path from the thrower's perspective would reveal a downward straight line relative to the background scenery, or opposite to the optical trajectory that occurs when intercepting an approaching airborne target.

Pilot Study for Assessing What the Flight Path of a Football Looks Like from the Perspective of the Person Throwing It

Participants

Four males ranging in age from 20-37 threw and caught Nike® college footballs. All participants had played football recreationally as quarterbacks, and one had also played starting quarterback at a high school varsity level.

Materials and Procedure

We mounted a Supercircuits® inline weather-resistant micro video camera (model no. PC75WR) on a bicycle helmet worn by the thrower that sent a signal to a Canon® GL1 camcorder, which recorded the flight of the football from the quarterback's perspective. The camera provided 380 lines of resolution with a field of view of 80°. A receiver who started 15 meters (m) to the side of the thrower ran in a straight line away from the thrower until catching the ball 25m away from their initial position. Fifteen trials in which the receiver caught the ball were analyzed for each thrower. The optical trajectory was measured by recording the ball position for each video frame onto a transparency taped to the video monitor. The transparency was moved frame-by-frame on a video monitor to keep thebackground aligned. Visual angle was calibrated by converting the pixel height of the thrower on the video image to the actual visual angle of the thrower that was observed at the time of recording. The initial location of the ball out of the thrower's hand was marked as the starting point, or (0,0) coordinate. The data were coded as pixel movement and then converted to degrees visual angle. This conversion produces very precise visual angles provided the ball is compared with background scenery that is distant and remains within a small visual angle of it. In this work, the comparison background scenery was always within 1° visual angle of the ball, well within the region of the law of small angles. We also had static test trials in which we varied the angle of the camera and verified that any errors in the optical angle were insignificant.

Results

Figure 1 shows four plots from each participant. There were about 10-20 frames where the ball had already been thrown, but did not yet come into the field of view of the camera.

That is, the ball is not even visible to the thrower for the first portion of the trajectory because of where the ball is displaced from the head when it is released, which is different for each thrower, and because throwers did not look at the football as it left their hand, but looked to where the ball was headed.

By the time the flight of the ball came into view, the ball was already at its highest point relative to where the thrower was looking. Cameras with wider fields of view might have shown more of the beginning of the flight of the ball, but we doubt this would accurately indicate the gaze direction of throwers.

The trajectories, like those shown in Figure 1, when analyzed as optical coordinates in the horizontal and vertical directions for all 60 trials were subjected to a principal components analysis. A descending straight line (the best fitting component) accounted for 95.85% of the total variance for all throwers across all trials.

In order to evaluate how many of the optical trajectories remained in downward straight lines as predicted, we counted how many had variance accounted for (or R^2) values = .90 or greater (this is equivalent to $r = .95$ or greater). A chi-square analysis confirmed that the large majority of optical trajectories remained in downward straight lines (trajectories with $R^2 = .90$ or greater = 48/60), $\chi^2(1) = 21.6$, $p < .001$.

Average variance accounted for by the best fitting component for each participant are listed in Figure 1 and were 91.36% (J.A.), 98.48% (D.S.), 96.76% (T.H.), and 95.47% (V.F.). work confirms that the football moves in a descending straight line relative to where throwers are looking.

The first 1/3-1/2s of the flight is not even seen by the thrower due to the aforementioned reasons resulting in a full three-dimensional experience in which the viewer only sees ½-2/3 of the entire flight path of the ball.

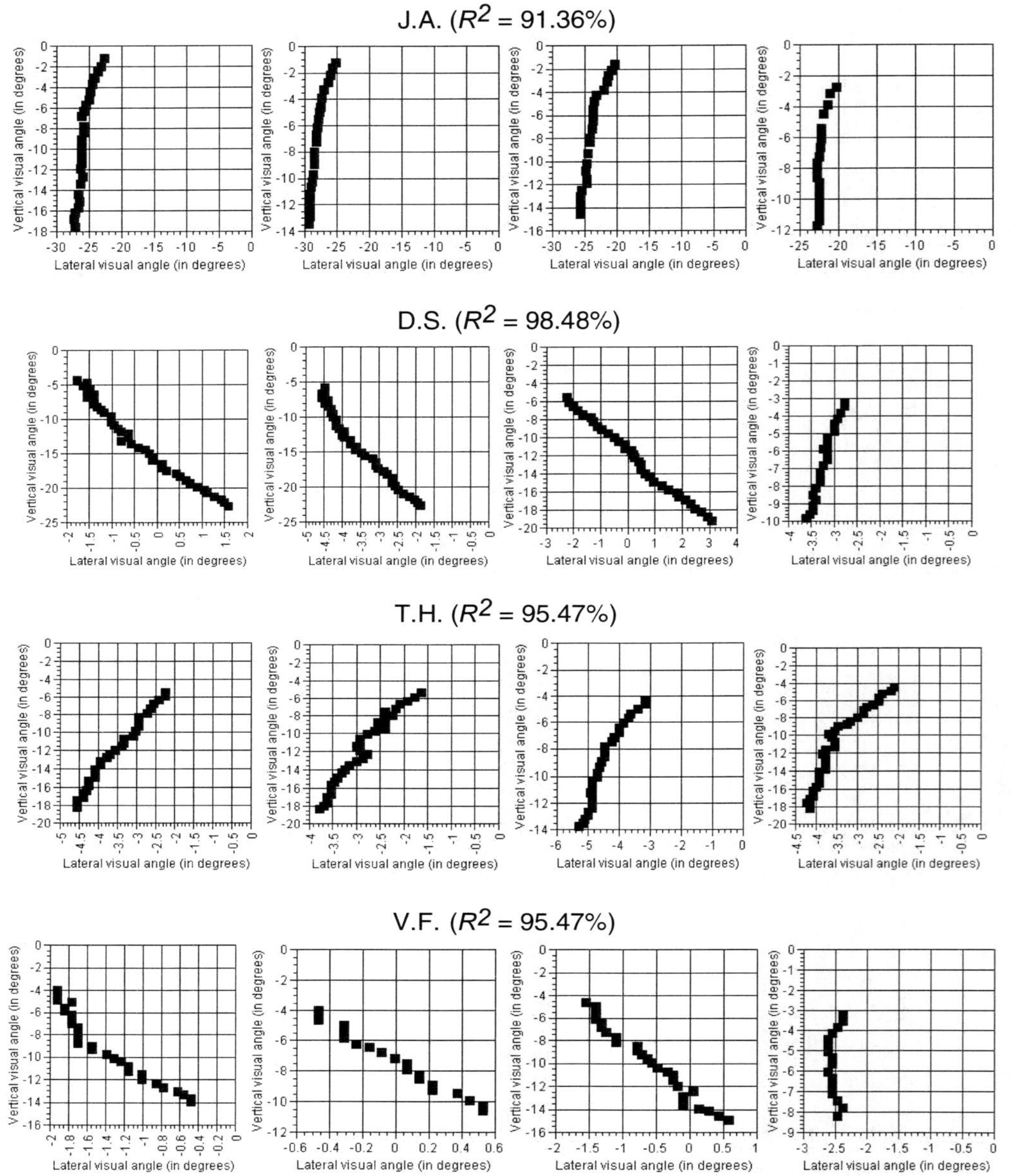

Figure 1. Shown are four representative optical trajectories from the perspective of each of the participants. The scales for individual trials and participants are different depending on where exactly each fielder was looking and how the ball was thrown.

Experiment 1

Our initial work confirms the counterintuitive finding that the optical trajectory of a football relative to the thrower is a descending straight line. In Experiment 1 we investigated whether people realize that the perspective of someone throwing a football is dramatically different from the up-down path the ball physically makes. While the downward optical straight line is what appears when video coding where the flight of the ball travels against the background scenery, the ball was thrown within parameters that allow optical depth cues to indicate that the ball is moving away from the observer. This might give rise to a conscious impression that does not exactly match a downward optical straight line.

So we first expect that observers will not indicate that the ball travels in a downward straight line. However, given the aforementioned slight mismatch between their gaze direction and conscious impression of the flight of the ball, this should not be surprising. We also hypothesize that observers do not take perspective into account, and so participants will indicate that the optical trajectory of the football for a thrower looks like the up-down flight path of the football one would see from the side orthogonal to the flight path of the ball if they stood far enough away.

This cannot be accounted for by the difference between a 2-D optical image versus a 3-D conscious impression of the flight of the ball. This would also suggest that observers believe that the perceived flight of the ball for someone away from whom the ball is traveling should appear similar to a side view of the physical flight of the ball. This interpretation is incorrect because the curvature in the physical ball flight does not occur perceptually from the throwers' perspective.

In order to elucidate how different the flight paths look for someone who throws the ball compared to someone who views it from the side, author (D.S.) threw a football either between 8-10m or ~26-38m. Figure 2 shows side-views of footballs thrown from the aforementioned distances (top to bottom panels, respectively).

The football moved in a relatively parabolic motion that peaks at a different height depending on the throw.

The perspective flight paths are dramatically different from those in Figure 1 due to the position one takes relative to the flight of the ball. Experiment 1 was next designed to investigate observer's mental representations concerning the flight path of a football from the perspective of someone throwing the ball. That is, we investigated whether observers understand how disparate the perspective is for someone who throws the football compared to someone who is standing far off to the side looking at the flight of the ball. We also investigated whether participants with more sophistication in physics or football throwing are any better at indicating what the flight path of the ball from the perspective of a thrower should look like.

Those with more experience with football throwing have more opportunities to see the flight of the ball from the perspective of a thrower. This might give them a distinct advantage over those with lesser experience. However, previous work has shown that more sophistication in areas like baseball playing and formal physics instruction leads to no difference in observers' conceptions concerning the flight paths of baseballs and a detrimental effect on people's conceptual beliefs concerning the effect of gravity on falling objects, respectively (Oberle, McBeath, Madigan, & Sugar, 2005; Shaffer & McBeath, 2005).

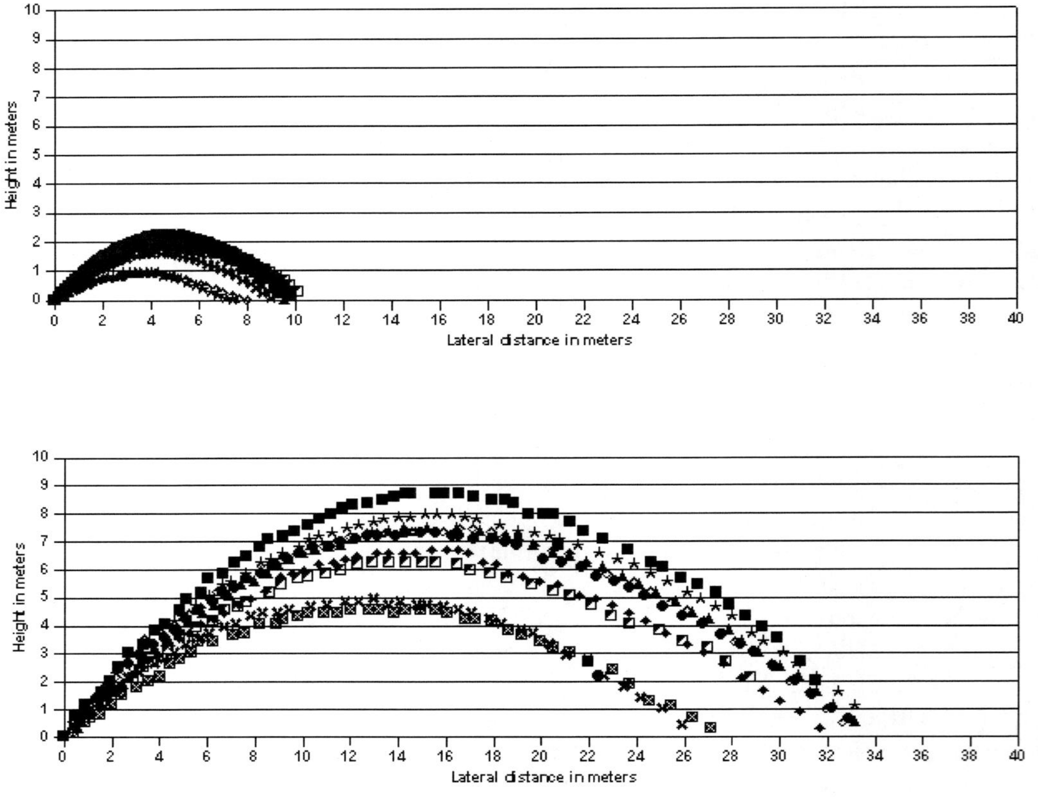

Figure 2. *(top panel)* Shown are eight physical trajectories of a football thrown between 8-10m and recorded from 35m away; *(bottom panel)* Shown are ten trajectories of a football thrown between 26-34m and recorded from 35m away.

Methodical Approach

Participants

One hundred twenty Ohio State University students (52 male, 68 female, average age = 21.47 years, *SD* = 6.32) participated in Experiment 1. All participants received credit toward an introductory psychology course for their participation.

Procedure

Participants were given a survey to fill out that asked them questions concerning how much experience they had with physics and football throwing. A 4-point Likert-type scale assessed participants' physics experience: None, one high school class, one college class, more than one college class. Another 4-point Likert-type scale was used to assess participants' football throwing experience: None, I have thrown a football, but rarely, I have thrown a football or played quarterback recreationally, and I have thrown a football or played quarterback competitively (i.e. played on a high school or college varsity or club team).

The corresponding figure participants used to answer the critical questions concerning the optical flight path of the ball is shown in Figure 3. All participants were reminded that the distance between the thrower and receiver was 50 yards (~46m). This was done because the figure does not quite capture this distance, and also at closer distances there is (on average) less curvature of the physical motion of the ball.

Participants completed the questionnaire one at a time. An individual was assigned to each participant to emphasize that we were interested in what they thought the flight of the ball looked like from the perspective of the person throwing the ball. This was done to make sure participants wouldn't simply revert to indicating the flight path the ball physically makes.

Results

Option (a), as determined by our analysis of thrown trajectories, is the correct flight path as viewed by the quarterback on Figure 3a, a downward straight line. Only 2.5%, or 3 participants out of 120 chose this answer. Almost 66% of participants chose one of two possible physical side-view trajectories for the ball (either option b -the high-arching trajectory- 10%) or option d -the flattened parabola- 55.83%). Most participants mistook what the flight path looks like from the perspective of the quarterback (i.e., option a) to be the physical up-down motion of the ball, or the flight of the ball as viewed from the side, $\chi^2(2, N = 120) = 32.45, p < .001$.

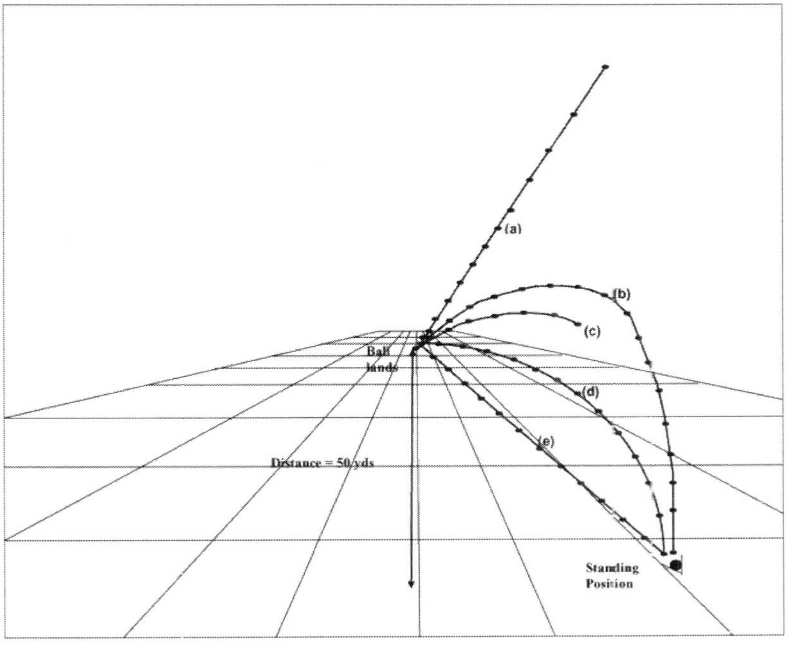

Figure 3. Questionnaire given to participants concerning what the flight path of a football looks like from the thrower's perspective. Participants were asked to indicate what the trajectory looks like from the perspective of the thrower throwing the football. Option (a) is the veridical optical trajectory and correct answer, while options (b) and (d) are what the flight path could look like from the perspective of someone standing off to the side, depending on the type of throw (and also represent the physical up-down motion of the ball). Option (c) is an optical compromise and option (e) is a straight line path from the thrower's hand to the receivers', which is an impossible flight path at that distance.

We also analyzed differences in flight path answers for the effects of sex, physics, and football throwing experience. We divided physics experience into expert-novice groups. Experts were those who had taken at least one course in physics (57%), while novices had no formal instruction in physics. We also divided football-throwing experience into novice-expert groups. Experts were those who had thrown a football recreationally or competitively on a high school/college team (31%), while novices were those who had rarely or never thrown a football. Option (a) was eliminated from the analysis, since only 3 participants chose that answer. We also collapsed options (b) and (d) as both represent what may be seen from a side-view. A multinomial logistic regression analysis revealed no significant differences among flight path answers for the factors of sex ($\chi^2(1, N = 120) = 1.79$, $p > .1$), physics expertise ($\chi^2(1, N = 120) = 0.12$, $p > .1$), or football throwing expertise ($\chi^2(1, N = 120) = 0.39$, $p > .1$). Option (a) was eliminated from the analysis, since only 3 participants chose that answer. We also collapsed options (b) and (c) as both represent side view perspectives. Multinomial logistic analyses revealed no differences for sex, $\chi^2(1, N = 120) = 1.79$, $p > .1$ or football throwing expertise, $\chi^2(1, N = 120) = 0.39$, $p > .1$.

Discussion

Experiment 1 documents a new perceptual-cognitive regularity -people mentally represent thrown footballs to rise and fall in a parabolic motion irrespective of where the observer is relative to the flight path of the ball. That only 3 participants out of 120 chose this answer is not surprising given that the correct answer is counterintuitive. However, what is surprising is that two-thirds of participants indicate that the flight path a thrower sees while throwing the football looks exactly like the physical trajectory a football makes, or what the flight path of the football would look like to someone standing off to the side of it. Participants do not acknowledge that their perspective relative to the football may influence what the flight of the ball looks like to them. Participants seem to mistake their reasonable understanding of what the ball physically does or what the flight path looks like from the side (similar to those shown in Figure 2) for the optical flight of the ball, or what the flight of the ball looks like from the thrower's perspective (similar to those shown in Figure 1). Sex and greater exposure to physics and football throwing do not lead to better (or different) understanding of how constrained the view of the flight path is to a thrower. One other interesting finding from this experiment is how many participants (almost 32%) chose the impossible trajectory (option e). In the top panel of figure 2 where footballs are thrown from only 10m away, the thrower on some throws purposely attempted to throw the football in a straight line with no arc. However, as can be seen from the figure, even at this short distance, there is always some curvature to the throw, although not as much as when the distance increases (e.g., middle and bottom panels). It is difficult to interpret why they might choose this answer. One possibility is that for people who have little or no experience with throwing a football they might either see it that way for very short throws and/or conceive that it could happen by virtue of where (what vertical height) it leaves the hand of the thrower and where it is caught by the receiver, irrespective of what is does in-between. Work on the "straight down belief" in intuitive physics—the perception that objects carried by a person, conveyor, or airplane are perceived to fall straight down by between ~one-third to one-half of participants—has shown that this (mis)belief is strengthened by everyday experience McCloskey, Washburn & Felch, 1983). Perhaps the same is true for participants choosing the "straight-ahead" trajectory in this work. In addition, typically more "physics-untrained" than "physics-trained" (at least one high school or college physics course) subjects than experts choose the "straight-down" option. To evaluate this, we looked at how many people chose option (e) (38 out of 120) and looked at how many of these participants fell in the novice category for throwing a football. Thirty-two out of thirty-eight, or 84% of participants who chose option (e) fell into the novice category. Another explanation for why so many people chose option (e) is that when throws are seen on television during football games, one seldom gets a view from the side or from the thrower's perspective. The view is usually from above, or from a position where the path looks flattened (perhaps to the extent of a straight line). Many times passes that are thrown very hard are even referred to by experts (players and coaches), fans, and announcers as "frozen ropes" because they appear to have traveled in a straight line. This may also influence how people think of football throws.

Experiment 2

Experiment 1 showed that people mentally represent thrown footballs to rise and fall in a parabolic motion irrespective of where the observer is relative to the flight path of the ball. This showed that when people rely on their memory or mental representation of the flight path of a football they do not seem to take perspective into account. Experiment 2 was designed to first assess how observers would respond when actually viewing a football throw and second whether making the downward motion of the ball more obvious to participants would cause participants to more frequently choose option (a), the correct answer on the questionnaire. Participants either saw a real time video of a throw or saw a real time video of a throw followed by viewing the same throw in slow motion. Using the video also made it more obvious as many of the depth cues that may give participants a conscious impression that is different from the downward optical straight line are absent or diminished by using a 2-D video.

In an indoor setting, like in a gymnasium, a video of a football throw would be perceived against the ceiling before being seen against a wall for the remainder of the throw, as was done initially in this paper creating the lines seen in Figure 1. Although the trajectories in the gymnasium still were inverted straight lines (even including the portion where the ceiling was the background) it might give the participants the false idea that there is a curve to the flight path toward the top. In order to make the downward motion more obvious to participants we recorded a person throwing the football outdoors, and against a tall building, so that throughout the trajectory the ball can be seen moving downward against the same uniform wall.

When coding the movement of the ball from when it is first seen on the video to when it is caught, it only moves downward similar to the straight lines shown in top panel of Figure 1. Thus, there is no ambiguity about the fact the ball is moving in a downward straight line the entire time the ball is in the field of view of the video camera.

Methodical Approach

Participants

Thirty-three Ohio State University students (22 female and 11 male, average age = 20.73 years, *SD* = 4.03) participated. All received credit towards an introductory psychology course for their participation.

Design and Procedure

We mounted a Supercircuits® inline weather-resistant micro video camera (model no. PC75WR) on a bicycle helmet worn by the thrower that sent a signal to a Canon® GL1 camcorder, which recorded the flight of the football from the quarterback's perspective. The camera provided 380 lines of resolution with a field of view of 80°. Author A.M. threw the ball to author D.S. who stood 25m away. D.S. stood stationary 25m away directly in front of the building against which the football could be seen from the moment it could be seen on the screen. The motion of the throw resembles one of the throws from J.A. (top panel) shown in Figure 1.

Participants viewed the real-motion video. Seventeen participants were allowed to slow down the video and replay the video as many times as they wanted. Sixteen saw the video in real time once and were allowed to see it again in real time if they so choose. Participants then completed the same questionnaire used in Experiment 1. We explicitly told participants to pick the flight path that best represented the motion of the ball they saw on the television screen. We did this because we wanted people to describe the flight path that they saw on the screen rather than to automatically revert to a memory or mental representation of the movement that they know a football makes. This also gave some indication to participants that what they were viewing might be different than what they were expecting.

Results

Only one participant chose option (a), the correct flight path answer. Most of the participants chose option (d) (the flattened parabola) (54.55%) or option (b) (the higher-arching path) (39.39%). Almost all (94%) of the participants chose one of two possible physical side-view trajectories for the ball (either option b or d). Most participants mistook the flight path seen by the quarterback (i.e., option a) to be the physical up-down motion of the ball one would see standing off to the side (i.e., either option b or d), $\chi^2(2, N = 33) = 25.48$, $p < .001$. A multinomial logistic regression analysis on flight path answers again revealed no differences for the factors of sex, physics or football throwing experience (all *p*'s > .1).

Discussion

Most participants again mistook the flight path seen by the quarterback to be the physical up-down motion of the ball one would see standing off to the side of the flight path, in spite of the fact that the only information they had available to them was that the ball was moving in a downward straight line relative to the building in the background. Watching the thrower throw the football in real time on video or in slow-motion made no difference in the distribution of flight paths participants chose, as only one participant chose the correct answer, and almost all participants chose one of the up-down physical motion alternatives.

What is amazing is that the majority of participants chose the flattened parabola option in spite of the fact that the ball appeared on the video screen virtually at the top of a 10-story high building. It seems as though the mental representation observers have of the up-down physical flight path of the football remains unchanged irrespective of constraining the perspective of the observer and making the downward motion more obvious to observers.

Experiment 3

In both previous experiments, participants were either asked about the flight of a football or could see that it was a football. Simply using the word football, though a seemingly subtle cue, may be enough to invoke a dynamic representation of a football physically moving up and down. This representation may overcome online perceptual characteristics of the flight of the ball observers are viewing. In order to test whether this judgment bias is due to top-down factors like the word "football" or the sight of a football invoking mental representations affecting or replacing online perception, we removed all domain-relevant context cues and systematically changed the way the motion was described in Experiment 3.

Methodical Approach

Participants

One hundred eighty-six Ohio State University students (103 female and 83 male, average age = 19.83 years, SD = 5.89) participated. All received credit towards an introductory psychology course for their participation.

Materials

A Vicon® eight-camera motion capture system with millimeter accuracy recorded a football throw of 20m to a receiver. We then used Vicon BodyBuilder™ software to remove the first 1/2s of the trajectory as well as all of the domain-relevant cues in the capture room, including the football, thrower, and receiver. The resulting trajectory is shown in Figure 4.

The Vicon BodyBuilder™ software also allows one to take the vantage point of virtually any position in the motion capture field. We used a view of the thrown ball that was directly in line with the thrower. The perspective participants saw was slightly more to the right (and in line with the thrower) than the one shown in the figure, where the slight curve seen toward the top was not visible to participants. In addition, in the real-time version the individual dots are seen as a continuous line for the duration of one second. The dots on the screen here simply reflect the path of the dot and do not represent dot positions at instantaneous time frames.

Trajectory Options

We bent 4 pipe cleaners that matched the color of the light blue colored dot on the screen in 4 different ways representing four possible trajectory options, including the straight downward line, the two up-down physical motion lines and the (relatively) straight outward line. The pipe cleaners were attached to a board representing the motion capture grid and are shown in Figure 5. We then took a picture of these against a black background to match what participants saw on the computer screen. The size of the picture exactly matched the size of the computer screen, and the distance the dot traveled along the computer screen was matched to the (perspective) length of the pipe cleaner.

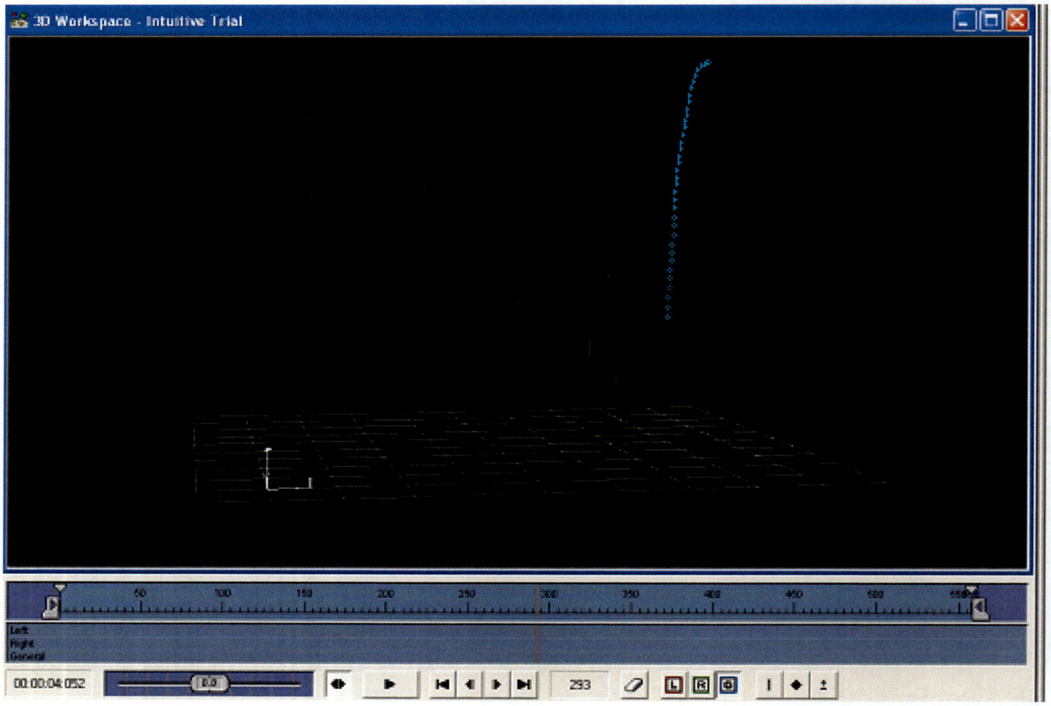

Figure 4. Shown is the trajectory that participants saw on the computer screen. This shows the path that the dot on the screen followed from the thrower's perspective (moving from the top down). The dots reflect the continuous path participants saw and do not represent dot positions at instantaneous time frames. The total time the trajectory was shown was for one full second.

Design and Procedure

Participants were randomly assigned to one of two conditions. In condition 1, participants were told that they would see a dot on a screen that was a reflective marker that was placed on a football that was thrown. We then told them that this software allows us to reveal the flight of the ball starting and ending at any two points in time, and the flight of the ball from any perspective within the screen. We then asked them to indicate the movement that the dot on the screen makes by choosing the option that best represents its movement. Participants were allowed to replay the trajectory. Ninety-six students participated in condition 1.

In condition 2, participants were simply told that they would see a dot move and to indicate the movement the dot on the screen makes by choosing the option that best represents its movement. The rest of the procedure was identical to that in condition 1. Ninety students participated in condition 2.

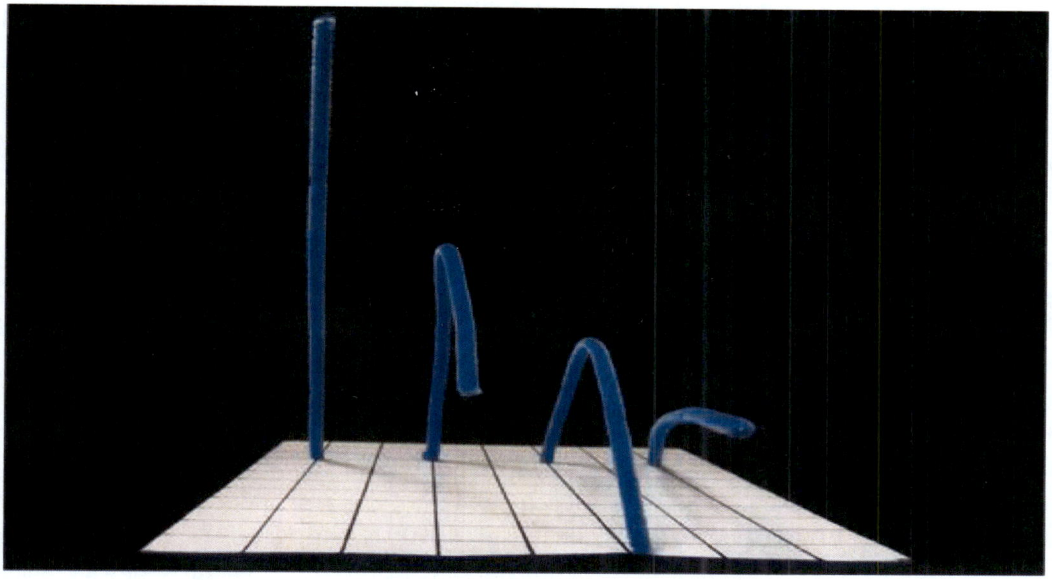

Figure 5. Shown are the four pipe cleaners that we bent to match four ways participants could report that the dot on the computer screen moved. Each is the same color of the light blue colored dot on the screen. The option furthest to the left is the downward straight line the football makes from the thrower's perspective. The middle two options represent the up-down motion the football physically makes, while the option furthest to the right is a straight line from the thrower to the receiver, which is an impossible flight path of the football from the thrower's perspective. The second option from the left and the option furthest to the right begin off the ground, and represent the approximate position the football would leave the hand of the thrower if the thrower were shown. The pipe cleaners were attached to a board representing the grid shown in Figure 4.

Results

Significantly more participants in the "football" condition chose one of the options indicating up-down movement than those in the "dot" condition, $\chi^2(1, N = 186) = 11.64$, $p < .001$. Sixty-nine percent of participants in the football condition chose one of the options representing the up-down movement versus forty-six percent in the dot condition, while fifty-three percent of participants in the dot condition chose the correct answer—the downward straight line--compared to only twenty-eight percent of the participants in the football condition. A multinomial logistic regression analysis on flight path answers again revealed no differences for the factors of sex or physics or football expertise (all p's > .1).

Discussion

Experiment 3 showed that the bias to mistake the flight path from the perspective of someone throwing the ball with the up-down motion the ball physically makes is largely due to the influence of top-down factors on online perception. Domain-relevant context cues that indicate a football is being thrown, even simply using the word "football" to describe a dot on the screen, overcame obvious perceptual information that showed the dot was only moving downward from a higher position on the screen. When we removed the domain-relevant cues, a majority of the "dot" condition (and almost twice as many as in the "football" condition) accurately indicated that the dot on the screen moved in a downward path only (i.e., this significantly reduced the judgment bias).

It is interesting that a substantial percentage of participants in the "dot" condition still chose one of the two up-down trajectory options (46%). As figure 4 shows, the portion of the trajectory shown to participants was when the ball was toward its physical apex and began to accelerate at a decelerating rate, or to slow down. This gives the impression that it is a portion of an entire trajectory that rises before it falls. Consistent with this, thirty-eight out of the forty-six percent of participants in the dot condition chose the second option in from the left in figure 5, which appears more like the dot is rising for a small portion of its flight before beginning its descent. In fact, the authors had a significant impression that it rose at least somewhat before descending. It took several trials before we could reliably discern that it was only falling. We feel that this might at least contribute to the large percentage of participants in the "dot" condition indicating that the dot appeared to rise somewhat before falling. Another explanation might be that the dot's slowing down implies gravitational and acceleration forces are acting on it. There are few objects in our environment that begin their descent from a higher position by slowing down before speeding up that do not first move in an upward direction. These factors have been shown to affect or induce apparent motion effects (Hubbard, 1997; Hubbard, 1995; Hubbard, 1990; Nagai, Kazai, & Yagi, 2002). It appears that the stimulus shown in Experiment 3 was powerful enough to induce such responses.

General Discussion and Conclusion

Observers overwhelmingly represent the flight path from the perspective of someone throwing the ball to be the physical up-down motion of the ball, or the flight path as seen from far off to the side. Observers' mental representations in Experiment 1 and the domain-relevant contextual cues that indicate up and down motion is to be expected in Experiments 2 and 3 overcame obvious perceptual information showing that a football (or dot on the screen) was only moving downward. In Experiment 3, simply using the word "football" caused almost 70% of participants to describe downward motion only of a reflective marker on the screen as a flight path that first ascended before descending. This perceptual-cognitive regularity is important for maintaining stability of our visual world, for while objects like footballs do not appear and disappear from existence, there are many situations in which objects remain physically present and traveling along a continuous path, but may only be intermittently visible. This is important to know where objects are going and where one should go relative to them to avoid or induce collisions with them, while the target may only be intermittently visible. So how else might not taking perspective into account affect interacting with objects in the 3-D world? This may also affect certainly expectations of and interactions with falling objects. Some of our work and others' work on dropping balls shows that people line up to intercept dropping objects from above as if they have more time to intercept them than actual (McBeath, Sugar, Morgan, Oberle, Mundhra, & Suluh, 2002). When asked to line up as far away as possible, while being close enough to catch a dropped ball comfortably, participants stand too far away to catch the ball. In fact, it is about the same distance away that would be correct to stand if the ball were to be first thrown upward from the ground, before falling from its initial dropping position. This has implications for people catching, or more importantly, avoiding falling objects.

Simply labeling the dot as a football may produce a dynamic perceptual representation of the physical motion of a football first moving upward before moving downward and may activate motion perception areas (e.g., MT) for upward movement. This may cause observers to perceive upward movement in the absence of any visual stimulus in the area in which upward movement is ostensibly perceived. For instance, work shows that using or changing the label of an object produces reported motion and systematic brain activation in motion perception areas for the induced motion label versus a label not inducing motion or inducing motion in a different direction or location (Fischer & Zwaan, 2008; Kaschak et al., 2005; Zwaan et al., 2004). This work serves as particularly compelling evidence that the conceptual knowledge of words is grounded in the perceptual system. For instance, the generation of action words has been found to activate a region in the middle temporal gyrus, just anterior to motion area MT/V5 (Martin, Haxby, Lalonde, Wiggs, & Ungerleider, 1995). This shows that object knowledge and identifying perceptual attributes and actions associated with them are stored close to the cortical regions that mediate perception of them. While we cannot be sure whether the verb "throw" or the noun "football" used in Experiment 3 might cause brain activation similar to that described earlier (as we used both), collectively it seems that this work could nicely explain the results of the football condition of Experiment 3.

One interesting direct test of this would be to use event-related fMRI to examine whether area MT is activated after hearing the word football, but before the trajectory is shown, and then to manipulate the difference in time from when the word football is heard to when observers see the movement for the first time.

In short, observers mentally represent balls thrown away from them to ascend and descend without awareness of how different their perspective view is from physical reality. Their mental representation of the physical up-down flight of the ball overcomes obvious perceptual information indicating the ball only moves downward from a higher position. Simply using the word football to describe the movement seems to invoke a dynamic perceptual representation of the physical up-down motion of its flight, which results in a phenomenon where observers believe that what goes down must first look like it's going up.

Acknowledgment

We would like to thank Laura McCartney, Bethany Briley, and Crystal England for their help in data collection.

References

Chapman, S. (1968). Catching a baseball. *American Journal of Physics, 36*, 868-870.

Dolgov, I., McBeath, M. K., & Sugar, T. (2009). Evidence for axis-aligned motion bias: Football axis-trajectory misalignment causes systematic error in projected final destinations of thrown American footballs. *Perception, 38*, 399-410.

Fajen, B. R., & Warren, W.H. (2007). Behavioral dynamics of intercepting a moving target. *Experimental Brain Research, 180*, 303-319.

Fischer, M.H., & Zwaan, R.A. (2008). The role of the motor system in language comprehension. *Quarterly Journal of Experimental Psychology, 61*, 825-850.

Gibson, J.J. (1979). *The Ecological Approach to Visual Perception*. Hillsdale, NJ: Lawrence Erlbaum Associates.

Hubbard, T.L. (1990). Cognitive representation of linear motion: Possible direction and gravity effects in judged displacement. *Memory & Cognition, 18*, 299-309.

Hubbard, T.L. (1995). Cognitive representation of motion: Evidence for friction and gravity analogues. *Journal of Experimental Psychology: Learning, Memory, and Cognition, 21*, 241-254.

Hubbard, T.L. (1997). Target size and displacement along the axis of implied gravitational attraction: Effects of implied weight and evidence of representational gravity. *Journal of Experimental Psychology: Learning, Memory, and Cognition, 23*, 1484-1493.

Kaschak, M.P., Madden, C.J., Therriault, D.J., Yaxley, R.H., Aveyard, M., Blanchard, A.A. et al (2005). Perception of motion affects language processing. *Cognition,* 94, B79-B89.

Martin, A., Haxby, J. V., Lalonde, F. M., Wiggs, C. L., Ungerleider, L. G, (1995, October 6). Discrete cortical regions associated with knowledge of color and knowledge of action. *Science*, 102-105.

McBeath, M.K., Shaffer, D.M., & Kaiser, M.K. (April 25, 1995). How baseball outfielders determine where to run to catch fly balls. *Science, 268*, 569-573.

McBeath, M.K., Sugar, T.G., Morgan, S. E., Oberle, C. D., Mundhra, K., & Suluh, A. (2002). Human and robotic catching of dropped balls and balloons: Fielders still try to make the image of the projection rise. [Abstract]. *Journal of Vision,* 2(7), 434a, http://journalofvision.org /2/7/434, doi: 10.1167/2.7.434.

McCloskey, M. Washburn, A., & Felch, L. (1983). Intuitive physics : The straight-down belief and its origin. Journal of Experimental Psychology : Learning, Memory & Cognition, 4, 636-649.

Nagai, M., Kazai, K., & Yagi, A. (2002). Larger forward memory displacement in the direction of gravity. *Visual Cognition, 9*, 28-40.

Oberle, C.D., McBeath, M.K., Madigan, S.C., & Sugar, T.G. (2005). The Galileo bias: A naïve conceptual belief that influences people's perceptions and performance in a ball-dropping task. *Journal of Experimental Psychology: Learning, Memory, and Cognition, 31*, 643-653.

Shaffer, D.M., & McBeath, M.K. (2005). Naïve beliefs in baseball: Systematic distortion in perceived time of apex for fly balls. *Journal of Experimental Psychology: Learning, Memory, and Cognition, 31*, 1492-1501.

Shepard, R. (2001). Perceptual-cognitive universals as reflections of the world. *Behavioral and Brain Sciences, 24*, 581-601.

Zwaan, R.A., Madden, C.J., Yaxley, R.H., & Aveyard, M.E. (2004). Moving words: Dynamic representations in language Comprehension. *Cognitive Science, 28*, 611-619.

In: Advances in Visual Perception Research
Editor: Thomas Heinen
ISBN: 978-1-63482-455-2
© 2015 Nova Science Publishers, Inc.

Chapter 8

Controlling Posture during Grasping with Different Optical Flow Conditions

***Sérgio Tosi Rodrigues*[1], *Gisele Cristina Bertoloni*[1], *Renato Moraes*[2], *Ana Maria Forti Barela*[3], *Geert Savelsbergh*[4] and *José Angelo Barela*[3,5,*]**

[1]State University of São Paulo, Bauru, SP, Brazil
[2]University of São Paulo, Ribeirão Preto, SP, Brazil
[3]Cruzeiro do Sul University, São Paulo, SP, Brazil
[4]Research Institute Move VU University, Amsterdam, The Netherlands
[5]State University of São Paulo, Rio Claro, SP, Brazil

Abstract

Many environmental aspects such as the optical flow and one's own movement can affect posture stabilization. However, little is known about how these two features can be combined as participants maintain upright stance during grasping actions. Therefore, the purpose of this study was to examine the effects of moving room discrete movements (approaching to or moving back from participants) combined with grasping an object on postural control stability. Twelve participants stood upright inside a moving room, moved discretely approaching or moving away from the participants, as they had to remain still or grasping a stationary or an approaching ball. Body displacement and correlation coefficient values were obtained during the movement of the moving room and mean sway amplitude were used to infer postural stability before and after room's movement. Results indicated that grasping and movement of the moving room disrupted and induced body sway, even after the grasping action, however in those conditions in which optical flow was created, due to the moving room and moving ball, postural sway was less pronounced. Based upon these results, we can suggest that in those conditions that structured optical flow is available, even when posture might be destabilized due to

[*] Corresponding author: Department of Physical Education, State University of São Paulo, Rio Claro, SP, Brazil. Email: jbarela@rc.unesp.br.

one's own movement, postural control takes advantage of the optical flow to maintain postural equilibrium.

Keywords: Posture, grasping, optical flow, moving room

Introduction

Reaching to grasp actions depend on whole-body postural stability (Voudouris, Radhakrishnan, Hatzitaki, & Brenner, 2013; Savelsbergh, Bennett, Angelakopolous, & Davids, 2005). Mechanical changes due to arm movements are anticipated by the postural system, affecting body segment dynamics and center of pressure displacement (Pozzo, Stapley, & Papaxanthis, 2002). However, the coordination process between postural and suprapostural tasks seems to involve mutual relationships among distinct body parts involved, favoring the environmental task goal (Stoffregen, Bardy, Bonnet, & Pagulayan, 2006). Although effects of arm movements on posture are well stablished (e.g., Patron, Stapley, & Pozzo, 2005), whole-body perturbations to grasping such as visual scene motion have been hardly explored.

Arm movements are known to affect balance in a variety of circumstances. Upper limb movements are classically considered as a disturbance to balance and the associated trunk displacements are compensated by an anticipatory or reactive strategy, suggesting that perturbations induced by arm motion are cancelled out in order to successfully reach the target, independently of balance constraints involved (Massion, 1992). It also could be that posture does not entirely compensate for the arm perturbation, but rather facilitates performance by adjusting the center of mass position within the area of support (Pozzo, Ouamer, & Gentil, 2001), accelerating towards the target (Pozzo et al., 2002).

Prior to contacting the goal object, manual prehension tasks are traditionally thought to consist of transport and grasp components. During the transport or reach component, the hand is moved toward the object; in the grasp component, the fingers and hand are prepared in anticipation of contact with the object (Jakobson & Goodale, 1991). The velocity of the wrist (transport component) shows a bell-shaped curve and its deceleration phase is assumed to represent the online use of sensory information to move the hand towards the object; the grip aperture between the index finger and thumb reaches its maximum approximately two-thirds of the reaching movement total duration and its value is proportional to object size (Jeannerod, 1984). These findings hold over different object sizes and distances, suggesting that wrist velocity and grip aperture are temporally coupled during hand movement towards the goal object (Hu, Osu, Okada, Goodale, & Kawato, 2005).

Constraints on postural stability while standing on foam have minimally affected a simultaneously executed arm movement during a reaching-to-grasp action, in particular, variables related to movements of the wrist but not of the fingertips (Voudouris, Brenner, Schot, & Smeets, 2010; Voudouris et al., 2013). How the digits move to suitable positions does not change when the whole-body posture was adjusted to cope with the surface stability. In this case, posture is modulated according to the type of surface without affecting the movement of the digits, which was interpreted as a consequence of the redundancy in the way movements can be performed, allowing participants to choose the most suitable changes in joint angles to achieve the desired movements of the digits under the prevailing conditions (Voudouris et al., 2013). Postural control of gait is also affected by the superposition of reach and grasp when both tasks are performed simultaneously (Rinaldi & Moraes, 2015).

Manipulations of visual information obtained through controlled continuous movement of a moving room create sensorial conflict and have strong effects on postural stability. Based on this clever experimental procedure, perception-action coupling between visual information and postural control has been extensively demonstrated in the literature (e.g., Barela, Godoi, Freitas Junior, & Polastri, 2000; Barela, Jeka, & Clark, 2003).

Particularly, the discrete movement of the moving room has been used to investigate the effects of more abrupt changes of visual scene on the posture of children and young adults. Eight year-old group showed greater body displacement than the other age groups when the room moved back from (but not when it approached) participants, suggesting a relationship between direction of the moving room movement and vision-posture coupling (Toledo, Rinaldi, & Barela, 2006).

In short, although the linkage between posture and arm movements has been vastly studied, the mutual effects between the reach to grasp action and body sway induced by discrete movements of a moving room are still open to debate. Therefore, the purpose of the present study was to examine the effects of moving room discrete movements (approaching to or moving back from participants) combined with grasping an object on postural control stability.

Methods

Participants

Twelve (six male and six female) young adults, mean age of 22.3 (SD = 2.3) years and mean height of 169.8 (SD = 7.1) cm, with normal or corrected to normal visual acuity, volunteered in the present study. All participants were asked about their manual preference for writing, following Corey et al. (2001) suggestion that this procedure is ideal for classifying hand dominance in 93% of the cases. Inclusion criteria were: right hand preference for writing and height in the range of 160-180cm due to size and position of equipment. All participants provided written consent prior to participation. The study was approved by the local institutional ethics committee.

Apparatus

The experiment was conducted inside of a moving room, consisted of three walls and a roof mounted on four wheels that slide on rails, allowing its back and forward movement, independently of the floor. The dimensions of the room were 2.1 x 2.1 x 2.1 meters (height, width, and length). The movement was produced by a servo-mechanism system consisting of a controller (Compumotor – Mod. APEX 6151), a controlled stepper motor (Compumotor – Mod. N0992GR0NMSN), and an electrical cylinder (Compumotor – Mod. EC3-X3xxn-10004A-MS1-MT1M). Movement was initiated by means of custom software (Compumotor

– Motion Architect for Windows). A pulley system (Figure 1A) was connected to the servo-mechanism in order to move simultaneously the room and a shaft (Figure 1B), which had a ball (6 cm of diameter) fixed in its end. Forward and backward movements of the room were associated with clockwise and anti-clockwise rotations of the pulley system, moving the shaft in speed and amplitude proportional to the movement of the room in the same or opposite directions.

Displacement data from participants' hand and body sway, room and shaft were recorded through a tridimensional movement analysis system (Optotrak 3020 – Northern Digital, Inc.) at the frequency of 100 Hz, using infra-red markers fixed to the participants' back between their scapulae, around the eight thoracic vertebra, right hand's thumb and index finger (a small support to the markers attached to each distal phalange was used to avoid occlusion), to the shaft (30 cm above the ball), and to the frontal wall of the room. A light bulb was attached to the room's back wall, 50 cm from the ceiling and aligned with the shaft, to indicate the starting time of the catching action.

Procedures

Each participant was centrally positioned inside the moving room facing the back wall at a distance of 1 meter. The starting position of the participant was with the left arm down at the side of the body and the right arm with the elbow joint at approximately 90 degrees, forearm horizontally placed and the palm directed forward; right hand's thumb and index finger were fully extended together and other fingers aligned to the index finger. Participants stood upright with their feet parallel and apart to one another, aligned to the shoulders' width. After familiarization period of ten trials in grasping the approaching ball without the movement of the room, participants performed a total of 45 trials, 5 trials in each of the 9 experimental conditions, combining movement/no movement of the room; stationary/approaching ball; grasping present/absent. A summary of all nine experimental conditions is depicted in Table 1.

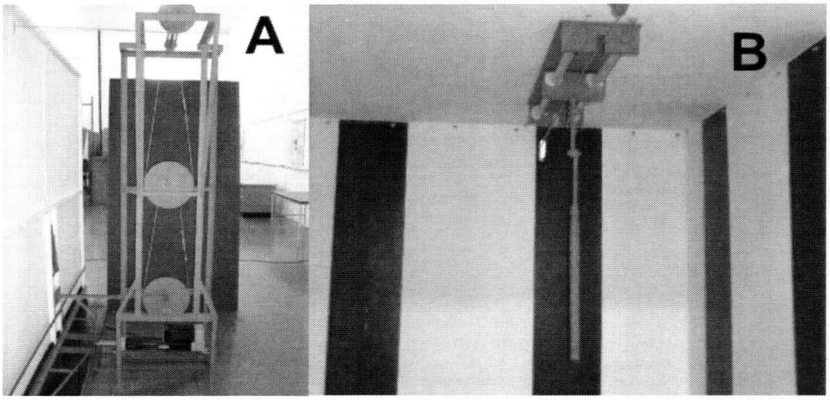

Figure 1. Pictures showing the moving room, the pulley (A, external view) and the shaft systems (B, internal view).

In all trials, participants were instructed to stay in the starting position as stable as possible and keep it through the end of the experimental trials with no grasping (conditions 1, 4, and 5), grasping the ball after the light being turned on with no movement of the room and of the ball (condition 2), and grasping the ball after the light being turned on simultaneously to the room and shaft movements initiation (conditions 3, 6, 7, 8, and 9).

Table 1. Experimental conditions combining conditions of the moving room, the ball, and the catching action

Condition	Room	Ball	Grasping
1	Stationary	Stationary	Absent
2	Stationary	Stationary	Present
3	Stationary	Approaching	Present
4	Approaching	Stationary	Absent
5	Moving back	Stationary	Absent
6	Approaching	Stationary	Present
7	Moving back	Stationary	Present
8	Approaching	Approaching	Present
9	Moving back	Approaching	Present

In the trial in which the room was moved, it was moved discretely, approaching or moving away from the participant's perspective, with approximate duration of two seconds, with peak velocity of 2.6 cm/s and amplitude of 2.5 cm (Prioli et al. 2005). The shaft approached the participant, being moved approximately during two seconds, with peak velocity of 74.8 cm/s, and amplitude of 53 cm. In the conditions with stationary ball, the position of the ball was set for all participants at 10 cm prior to the end of its trajectory.

During all conditions, participants were required to stand upright for 18 seconds, maintaining fixation with their eyes on the ball. Each trial was divided into four time windows: prior to room movement initiation (four seconds), during room movement (two seconds), after room movement – first and second periods (four seconds each), totalizing 14 seconds; the remaining time was excluded from analysis. The order of conditions was randomized to controlling for possible order effects according to a Latin Square Design (Maxwell & Delaney, 1990). Rest intervals were given to participants after five trials or as they requested.

Data Processing

The entire 14-s recorded signal was used for further analyses after being filtered using a digital Butterworth filter. Data relative to postural control was filtered with a second order filter with a cutoff frequency of 5 Hz and data relative to catching action was filtered with a fourth order filter with a cutoff frequency of 4 Hz. The variables below were obtained using custom software written in Matlab (Version 7.10, Math Works, Inc.). The dependent variables used to verify the maintenance of the upright stance were:

Mean sway amplitude (MSA). This variable was obtained for the previously referred time windows relative to the room movement initiation, in the anterior-posterior direction, and named accordingly: MSApre, MSApost1, and MSApost2. In the conditions 1 and 2 (without room and shaft movements), the time windows were, respectively, the initial four seconds of the trial and the final eight seconds of the trial divided into two halves; in the condition 3 (only shaft movement), the time windows were, respectively, the four seconds immediately prior to the shaft movement initiation and a period of eight seconds divided into two halves defined after the instant of maximum trunk displacement plus two seconds. MSA is obtained from the calculation of standard deviation after subtracting the mean values; it quantifies the amplitude of body sway and it corresponds to the variance of the data. Smaller values indicate reduced body sway and a better performance of the postural control system, and vice-versa (Toledo et al., 2006).

Body displacement. It verifies the effect of visual information as a consequence of the room movement on the participants' body displacement. It corresponds to the displacement between the beginning and the end of the body displacement due to the movement of the room. Small values of displacement indicate smaller influence of the visual manipulation and a quick resolution of the sensorial conflict generated by the moving room (Toledo et al., 2006).

Correlation coefficient and temporal difference. These variables result from a cross-correlation analysis between body sway and moving room position. It indicates how associated were room and participant's body sway. Values close to 1.0 indicate that both were highly related and values close to zero, the opposite.

Statistical Analysis

The data of all participants were submitted to analyses of variance regarding two types of effects on postural dependent variables: *Grasping effect on posture*: Room movement (Stationary, Approaching, Moving back) x Grasping (Present, Absent) ANOVA, with repeated measures in both factors; *Moving room and ball effects on posture*: Room movement (Stationary, Approaching, Moving back) x Ball movement (Stationary, Approaching), with repeated measures in both factors. Dependent variables which calculation depended on room movement (body displacement, correlation coefficient, and temporal difference) used only two levels (Approaching and Moving Back) for the Room factor. Tukey HSD tests, Greenhouse-Geisser degrees of freedom adjustments, and Bonferroni multiple comparisons probability adjustments were conducted as necessary (Maxwell & Delaney, 1990). The significance level adopted was 0.05 for all analyses.

Results

Results were organized and presented in two groups based upon the manipulations performed in the study: grasping affecting posture and movement of the room and of the ball affecting posture. Following, the main results from these analyses are depicted.

Grasping Affecting Posture

Body Displacement. Figure 2 depicts body displacement with and without grasping in the approaching and moving back movement of the moving room. ANOVA revealed significant effect of grasping, F (1, 11) = 41.773, p < 0.001. Body displacement was larger when participants had to grasp (M = 1.680 cm, SE = 0.144) than when they did not have to grasp the ball (M = 0.782 cm, SE = 0.105).

Correlation coefficient and temporal difference. Figure 3 depicts the correlation coefficient values between the movement of the room and body displacement with and without grasping in the approaching and moving back movement of the moving room. ANOVA revealed that the correlation coefficient was significantly higher in those trials when the room moved back from participant (M = 0.635, SE = 0.045) than in those trials when the room was approaching the participant (M = 0.463, SE = 0.044), F (1, 11) = 5.217, p=0.043. No significant difference was observed for temporal difference between the movement of the moving room and the induced body sway (M = 0.065, SE = 0.032).

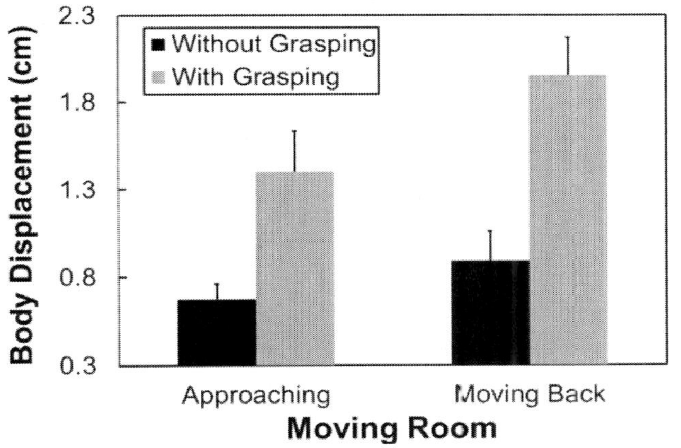

Figure 2. Mean and standard errors of the body displacement, due to the approaching and moving back movement of the moving room, with and without grasping.

Mean Sway Amplitude: Figure 4 depicts the mean sway amplitude, for the period of four seconds after the movement of the room, in the conditions in which the ball remained stationary (conditions 1, 2, 4, 5, 6, and 7). ANOVA revealed significant grasping effect, F(1,11)=8.031, p=0.016, and room movement by grasping interaction, F(2,22)=18.335, p<0.001. Pairwise comparisons showed that, when the room was stationary, mean sway amplitude was larger with grasping. Mean sway amplitude was not different with and without grasping when the room approached or moved away from the participant.

ANOVA did not revealed any difference regarding mean sway amplitude, for the period previously to the movement of the room and from 4 to 8 seconds after the movement of the moving room. Therefore, previously and after a period of 4 seconds, postural sway performance was already established.

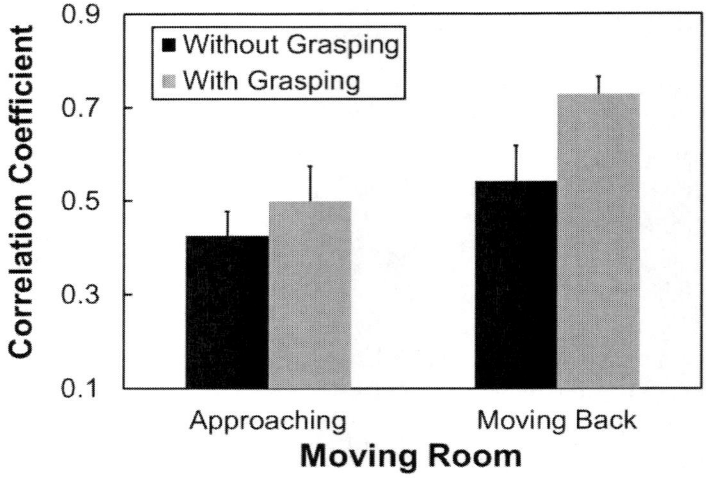

Figure 3. Mean and standard errors of the correlation coefficient during the approaching and moving back movement of the moving room, with and without grasping.

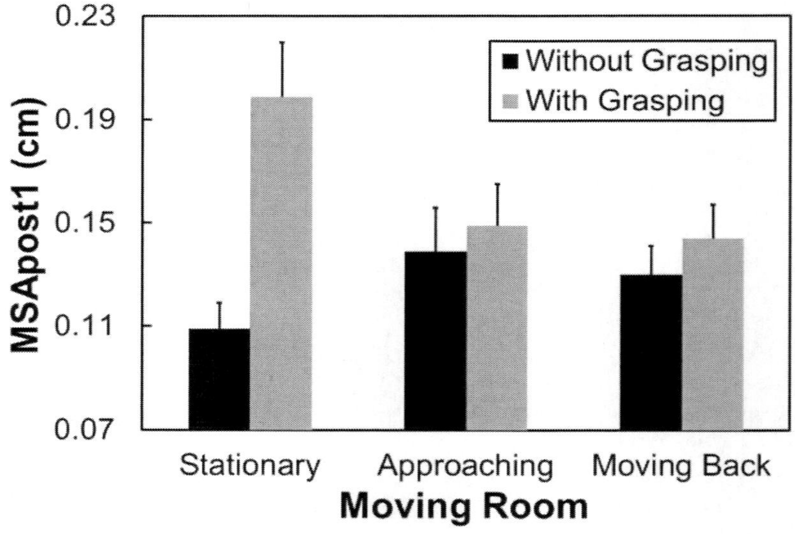

Figure 4. Mean and standard errors of the mean sway amplitude, period of four seconds after the movement of the room, for the conditions with and without grasping, with stationary, approaching, and moving back moving room.

Stationary and Moving Ball Grasping Affecting Posture

Body displacement. Figure 5 depicts body displacement due to the movement of the room in stationary and moving ball conditions. ANOVA revealed ball movement effect, $F(1, 11)=35.174$, $p<0.001$, and room by ball movement interaction, $F(1, 11)=5.746$, $p=0.035$. Pairwise comparisons involving the room by ball movement interaction showed that, when the room approached the participant, body displacement was significantly greater when the participant grasped the stationary ball (M = 1.407 cm, SE = 0.228) than when the participant grasped the approaching ball (M = 1.087cm, SE = 0.173), F (1, 11) = 8.310, p= 0.015. When the room moved back from the participant, the effect of the movement of the ball was stronger, with greater body displacement for stationary ball (M = 1.952 cm, SE = 0.223) than for approaching ball (M = 1.085cm, SE = 0.209), F (1, 11) = 22.240, p= 0.001.

Correlation coefficient and temporal difference. Figure 6 depicts correlation coefficient between the movement of the room and body displacement induced by the moving room. ANOVA revealed a room by ball movement interaction, F(1, 11)=6.469, p=0.027. Pairwise comparisons revealed that, when the room was moving back, the correlation coefficient was significantly greater than when the participants grasped the stationary ball (M = 0.729, SE = 0.037) than when they grasped the approaching ball (M = 0.503, SE = 0.019), F (1, 11) = 47.158, $p < 0.001$. When the room approached the participant, there was no significant effect of the ball movement (M = 0.510, SE = 0.049). Finally, no significant differences were observed for the variable temporal difference (M = 0.057, SE = 0.032).

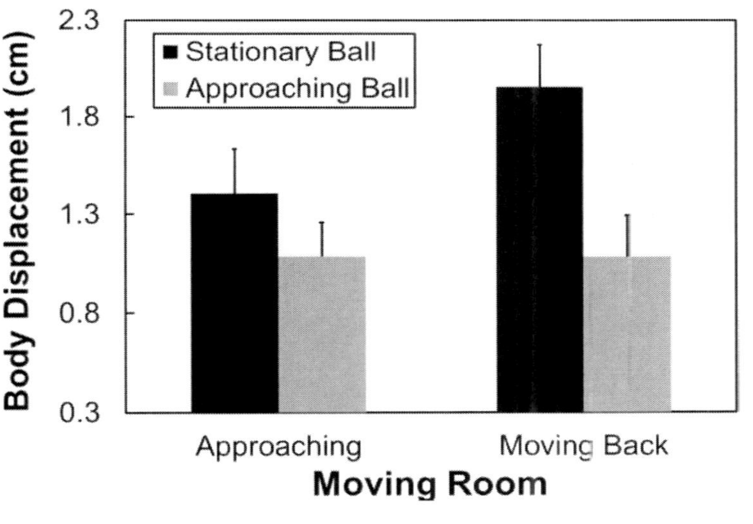

Figure 5. Mean and standard errors of the variable body displacement due to the approaching and moving back movement of the moving room, in grasping a stationary and an approaching ball.

Mean Sway Amplitude: Figure 7 depicts the mean sway amplitude, for the period of four seconds after the movement of the room, in the conditions in which the ball was moved together with the room (conditions 2, 3, 6, 8, 7 and 9). ANOVA revealed room by ball movement interaction, F (2, 22)=5.987, p=0.010. Pairwise comparisons revealed that, when room was stationary, participants showed larger body sway magnitude than when they had to grasp the approaching ball. No significant differences were observed in the other two pairwise comparisons, when the room was approaching or moving back.

ANOVA did not revealed any difference regarding mean sway amplitude, for the period previously to the movement of the room and from 4 to 8 seconds after the movement of the moving room. Therefore, previously and after a period of 4 seconds, postural sway performance was already established.

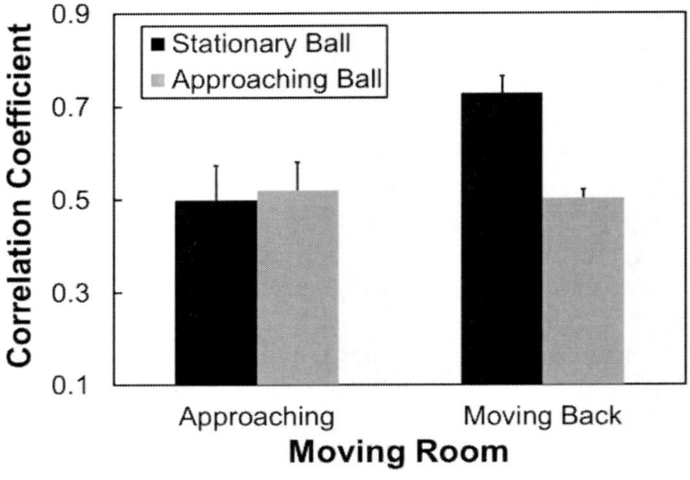

Figure 6. Mean and standard errors of the variable correlation coefficient during the approaching and moving back movement of the moving room, in gasping a stationary and an approaching ball.

Discussion

The purpose of the present study was to examine the effects of moving room discrete movements (approaching to or moving back from participants) combined with grasping an object on postural control stability. Our results showed that grasping leads to increased effect of moving room on induced body sway, as body displacement is larger during grasping. However, body sway is more related to room movement when the room is moved back compared to the approaching movement.

Despite inducing larger body sway during the movement of the moving room, grasping disruption of postural equilibrium is even larger when there is no moving room visual flow. Our results also showed that grasping an stationary ball in a moving scenario is worse, leading to larger body sway induced by the moving room and such effect is even larger in the moving back movement of the room. Such postural equilibrium disruption is still observed after the grasping has ended (following four seconds).

The observation that moving room discrete movement induces correspondent body sway has already been observed in children (Perotti Júnior, Barela, Polastri, & Tani, 2007), adults (e.g., Prioli, Freitas Júnior, & Barela, 2005), and even in elderlies (Wade, Lindquist, Taylor, & Treat-Jacobson, 1995), but the observation that grasping in such condition leads to a larger sway is new and surprising. One possible explanation is that when adults have to gather information about the ball position, they are more influenced by the peripheral flow. In the context of a moving room with no arm movement involved, it is known that flow with large lamellar (peripheral) structure generates stronger sway response than more radially (centrally) structured flow (Stoffregen, 1985). However, under random dots stimuli condition, young adults exhibited greater anterior-posterior sway during central vision as compared to the peripheral vision, in addition to evidence of a viewer-centered frame of reference characterized by the head/gaze direction (Berencsi, Ishihara, & Imanaka, 2005). It could be that, as participants attentionally reduced their area of interest to central vision fixating the ball, balance was influenced by a combination of these two disrupting effects. In line with this reasoning is that, although vision of the hand in our experiment is peripherally available during its initial movement, the use of central vision during the later stages of grasping is advantageous for controlling movement amplitude as the limb decelerates (Lawrence, Khan, Buckolz, & Oldham, 2006).

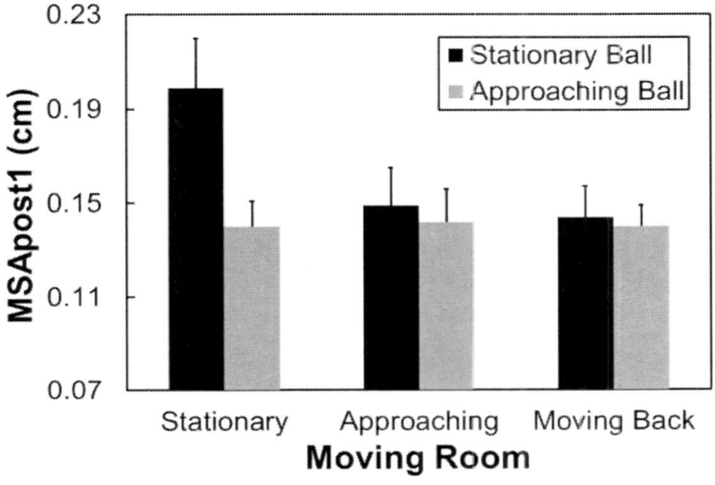

Figure 7. Mean and standard errors of the mean sway amplitude, period of four seconds after the movement of the room, for conditions of stationary and approaching ball with stationary, approaching, and moving back moving room.

Interestingly, however, optical flow used by the participants was dependent of the direction that the flow was created. The relationship between moving room and body sway was stronger in the condition of backward optical flow (correlation coefficient in the moving back condition – Figure 3), with the room moving away from the participant. It is well-known that infant rhesus monkeys (Schiff, Caviness, & Gibson, 1962) and infant humans (Bower, Broughton & Moore, 1970) show defensive reactions to approaching (looming) patterns of optic flow; these responses were in clear contrast to those related to objects approaching on a non-collision path or a shrinking (as opposed to a looming) pattern (Bruce & Green, 1990). In the moving room paradigm, the room approaches the observers who respond to the optical flow (looming) as if it arose from their own postural sway (Stoffregen & Riccio, 1990), attempting to keep a constant relation with the room's walls. As in our experiment a grasping action was required, the postural adjustment in response to the approaching movement of the room would result in increase of hand-ball distance; instead, a sway stabilization took place to allow a proper grasping movement. Differently, the room moving back from participants seemed to have facilitated grasping as they both were in the same direction.

Despite being disrupted by the moving room, grasping without the optical flow is more detrimental. Clearly our results showed that after grasping with the stationary room, body sway was larger than in any other condition. Therefore, although moving room induces body sway and this sway still remains after the grasping action, optical flow seems to be more informative to control sway after the action. When no optic flow is available, such as during catching in a dark environment (Savelsbergh & Whiting, 1988), catching is clearly affected; it seems that posture might be stabilized and catching enhanced due to the optic flow availability even in a moving room context. In a situation where the perturbation was induced by a foam, Voudouris et al. (2013) found that prior to reaching movement initiation participants exhibit more body sway and greater fluctuations in the center of pressure. However, during reaching to grasp action, overall body posture was less affected when standing on foam than when standing on a stable (control) surface; variables related to digits and wrist movements did not differ between these two types of surface. Authors interpreted these responses as a way of participants to ensure that they could cope with the destabilizing effect of the arm movement, suggesting that postural considerations are fully integrated in planning the upcoming arm movement (Voudouris et al., 2013). In the present study, in the stationary (no perturbation) room condition, participants could adapt posture to favor a less constrained grasping action towards a stationary ball (Figure 4). Interestingly, when the room was stationary and the ball approaching, the movement of the ball seemed to have limited body sway adjustments as compared to the stationary ball condition (Figure 7), similarly to the effect of room movement in both directions.

Conclusion

The present study showed that grasping leads to increased effect of moving room on induced body sway. In this context, posture was more affected when the room was moved back compared to the approaching movement. Based upon these results, we suggest that postural control takes advantage of the structured optical flow available due to room movement, even when posture might be destabilized due to one's own movement, to maintain postural equilibrium.

References

Barela, J. A., Godoi, D., Freitas Júnior, P. B. & Polastri, P. F. (2000). Visual information and body sway coupling in infants during sitting acquisition. *Infant Behavior and Development*, *23*, 285-287.

Barela, J. A., Jeka, J. J. & Clark, J. E. (2003). Postural control in children. Coupling to dynamic somatosensory information. *Experimental Brain Research*, *150*, 434-442.

Berencsi, A., Ishihara, M. & Imanaka, K. (2005). The functional role of central and peripheral vision in the control of posture. *Human Movement Science*, *24*, 689–709.

Bower, T. G. R., Broughton, J. M. & Moore, M. K. (1970). Infant responses to approaching objects: An indicator of response to distal variables. *Perception and Psychophysics*, *12*, 171-179.

Bruce, V. & Green, P. R. (1990). *Visual perception: Physiology, Psychology and Ecology*. Hove: Lawrence Erlbaum.

Hu, Y., Osu, R., Okada, M., Goodale, M. A. & Kawato, M. (2005). A model of the coupling between grip aperture and hand transport during human prehension. *Experimental Brain Research*, *167*, 301–304.

Jakobson, J. S. & Goodale, M. A. (1991). Factors affecting higher-order movement planning: A kinematic analysis of human prehension. *Experimental Brain Research*, *86*, 199–208.

Jeannerod, M. (1984). The timing of natural prehension movements. *Journal of Motor Behavior*, *16*, 235–254.

Lawrence, G. P., Khan, M. A., Buckolz, E. & Oldham, A. R. H. (2006). The contribution of peripheral and central vision in the control of movement amplitude. *Human Movement Science*, *25*, 326–338.

Massion, J. (1992). Movement, posture and equilibrium: interaction and coordination. *Progress in Neurobiology*, *38*, 35–56.

Maxwell, S. E. & Delaney, H. D. (1990). *Designing experiments and analyzing data: A model comparison approach.* Belmont, CA: Wadsworth.

Perotti Júnior, A. P., Barela, J. A., Polastri, P. F. & Tani, G. (2007). Influência de diferentes informações comportamentais na dinâmica intrínseca entre informação visual e oscilação corporal. *Brazilian Journal of Motor Behavior*, *2*(1), 40-50.

Patron, J., Stapley, P. & Pozzo, T. (2005). Human whole-body reaching in normal gravity and microgravity reveals a strong temporal coordination between postural and focal task components. *Experimental Brain Research*, *165*, 84–96.

Prioli, A. C., Freitas Júnior, P. B. & Barela, J. E. A. (2005). Physical activity and postural control in the elderly: coupling between visual information and body sway. *Gerontology*, *51*(3), 145-148.

Pozzo, T., Ouamer, M. & Gentil, C. (2001). Mechanical effect of voluntary arm lifting movement on whole body equilibrium: a simulation study. *Biological Cybernetics*, *85*, 39–49.

Pozzo, T., Stapley, P. J. & Papaxanthis, C. (2002). Coordination between equilibrium and hand trajectories during whole body pointing movements. *Experimental Brain Research*, *144*, 343–350.

Rinaldi, N. M. & Moraes, R. (2015). Gait and reach-to-grasp movements are mutually modified when performed simultaneously. *Human Movement Science*, *40*, 35-58.

Savelsbergh, G. J. P., Bennett, S., Angelakopolous, G. T. & Davids, K. (2005). Perceptual-motor organization of children's catching behaviour under different postural constraints. *Neuroscience letters*, *373*, 153-158.

Savelsbergh, G. J. P. & Whiting, H. T. A. (1988). The effect of skill level, external frame of reference and environmental changes on one handed catching. *Ergonomics*, *31*, 1655-1663.

Schiff, W., Caviness, J. A. & Gibson, J. J. (1962). Persistent fear responses in rhesus to the optical stimulus of "looming". *Science*, *136*, 982-983.

Stoffregen, T. A. (1985). Flow structure versus retinal location in the optical control of stance. *Journal of Experimental Psychology: Human Perception and Performance*, *1*, 554-565.

Stoffregen, T. A., Bardy, B. G., Bonnet, C. T. & Pagulayan, R. J. (2006). Postural stabilization of visually guided eye movements. *Ecological Psychology*, *18*, 191-222.

Stoffregen, T. A. & Riccio, G. E. (1990). Responses to optical looming in the retinal center and periphery. *Ecological Psychology*, *2*, 251-274.

Toledo, D. R., Rinaldi, N. M. & Barela, J. A. (2006). Controle postural em crianças: Efeito da manipulação da informação visual discreta. *Brazilian Journal of Motor Behavior*, *1*, 82-88.

Voudouris, D., Brenner, E., Schot, W. D. & Smeets, J. B. J. (2010). Does planning a different trajectory influence the choice of grasping points? *Experimental Brain Research*, *206*, 15–24.

Voudouris, D., Radhakrishnan, S. Hatzitaki, V. & Brenner, E. (2013). Does postural stability affect grasping? *Gait & Posture*, *38*, 477–482.

Wade, M. G., Lindquist, R., Taylor, J. R. & Treat-Jacobson, D. (1995). Optical flow, spatial orientation, and the control of posture in the elderly. *The Journals of Gerontology Series B: Psychological Sciences and Social Sciences*, *50*(1), 51-54.

In: Advances in Visual Perception Research
Editor: Thomas Heinen

ISBN: 978-1-63482-455-2
© 2015 Nova Science Publishers, Inc.

Chapter 9

Precision in Matching Oriented Lines Is Influenced by Perspective and Viewing Frames

***Laura Pérez Zapata*[1,2], *J. Antonio Aznar-Casanova*[1,2,*], *Manuel Moreno*[1], *Matthias Keil*[1,2] *and Hans Supèr*[1, 2,3]**

[1]Department of Basic Psychology, Faculty of Psychology, University of Barcelona

[2]Institute for Brain, Cognition and Behaviour (IR3C)

[3]Catalan Institution for Research and Advanced Studies (ICREA)

Abstract

Orientation is one of the main elements that form our perceptual space. Many studies have shown that people misjudge orientation in the frontoparallel plane. Here we examined precision in matching oriented lines in a 3D environment. In Experiment 1 we used perspective as a pictorial cue to provide the impression of a surface inclined in depth. In the first task we applied "direct perspective" where observers had to draw lines on apparently inclined surfaces, in the second task we applied "inverse perspective" where observers had to transform a perspective drawing onto a frontoparallel surface. Results showed two patterns, one related to inverse perspective, where precision matching oriented lines (PMOL) were modulated by the inclination of the surface. Here the observers had to perform more than one spatial transformation to solve the tasks. Another different pattern was found for direct perspective, in which observers had to perform only one spatial (cognitive) transformation. In Experiment 2, we studied how PMOL is affected by the surrounding surface contours (global shape) of an apparently inclined surface. Three rectangular surfaces (square, portrait and landscape), circles and star-like-shaped surfaces were studied. The data described in this chapter suggest that

[*] Corresponding author: Department of Basic Psychology. Faculty of Psychology University of Barcelona. Passeig Vall d'Hebron, 171. 08035-Barcelnona (Spain). Email: jaznar2@ub.edu.

rectangular surface contours improve orientation judgment at corresponding cardinal orientations.

Keywords: Orientation perception, pictorial depth cues, figure shape, visual psychophysics

Introduction

A major finding in attempting to account for shape perception in the early sixties was the discovering of neurons in the visual system that responded selectively to lines with specific orientation. Hubel and Wiesel (1959) described receptive fields of neurons in the cat striate cortex by claiming “the particular arrangements within receptive fields of excitatory and inhibitory regions seem to determine the form, size and orientation of the most effective stimuli” (p. 588). This discovery was followed by a series of articles in which they described the properties of receptive fields of single neurons in the cat cortex (Hubel & Wiesel, 1962, 1968).

Later, from the psychophysical approach, Campbell and Kulikowski (1966) found evidence of such orientation detectors by showing that also in men, like in the visual cortex of the cats, many of the cells responded only to lines with a certain orientation. Many other psychophysical and physiological studies (Blakemore & Campbell, 1969; Blakemore & Sutton, 1969; Campbell & Kulikowski, 1966; Campbell & Robson, 1968; De Valois, Yund & Hepler, 1982; Gilinsky, 1951), the most of them by using the selective adaptation procedure to oriented lines arranged in the frontal plane, demonstrated the existence of orientation and spatial frequency channels in humans. So, the experimenters examined the impact of an adapting exposure to a particular orientation or spatial frequency on subsequent sensitivity to that feature. The resulting decrease in sensitivity, which usually occurred across a narrow band of orientations or frequencies, was taken as an indication of the tuning of the relevant detector.

Precision in orientation perception has been widely studied in the frontoparallel plane, but neuronal and behavioral performance on inclined planes receding in depth or in images using perspective representing them, remind almost unstudied (these are the studies previously performed in the topic: Ellis, Smith, Grunwald, & McGreevy, 1991; Tharp, & Ellis, 1990). This is an important topic because it can help to best understand how 3D orientation is coded in the brain and then to account for how this knowledge could be used in a multiplicity of real life activities.

From the psychophysical approach previous studies (see Wagner, 2006, for a review) have assessed the precision in matching oriented lines (PMOL) by relating the perceived orientation (α') with its physical orientation (α). Several studies suggest that orientation of lines that subtend acute angles are over-estimated ($\alpha'/\alpha>1$), while orientation of lines subtending obtuse angles are under-estimated ($\alpha'/\alpha<1$). These distortions in orientation perception imply an approaching of the perceived angle to a right one (Carpenter & Blakemore, 1973; Greene, 1993; Greene & Fraweley, 2001; Nundy, Lotto, Coppola, Shimpi, & Purves, 2000; Predebon, 1994; Wenderoth, Parkinson, & White, 1979).

Most studies agree in that the highest PMOL is at cardinal orientations (0° and 90°), what can be attributed to the average intrinsic structure of visual scenes (e.g. Keil & Cristóbal,

2000) or to the amount of neurons representing each orientation in primary visual cortex (V1) or middle temporal visual area (MT) (Li, Peterson & Freeman, 2003; Xu, Collins, Khaytin, Kaas, & Casagrande, 2006). The enhanced PMOL at cardinal versus tilted orientations is referred to as the oblique effect (Appelle, 1972).

Most of these results were obtained from psychophysical experiments using frontally oriented surfaces (Howard, 1982; Morgan & Baldassi, 1997; Dakin, Williams & Hess, 1999; Borra, Hooge & Verstraten, 2007; Westheimer, 1984, 2003). In natural viewing conditions, however, we find often structures embedded in arbitrarily oriented planes and surfaces where depth dimension plays a relevant role in perception of orientation and size (Foley, 1980; Foley, Ribeiro-Filho & Da Silva, 2004; Loomis & Philbeck, 1999; Witkin & Asch, 1948). The interpretation of orientation on depth oriented devices seems to imply some spatial transformation which is related to participants response time (RT). It has been probed that the more complex the required spatial transformation, the more longer RT (Shepard & Metzler, 1971),

This chapter aims to present two experiments which test RT and PMOL in the context of a 3D environment created by using perspective cues (as textures and global distorted shapes).In order to test the influence of depth on PMOL and RT, we studied how participants applied two spatial transformations: "direct perspective" and "inverse perspective". Direct perspective is the forward transformation, where an observer views a frontoparallel scene and compiles a corresponding 3D drawing (or pictorial representation). Inverse perspective is the transformation that proceeds in the opposite direction, where an observer looks at the pictorial representation and reproduces it on a frontoparallel scene.

The aim of this first experiment is to describe the amount of spatial transformations under direct and inverse perspective tasks and to analyze the modulation of the oblique effect derived of depth perception. By comparing the observer's performances in these two transformations, we could look for asymmetries, which reveal how encoding of depth, for the tasks implying direct perspective, or decoding of depth, for the tasks implying inverse perspective, affects PMOL and RT differently.

The second experiment studies variations of surface shape, for example portrait versus landscape orientation, or circular or irregular shapes. Specifically, we tested whether an observer uses the same pictorial depth cues for the various shapes, and our goal is to determine if some informative cues derived from the global surrounding shape influenced the PMOL.

Experiment 1

Methods

Participants

Six volunteer observers took part in Experiments 1 and 2 (3 men, age ranged from 29 to 55 years, and 3 women, age ranged from 24 to 27 years). Four of them were experienced psychophysics observers and naive to the purpose of the study. All had normal or corrected-to-normal vision, as well as normal stereo acuity (60 min arc, assessed by the Titmus test). These studies were approved by the Ethics Committee of the Faculty of Psychology of the

University of Barcelona, in accordance with the ethical standards laid down in the 1954 Declaration of Helsinki.

Stimuli and Apparatus

Each stimulus consisted of a flat picture (see Figure 1) that showed the end-points of an implicit line, which is subjected to perspective transformation. Line-end-points were drawn in the center of a surface with rectangular shape at some inclination. The orientation of the implicit lines was 22.5°, 45°, 67.5°, 90°, 112.5°, 135° and 157.5°, where 0° defines a horizontal line and 90° a vertical one. Surface inclination angles were 10°, 30°, 50°, 70° and 90° (the frontoparallel plane) relative to the observer's viewpoint. Previously Saunders and Bakus (2006) showed in a similar gradients of surface inclination that observers were able to realiably judge surface aspect ratios from the monocular images. The size of the rectangular surface was 30 cm x 40 cm and it was textured with a white (79.8 cd/m^2) grid (square cells with side length 2.4 mm) against a black (<0.008 cd/m^2) background. The endpoints of the virtual lines consisted of yellow dots with diameter 3.6 mm. When the frame was frontoparallel (90°), the relative distance between each pair of endpoints was changed randomly from trial to trial, in a range from 14 to 21 cm (subtended visual angles between 1.6° and 2.5°), and the global area in which stimuli were displayed subtended a visual angle of 3.4° x 4.6°.

In total 40 perspective projections were generated, resulting of combining 5 inclinations with 8 orientations. The first step for rendering the stimulus was to generate the (implicit) line with length r and orientation α in the frontoparallel plane:

$$x = r \cdot \cos(\alpha) \qquad \text{[Eq. 1]}$$

$$y = r \cdot \sin(\alpha) \qquad \text{[Eq. 2]}$$

The second step introduces perspective by means of a 3D rotation around the x-axis:

$$x' = x \qquad \text{[Eq. 3]}$$

$$y' = y \cdot \cos(\varphi) - z \cdot \sin(\varphi) \qquad \text{[Eq. 4]}$$

$$z' = y \cdot \sin(\varphi) + z \cdot \cos(\varphi) \qquad \text{[Eq. 5]}$$

where surface inclination is denoted by φ.

A chinrest fixed the observers' vantage point at 5 m viewing distance and 110 cm height. In this way, the mid-point of the screen, in which stimuli were presented, was at the eye level. The stimuli were presented on a 22" Philips Brilliance color display monitor with a 1024 x 768 pixels display resolution (0.30 mm pitch dot) connected to a Pentium IV 3.0 GHz computer. The images of the reference stimuli and subject responses were controlled by a computer program (OpenGL with glut32 library) developed *ad hoc* for this experiment. Observers responded by clicking on one of the end-points with the left and right mouse button, respectively (corresponding coordinates were recorded). Mouse position was available for participants when the response had to be drawn, it was not available when stimuli were shown.

Procedure

The experiment was carried out in a dimly lit laboratory (4 cd/m^2) where participants looked at a computer monitor on which the stimuli were displayed. Two stimuli were successively presented at each trial: (1) the *reference stimuli* (i.e. the planes with the line end-points) and (2) the *test stimuli* (i.e. the frames where the first end-point was presented and observers had to draw the second one; see Figure 1). Observers were asked to geometrically transform the endpoint locations from a *reference stimulus* to a *test stimulus* as accurately and fast as possible.

The experimental sequence for each trial started with showing the reference stimulus for 3 sec, followed by a white mask (100 cd/m^2) for 500 ms, in order to avoid after-images. The mask was then replaced by the response frame (test stimulus), showing a picture of an inclined surface with the near end-point. Observers then had to draw the far endpoint (i.e., the one with the highest elevation), correcting orientation and size in accordance with the inclination of the reference. Finally, for each response, feedback was given by showing the true physical location of the endpoint, allowing participants to verify their task performance. An analysis revealed no perceptual learning-based improvement (data not shown). Subsequently a white mask (duration 500 ms) and a sound (200 Hz, 100 ms) indicated the onset of the next trial.

We defined four conditions (C1 to C4) as illustrated in Figure 1.

In C1 (Direct Perspective), two dots as the endpoints of an imaginary line were displayed, which was embedded in a rectangular, frontoparallel surface (here "frontoparallel" means inclination angle 90º). The participants then had to re-draw this line on a second surface with inclination between 10º and 90º. In C2 (Inverse Perspective) we asked observers for the inverse spatial transformation: endpoints of an implicit line were shown on an apparently inclined surface (from 10º to 90º), and we asked them to re-draw the endpoints on a frontoparallel surface (i.e. at inclination 90º). The comparison between C1 and C2 could be affected by the fact that C1 implies transformations into a no tilted space (which implies a perceptual expansion of the canvas to draw on), and C2 into a foreshortened one (which implies a perceptual compression of the canvas to draw on). In order to exclude as an explicative factor the change of the perceptual canvas (compression or expansion), we designed a third condition (C3), where reference stimuli were presented on a 45º inclined surface, and the observer had to respond on a second surface being more or less inclined than the first (inclination range 45º±40º). As far as observers performance for this condition results in no differences with one of the previously tested we could exclude changes in perceptual dimensions of the canvas as an explicative factor. Also this C3 condition combined the direct and inverse perspective tasks, we hypothesized observers did a first direct transformation completed by a second inverse one in order to respond the asked task. Finally, PMOL could be different dependent on whether orientations were encoded on a flat surface or on a volumetric piece. We therefore need to discard whether encoding was done like on the frontoparallel plane, and this is why control condition (C4) was included, in which inclination of the reference and the response surface was the same. In order to solve this particular task observers could not decode and encode depth but work in a fronto-parallel surface, in such a case PMOL would show the traditionally found modulation, that is the oblique effect (Appelle, 1972).

Each participant completed all conditions on separate days ordering in a random sequence. Conditions were counterbalanced across the subjects. They did 120 trials for each condition, (5 inclinations x 8 orientations x 3 repetitions). Trials were randomized across orientations and inclination angles. On the average, it took subjects about 20 minutes to complete each condition. Relative PMOL was measured by the ratios between the perceived orientations and the corresponding true orientations (α'/α), both drawn on the screen's projection of the slanted plane.

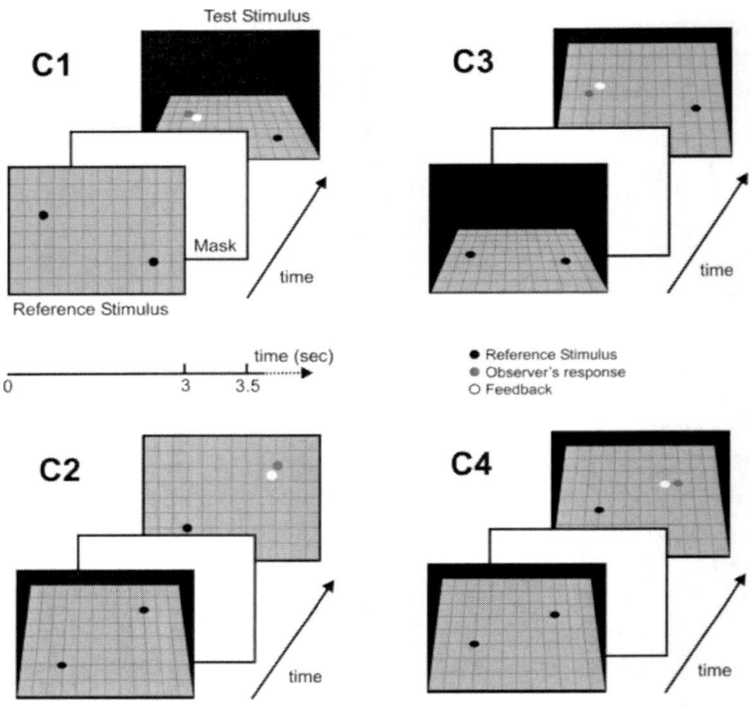

Figure 1. Experimental conditions in Experiment 1. In C1 observers were asked to perform a spatial transformation from a virtual line on a frontal surface used as a reference onto an inclined response surface. In C2 they were asked to perform a spatial transformation from an inclined reference surface onto a frontal one. In C3 they had to transform the oriented segment from a 45° inclined surface by drawing it on a surface with another inclination (in a range of 45°±40°). In C4 they were asked to transform the oriented segment from an inclined reference surface onto a response surface with the same inclination.

Results and Discussion

First, we verified the extent as to whether orientation perception was as expected in accordance with projective geometry rules. In doing so, we quantified the strength acting perspective geometry to generate the illusion of a surface inclined in depth. Therefore, we applied two different statistical analyses. On the one hand, we calculated the goodness-of-fit values (R^2) between the true geometrical orientations values (trigonometrically computed) and the orientation implicit in the observers' response. On the other hand, the response times (RT) of the participants were analyzed. As has been stated at the introduction section, it has been assumed that the longer RT, the more complex the required spatial transformation. Thus, t-test pairs using the RT as measure were performed for each couple of the four conditions. Further, the influence of orientation and inclination, as experimental factors, affecting RT variances where also analyzed by repeated measures ANOVA. Finally, the PMOL of implicit lines (between the endpoints) in the test stimulus with those in the reference stimuli was contrasted for the four conditions. This is why we compared (by repeated measures ANOVA) the orientation ratio between the perceived orientation of the endpoints and the true geometrical orientation (α'/α).

Strength of Perspective in Promoting 3D Illusion

To verify whether the observers perceived an apparently inclined rectangular surface we looked for the best fitting function relating the physical orientation and the perceived one for each particular inclination. Linear functions were the best fit to the data (R^2 between 0.978 and 0.993) and the high value of the coefficient of determination (R^2) suggested that the pictorial depth cues promoted efficiently the impression of a surface inclined in depth.

We defined RT as the elapsed time between the appearance of the test stimuli and the observer clicking the mouse button to locate the requested point. Given that a greater RT imply more mental rotation (Shepard & Metzler, 1971), we conjectured that relative RT was a correlate of the observers' cognitive costs in performing the required spatial transformation. Longer RTs were expected for those conditions, which involved a higher amount of spatial transformations. We computed a temporal cost as the mean RT, across trials and subjects (Figure 2).

The mean RT associated with each condition showed significant differences: Mean RT for C1 was 4.16 s (± 0.4 s S.E), for C2 it was 3.73 s (± 0.3 s), for C3 it was 6.74 s (± 0.4 s), and for C4 it was 4.8 (± 0.3 s). At table 1 can be seen the t-test for paired groups showed significant differences in mean RT between all conditions ($p<0.001$).

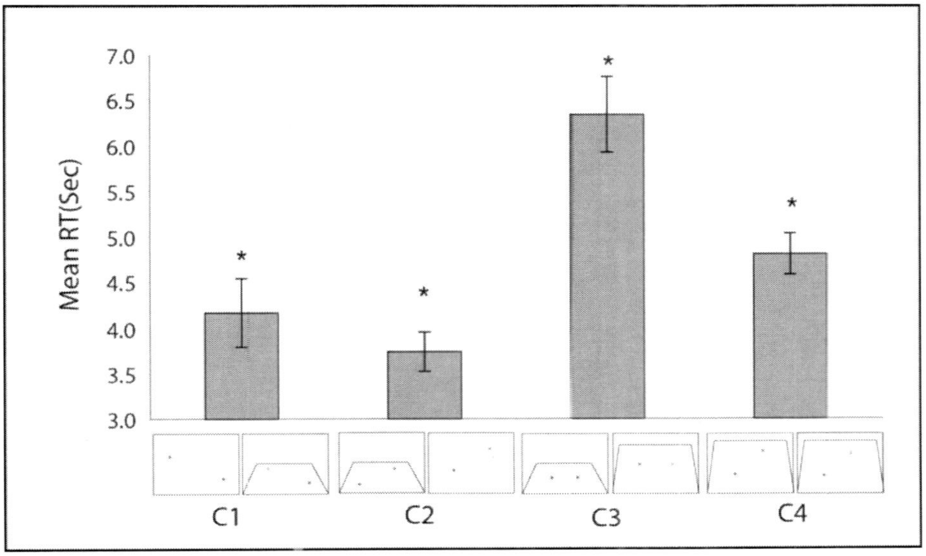

Figure 2. Mean response times by observers, inclinations and orientations as an indicator of the cognitive component of the psychophysical response (decision making). Error bars represent standard errors, while * indicates significant differences on the t-test.

Table 1. T-test pairwise comparisons of mean reaction time (RT) by condition (Experiment 1)

	Mean	Standard deviation	Mean standard error	t (239 DoF)	Sig.
MeanRT C1					
MeanRT C2	.426	.48	.03	13.87	
MeanRT C3	-2.17	.50	.03	-67.07	<.001
MeanRT C4	-.64	.75	.05	-13.26	<.001
MeanRT C2					
MeanRT C3	1.53	.78	.05	30.49	<.001
MeanRT C4	-1.07	.67	.04	-24.52	<.001
MeanRT C3					
MeanRT C4	-2.59	.54	.03	-74.53	<.001

Thus there seems to exist an asymmetry between the RT for making a spatial transformation from an inclined plane to a frontal plane (C2, Inverse Perspective) and vice versa, the RT for making a spatial transformation from frontal plane to an inclined plane (C1, Direct Perspective). Curiously, in conditions C3 and C4 (that require observers to perceived and respond on inclined planes) the temporal cost of matching orientation is higher than with conditions involving only one spatial transformation. Interestingly, observers needed more time for C4 than for C1 & C2. Results indicate that depth in perspective-inclined surfaces was encoded as if the lines were not in the frontoparallel plane. The reaction time was modulated by the difference of a plane to the frontoparallel, which serves as (mental) reference. This could explain the observed gradient of RTs between C2, C1 and C3.

We then carried out a repeated measures ANOVA with RT as dependent and inclination as a factor. It showed that inclination was significant for each condition, except C2 (C1: F (4, 68) =5.27, p <.001, ε = .835; C3: F (4, 68) =17.46, p <.001, ε = .530; C4: F (4, 68) =8.72, p <.001, ε = .325). This RT analysis revealed that inclination where stimuli were presented play not a role in observer's RT, but changes in inclinations where stimuli had to be reproduced played a modulating role in observer's RT.

Precision in Matching Orientation (PMOL)

Precision in matching oriented lines (α'/α) was analyzed for each condition using a 5 (inclinations) x 8 (orientations) repeated-measures ANOVA. Figure 3 shows PMOL for each inclination as a function of the real orientation, where each arc shows a different inclination, the angle of the graphs indicates the true geometrical orientation, and the color indicates the value of the α'/α ratio (i.e., precision).

The main effect for inclination was found to be significant (F (4, 68) = 4.211, p = .007, ε = .835) in condition 1 (see Figure 3, C1), as was the main effect of orientation (F (7, 119) = 37.918, p < .001, ε = .530). We observed also a significant interaction between inclination and orientation (F (28, 476) = 10.167, p < 0.001, ε = .325). Only the main effect of orientation was significant (F (7, 119) = 37.614, p < .001, ε = .449) in condition 2 (see Figure 3, C2) indicating (as in the RT analysis) that the processes for encoding orientation seem not to be affected by different pictorial inclinations (transformations from 2D to 3D), whereas, it seems to be affected by transformations from 3D to 2D. In condition 3 (see Figure 3, C3) we found significant single effects for inclination (F (4, 68) = 3.989, p = .006, ε = .847), for orientation (F (7, 119) = 24.787, p < .001, ε = .395), but also for the inclination x orientation interaction (F (28, 476) = 12.574, p < .001, ε = .317). Figure 3 shows the PMOL (α'/α) for all conditions (C1, C2, C3 and C4). Comparing the functions obtained in C1 and C2 with that of C3, the data revealed that the "precision function" for smaller differences in inclination between the reference and test stimulus ($\varphi_1 - \varphi_2 < 20°$) varied in a different way for spatial compression than for expansion. However, such differences were not significant when differences in inclination were higher than 20º. Figure 4 show an extreme case of difference in inclination ($\varphi_1 - \varphi_2 > 60°$).

Finally, in condition 4 (Figure 3, C4), which implied no changes in inclinations between reference and test stimuli, both a main effect for orientation (F(7, 161) = 12.933, p < .001, ε = .393), and a marginally but significant effect for inclination (F(4, 92) = 3.27, p = .058, ε = .411) were found. The 'orientation x inclination' interaction however did not reach significance (F(28, 644) = 2.808, p = .074, ε = .68). Given the invariance of inclination inherent to this condition, the observers could have done the task by encoding the end-points in a 2D coordinates system. However, this seems unlikely because the RT analysis revealed that observers spent more time on completion of task C4 (where both planes, reference and response, were inclined) than in those where only the response (C1) or the reference (C2) were inclined. It seems that for this condition 4 observers perceived orientation in 3D, transform it to an orthogonal codification and draw this particular orientation on the inclined surface as if it were a new one.

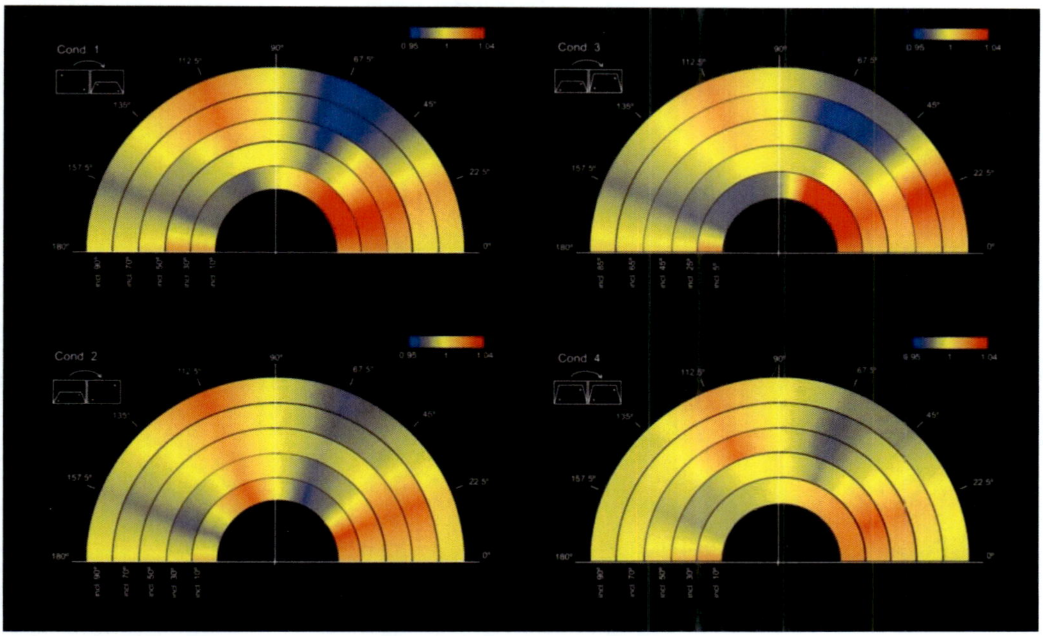

Figure 3. Polar graphs of precision in perceived orientation for each condition of Experiment 1. PMOL for each combination of inclination by orientation (angle) is depicted in a different arc. The mean precision in matching oriented lines (α'/α), i.e. PMOL, is indicated by the color scale. Changes in mean precision are depicted in different color from under-constancy (α'/α<1, blue color) to over-constancy (α'/α>1, red color), being used the yellow color for constancy (α'/α=1).

In the same direction data relative to PMOL shows that PMOL was more precise when observers responded in a frontoparallel plane (C2) than when observers responded in an inclined surface (C1 and C3) no matter where the stimulus were presented in a frontoparallel or inclined plane (Figure 3). However C4 was a particular condition where observers responded in an inclined plane as well as they do on the frontoparallel but involving more temporal cost.

These results suggested that two different spatial transformations are involved: The 'Direct Transformation' (DT) and another that could be called 'Inverse Transformation' (IT). And two processes are involved: one related with encoding/storing the stimulus by the spatial memory and another related with the motor response.

Could be said that for C2 (Inverse perspective task) data show that DT was necessary and the motor response seems not to decrease the PMOL. C1 (Direct perspective task) seems to be based on the IT and seems the motor response modulated PMOL. For C3 both spatial transformations (DT and IT) seem to be involved, observers seems to codified depth related data and construct a representation in the frontal plane, after this, they responded in another inclined plane, but with a new inclination (a new compression rate), resulting in a decrease in PMOL similar to that observed for C1. An asymmetry was found for C1 and C3 (tasks which involved make an orientation transformation from a plane to another and draw the resultant in an inclined surface) which could be explained in base to the observers' handedness. Finally, for C4, PMOL seems to indicate only DT, however, RT analysis indicated two different processes are having a role increasing the temporal cost. In short, these data suggest that in conditions C1 and C3 observers responded on a 3D coordinates system, while in conditions C2 and C4 observers responded on the frontoparallel plane.

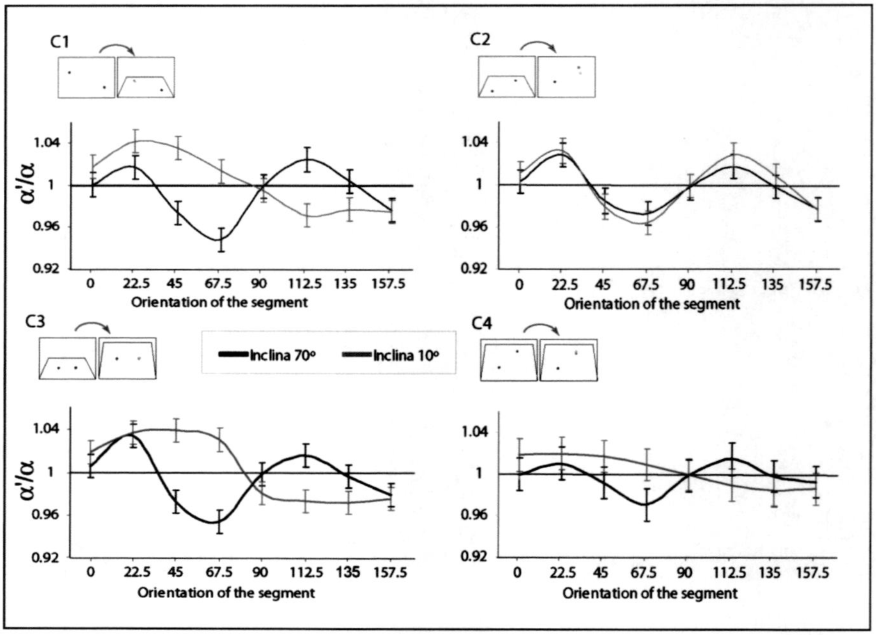

Figure 4. Comparing precision in matching oriented lines between spatial transformations in all conditions: C1, C2, C3 and C4. For clarity in the figure, only the most extreme changes in inclination are depicted (70° and 10°). Error bars represent the standard errors of the observers' response distribution.

The study also allows us dissociate between orientation and inclination processing. Two of the proposed tasks (C1 and C3) resulted in an interaction between both variables whereas the other two tasks (C2 and C4) didn't show that interaction.

Strength of the Diagonals of the Contour of the Surface As a Slant Cue

In general, the most precise perceived orientations varied as a function of current orientation (Figure 3 & 4). However, the corresponding PMOL with $\alpha'/\alpha = 1$ (perceptual constancy) did not exactly match those orientations predicted by the well-known oblique effect (see 'zero crossing' in Figure 4). Certainly, we found a higher precision for horizontally and vertically oriented segments, but this can be affected by other factors (Daini, Wenderoth and Smith, 2003; Meng & Quian, 2005). Specifically, these authors showed that the shape of the global frame (contour of the surface) can be a crucial factor for causing an additional modulation in perceived orientation. To verify this hypothesis, we adjusted a set of periodical functions[1] to the observers' data (Equation 6) which enabled us to predict the observers' PMOL for any geometrical orientation between 0º and 180º:

$$\alpha'/\alpha = a_1 \cdot \sin(b_1 \cdot \alpha_{frontal} + c_1) + a_2 \cdot \sin(b_2 \cdot \alpha_{frontal} + c_2) + a_3 \cdot \sin(b_3 \cdot \alpha_{frontal} + c_3) \qquad \text{[Eq. 6]}$$

where α' and α are perceived and true geometrical precision, respectively, $\alpha_{frontal}$ is the true orientation in the frontal plane, a_1, a_2, a_3, b_1, b_2 and b_3 are coefficients which vary according to inclinations, and c_1, c_2, and c_3 are additive constants in the function. Table 2 shows the coefficients for each of the adjusted functions.

Table 2. Specific parameters (ai, bi, and ci) in equation 6 for each condition and inclination of Experiment 1; these parameters allow us to predict constancy in orientation. The final row shows the correlations between geometrical predicted and empirical data

		Condition 1					Condition 2					Condition 3					Condition 4				
	Slant	10°	30°	50°	70°	90°	10°	30°	50°	70°	90°	5°	25°	45°	65°	85°	10°	30°	50°	70°	90°
Coefficients	a_1	1.88	2.3	1.41	2.09	1.43	2.02	1.91	4.10	2.01	2.58	2.83	1.92	2.52	3.23	2.74	2.03	2.09	2.02	2.02	2.02
	b_1	0.01	0.01	0.01	0.01	0.01	0.02	0.01	0.01	0.01	0.00	0.00	0.01	0.01	0.02	0.02	0.01	0.01	0.01	0.01	0.01
	c_1	0.41	0.72	0.93	0.73	0.48	0.03	0.05	0.69	0.27	0.11	0.2	0.64	0.92	-0.26	0.00	0.78	0.81	0.93	0.93	0.93
	a_2	0.95	1.32	0.43	1.12	0.47	1.19	1.07	3.11	1.05	0.7	0.54	0.93	1.54	2.46	1.83	1.04	1.10	1.03	1.03	1.0
	b_2	0.02	0.02	0.02	0.02	0.03	0.03	0.02	0.01	0.02	0.02	0.01	0.02	0.01	0.02	0.02	0.01	0.02	0.02	0.02	0.02
	c_2	2.78	3.53	3.36	3.49	2.43	2.19	2.11	3.69	2.71	1.5	2.15	3.3	3.83	2.28	2.58	3.53	3.61	3.76	3.76	3.76
	a_3	0.08	0.01	0.03	0.02	0.01	0.19	0.18	0.01	0.04	0.18	0.01	0.01	0.01	0.24	0.10	0.02	0.01	0.02	0.02	0.02
	b_3	0.04	0.09	0.09	0.09	0.05	0.04	0.04	0.07	0.05	0.04	0.1	0.08	0.09	0.04	0.05	0.04	0.1	0.09	0.09	0.09
	c_3	4.47	-0.6	-1.5	-1.1	2.59	3.38	3.22	-0.1	2.77	3.02	1.29	0.09	-0.9	3.26	2.97	5.15	-1.5	-1.1	-1.1	-1.1
Goodness of fit	SSE	0.00	0.00	0.00	0.00	0.00	0.00	0.00	0.00	0.01	0.00	0.00	0.00	0.00	0.00	0.00	0.00	0.00	0.00	0.00	0.00
	R^2	0.98	1	1	1	0.96	0.98	0.99	1	0.82	0.93	0.99	1	1	0.99	0.99	0.98	1	1	1	1
	Adj. R^2	0.98	1	1	1	0.96	0.98	0.99	1	0.81	0.93	0.99	1	1	0.99	0.99	0.98	1	1	1	1
	RMSE	0.00	0.00	0.00	0.00	2.58	0.00	0.00	0.00	0.01	0.00	0.00	0.00	0.00	0.00	0.00	0.00	0.00	0.00	0.00	0.00

From the coefficient values in equation 6, we obtained the particular orientations at which the observers' precision reached orientation constancy (ratio $\alpha'/\alpha = 1$). This would be equivalent to calculate the zero crossing for each sinus wave function. Notice, the true orientation of the diagonal in the geometrical projection of the rectangular surface gets increasingly distorted with growing inclination

[1] Firstly, we identified the best fitting function for all data. Secondly, we adjusted the values of the coefficients of these functions for each one of the twenty resulting sinusoidal functions (4 Conditions x 5 Inclinations).

Table 3. Pearson's coefficients obtained for the correlations between the orientations defined by the surface diagonals and those showing the observer's best PMOL (orientation constancy) in Experiment 1

	Conticion 1					Condition 2					Condition 3					Condition 4				
Slant	10°	30°	50°	70°	90°	10°	30°	50°	70°	90°	5°	25°	45°	65°	85°	10°	30°	50°	70°	90°
a	X	0.85	1.02	0.97	1.06	1.16	0.99	0.95	1.05	1.21	1.16	0.84	0.95	1.13	1.13	0.3	0.69	1.01	1.01	0.90
b	X	12.8	2.25	1.92	- 3.81	-9.1	0.24	8.72	5.02	- 10.1	- 20.7	18.3	5.73	-9.2	-8.5	60.86	24.61	2.85	2.85	15.09

We calculate the orientation of the diagonals of the trapeziums (α'') representing the inclined rectangular surface for each of the five inclinations (10°, 30°, 50°, 70° and 90°) by equation 7.

$$\alpha'' = \text{arc tan } (2h / (b_l + b_u)) \qquad \text{[Eq. 7]}$$

where h is height, b_l is the lower base and b_u is the upper base of the projection on a plane of an inclined rectangular surface.

Finally, we calculated the momentum-Pearson correlation between: 1) the true geometrical orientation of the trapeziums-diagonals (as predicted by Eq. 7); and 2) the predicted values (by applying Eq. 6 for each particular case) where observers reached orientation constancy. Correlation between the orientations of the trapeziums-diagonals and predicted values corresponding to orientation constancy, for each experimental condition and inclination, were between 0.97 and 0.99 (except in case of 10° inclined surface in C1 and C4; Table 2 & 3).

Therefore, orientation of the diagonals to the presented contour operated like "attractors" biasing the responses of observers and neutralizing the "oblique effect". This is in agreement with the studies of Saunders and coworkers (Saunders & Knill, 2001; Saunders & Backus, 2006, 2007), who investigated the ability to use linear perspective to perceive depth from monocular images. They used 2D perspective images of a slanted rectangular object, which were sufficient to create a strong 3D percept. Thus, they demonstrated that participants could infer inclination from the "skew" of the contour (angle subtended between the diagonals and the horizontal side of the rectangle). Subsequently (Saunders & Backus, 2006), concluded that both parallelism and orthogonality constraints are used to perceive depth from linear perspective. Our results corroborate this finding and suggest that observers use diagonals of the frame (i.e., rectangle in frontal surfaces or trapeziums in inclined surfaces), but not the bisectors, as attractors which bias responses towards orientation constancy. This tendency is subject to modulation in C1, C3 and C4, but not in C2. This is because (except in C2) two frames were shown in the response frame: i) the projected contour of the inclined surface, and ii) the viewing window (shape of the screen).

Several studies had addressed the question how the use of more than one frame of reference modifies perceived orientation (Daini, Wenderoth and Smith, 2003; Meng & Quian, 2005). To analyze this effect we conducted Experiment 2.

Experiment 2

Here we examined whether the external viewing frame (shape of the surface's contour), in which the *test stimuli* were embedded could modulate the observer's PMOL of implicit lines. To this end, two factors were manipulated: (i) the presence/absence of an orthogonal frame such as contour of the viewing windows. (ii) the aspect-ratio (AR) between the base and height of such frame, which varied in the range $1 \leq AR < 1$, only in the case of using orthogonal frames. From the two factors we expected to verify whether the bias observed in Experiment 1 was caused by the so-called "carpentered-world effect[2]".

Methods

The method used in this experiment was largely adopted from Experiment 1. In what follows we will only describe the differences.

Participants

The same six volunteer observers of Experiment 1 took also part in Experiment 2.

Procedure

Experimental setting, basic task asked for the participants, trial sequence and structure of the experimental test was identical with Experiment 1. Only two main differences have to be highlighted. First, only one spatial transformation (C2) was required in experiment 2 (inverse perspective; like an *observer* when decode a perspective painting). Second, five different viewing frames (experimental conditions) were designed by changing both the area of the inclined surface (presented to the participants) and the shape of the attached black cardboard occluding the screen (viewing window). The conditions were: landscape rectangle (40 cm x 30 cm) (Figure 5, C1), portrait rectangle (30 cm x 40 cm; figure 5, C2), square (34.64 cm x 34.64 cm) (Figure 5, C3), circle (radius = 19.54 cm) (figure 5, C4), and star-like-shaped, which was built by adding or subtracting a random length to or from the coordinates of an 24-sided polygon (Figure 5, C5). This star-shaped contour was viewed through a circular piece of black cardboard.

Three repetitions for each condition were required. Each repetition consisted of 40 trials (5 inclinations x 8 orientations). The order of order presentation for the different orientations was randomized across each condition. Each condition was conducted on successive days for all observers, taking around 20 min each. Analogously to Experiment 1, we use PMOL as dependent variable in Experiment 2, i.e.: α'/α.

---

2 According to the 'carpentered-world' hypothesis (Segall, Campbell & Herskovits, 1966), people living in cultures in developed Western societies (where rectangular shapes, straight lines, square corners abound) are more susceptible to interpret oblique and acute angles as displaced right-angles and to perceive two-dimensional drawings in terms of depth. On the contrary, people living in cultures in which right-angled structures are less prone, for instance, to the Müller-Lyer illusion.

Results and Discussion

First, we verified the influence of inclination on the PMOL for each of the five '*viewing windows*' by a repeated-measures ANOVA, taking both orientation and inclination as repeated measure factors. The results showed that the main effect of orientation was significant for all five conditions (Landscape: $F(7, 119) = 37.614, p < .001, \varepsilon = .449$; Portrait: $F(7, 119) = 43.638, p < .001, \varepsilon = .426$; Square: $F(7, 119) = 22.897, p < .001, \varepsilon = .499$; Circle: $F(7, 119) = 15.025, p < .001, \varepsilon = .379$; Star-shaped: $F(7, 119) = 19.959, p < .001, \varepsilon = .321$) (see Figure 6 and Figure 3, C2 for Landscape condition). However, neither the main effect of inclination nor the "orientation by inclination" interaction was significant. This lack of significance was expected on the basis of the results from C2 in Experiment 1 and also supports the fact that the effect of the inclination was not linked to the encoding of orientation but can be derived from the transformation as required in the task.

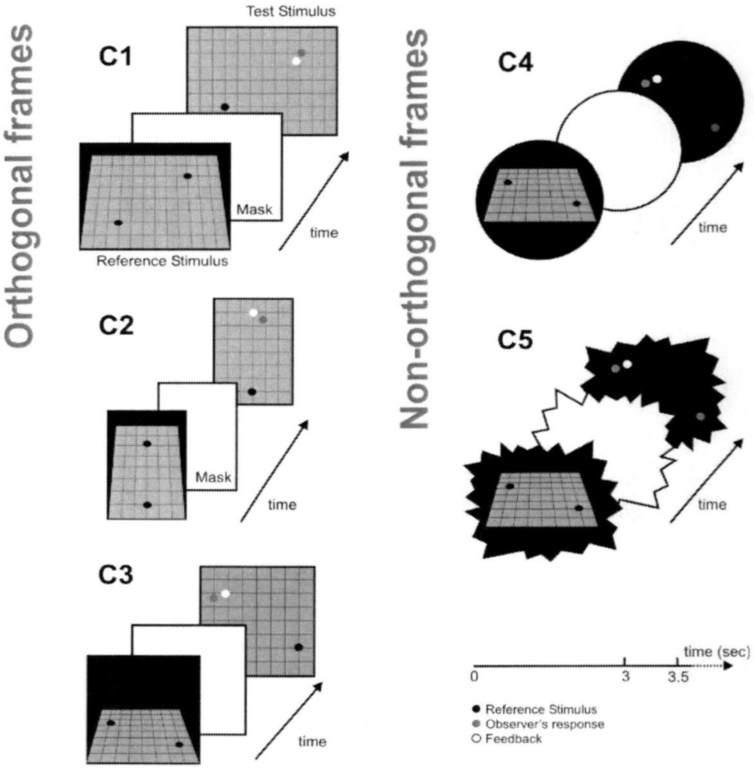

Figure 5. Diagram of the conditions used in Experiment 2. In Condition 1 (C1) the viewing window (viewing frame) was a rectangular landscape, through which the observers saw the test stimuli. In Condition 2 (C2) the viewing window was a rectangular portrait frame. In Condition 3 (C3) the viewing window was a square frame. In Condition 4 (C4) the viewing window was a circular window, with some orthogonal elements therein. In Condition 5 (C5) the viewing window was a star-like-shaped frame, without any orthogonal references.

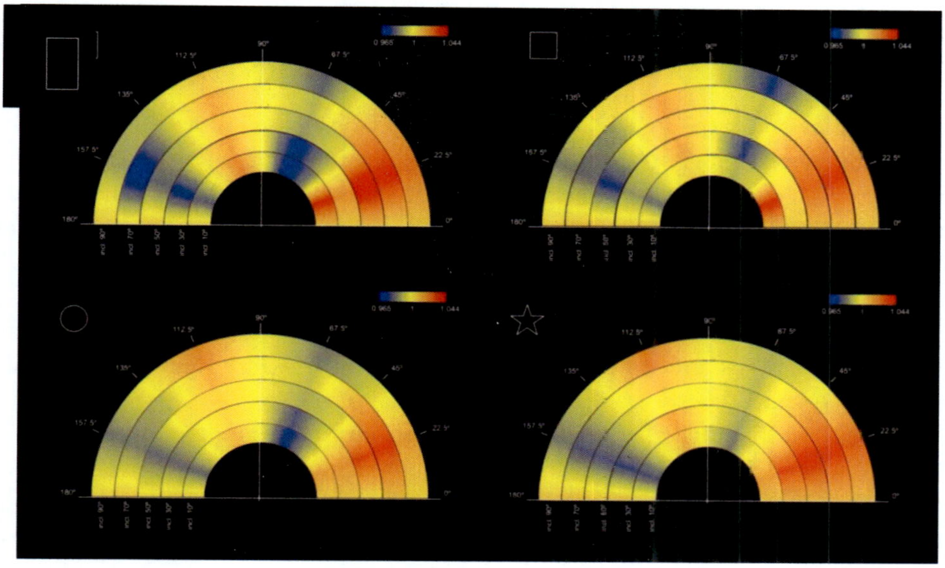

Figure 6. Polar graphs of precision in perceived orientation for each condition of Experiment 2. PMOL for each combination of inclination by orientation (angle) is depicted in a different arc. The mean precision in matching oriented lines (α'/ α), i.e. PMOL, is indicated by the color scale. Changes in mean precision are depicted in different color from under-constancy (α'/ α < 1, blue color) to over-constancy (α'/ α > 1, red color), being used the yellow color for constancy (α'/ α = 1).

Table 4. Parameter values (a_i, bi, and c_i) of equation 6 for each condition of experiment 2

		Landscape	Square	Portrait	Circle	Random
Coefficients	a_1	2.438	1.672	3.348	4.401	2.746
	b_1	0.011	0.010	0.010	0.013	0.012
	c_1	0.011	0.506	0.759	0.608	0.101
	a_2	1.506	0.689	2.35	3.408	1.795
	b_2	0.017	0.017	0.012	0.015	0.016
	c_2	2.424	2.901	3.727	3.6	2.743
	a_3	0.102	0.031	0.013	0	0.059
	b_3	0.044	0.057	0.072	0	0.046
	c_3	2.728	1.506	-0.015	0	2.553
Goodness of fit	SSE	0.001	0.00	0.00	0.025	0.001
	R^2	0.993	0.999	1	0.75	0.992
	Adj. R^2	0.993	0.999	1	0.748	0.992
	RMSE	0.001	0.00	0.00	0.006	0.001

Second, we verified whether cardinal axis and/or diagonals in the contours acted as a bias for perceived orientation. We first determined for each of the five conditions the best fitting function between PMOL and real orientations. Since no significant effect of inclination was found (see ANOVA of Experiment 1), we pooled the different inclinations for the subsequent analysis. We obtained five periodical functions with three sine wave components. Table 4 shows the coefficients found for each of these functions, allowing us adapting equation 6 to these new frames.

Figure 7 shows the experimental data, which are associated with these functions for the orthogonal contoured frames (C1, C2 and C3, in experiment 2). Points in the function defining better PMOL, orientation constancy ($\alpha'/\alpha = 1$), are placed at the cardinal orientations (0 ° and 90 °). However, they can also be seen at other orientations, which vary according to the diagonal of the shape of the viewing window used in the different conditions.

Results indicated that the diagonals (36.86° for the landscape frame, 45° for the square landscape and 53.13° for the portrait frame) are used by observers as valid references to match the orientation by correcting the inclination of the surface (see figure 6). This holds in particular when oriented lines were drawn on rectangular ones.

Finally, we verified whether the angles subtended between the lower base of the orthogonal contoured frame and their diagonal [Eq. 7] modulated the perceived orientation, we calculated the correlation between the orientation constancy points and their true geometrical angles (cardinal and diagonal references for orientation; Table 3 and Table 5).

No orthogonal contours in C4 and C5 lead to a better mean PMOL than in conditions with orthogonal contours. This latter finding suggests that the observers used something like 'a by default contour-frame' for applying the requested spatial transformation of the orientations.

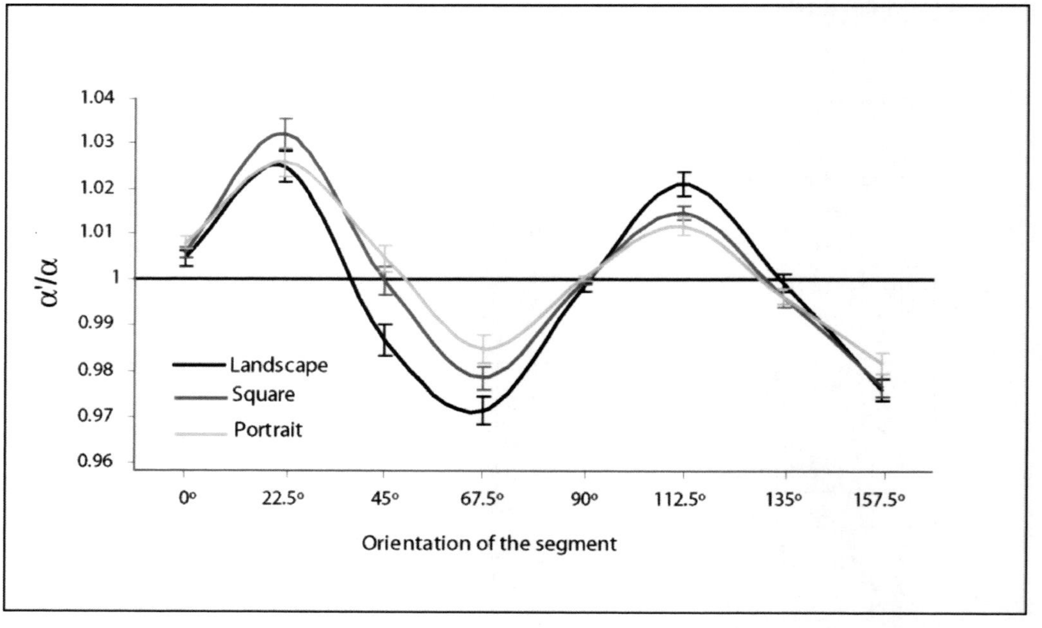

Figure 7. Precision in orientation for conditions used in Experiment 2. Only those conditions with orthogonal frame are depicted (different grey lines). Note that as the inclination has no significant effect, the averages were computed. Error bars indicate the standard errors for the response distribution.

Table 5. Coefficients defining Momentum-Pearson correlation for those conditions involving an orthogonal frame in Experiment 2

	Landscape	Square	Portrait	Circle	Random
a	1.066	0.841	1.115	X	X
b	-2.97	15.153	-9.89	X	X
R^2	0.995	0.992	0.991	X	X

General Discussion

Our results address how PMOL is modulated by apparently (perspective drawings) inclined surfaces. Specifically, we studied how linear perspective promoting illusory slopes affects PMOL. To this end, we designed two tasks: In one task observers had to replicate the orientation of a line presented on a frontoparallel surface onto an inclined surface (direct perspective) and in the other task observers had to retrieve the line orientation presented in a representation of a 3D environment in a frontoparallel plane (inverse perspective). Experiment 1 allowed us to compare these tasks as well as to postulate which spatial transformations influenced PMOL. Experiment 2 addressed how the shape of the viewing window can bias PMOL.

In agreement with the findings by Saunders & Backus (2006, 2007), we found a significant influence of "apparent inclination" on the PMOL. The RT analysis revealed a significant difference between conditions C1 and C2, showing an asymmetry between making a spatial transformations from an inclined plane to a frontal one (C2: inverse perspective) and vice versa (C1: direct perspective). The results provide therefore support for the hypothesis that orientations were encoded as they were in a 2D system with orthogonal axes, (Saunders & Backus, 2006, 2007). It seems as if orientation of lines was tuned to an orthogonal coordinate system that is aligned with the frontoparallel plane. In fact, the conditions that require observers to operate onto two apparent inclinations (C3 and C4), yielded higher latencies for matching orientation than those conditions where was presented the frontal rectangle (C1 and C2). This finding supports the notion of a frontoparallel encoding of orientations.

Furthermore, we have shown that PMOL was mainly affected by the true physical orientation, being the higher precision observed for the cardinal orientations (eg. Apelle, 1972; Keil & Cristóbal, 2000, Xu et al., 2006) and, as we mentioned below, also for some particular oblique orientations, such as those near to the tilt of the diagonal of the frame (contour of the surface). PMOL was also modulated by the apparent inclination of the surface in which the line was drawn. This effect was clearly visible in C1 and C3, but not in C4 and C2. The result was reinforced by a lack of a significant effect of the inclination factor and the absence of any interaction between 'inclination' and orientation, in any of the conditions of Experiment 2. It seemed that apparent inclination was only relevant for those conditions, which involved some change in the apparent inclination of the tested surface. An explanation for this result could be related to the change in the expansion/compression rate (variation in the spatial scale) associated with the retinal image, at which the surface was projected. Indeed, responses in the frontoparallel plane imply to operate at an almost linear scale. This stands in contrast to inclined surfaces, where a non-linear scale is associated with each slope (Wagner 2006). Therefore, linear perspective modulates PMOL due to an uncertainty associated with apparent inclination: PMOL decreases with increasing surface inclination.

In order to become more efficient, the visual system must operate preferentially in a plane aligned to the frontoparallel, what implies a translation of each input (inclined surface) into an orthogonal 3D system. This is probably the cause why in C2 inclination did not affect the PMOL. The oblique effect disappeared when expansion took place and appeared when compression increased, due to the inclination of the surface (see figure 3 and 4). It seems that the diagonal of the surface contour (or whatever equivalent factor) could help to reduce the oblique effect. In summary, PMOL varied as a function of the current orientation (see figure 3 and figure 4). However, perceptual constancy ($\alpha'/\alpha = 1$) did not exactly match those predicted by the well-known oblique effect, given that diagonals of the surface contour seems to operate as reference axes.

Our data suggest that perceptual constancy ($\alpha'/\alpha = 1$) was found for those orientations which were close to that of the diagonals in the projected contour of the response frame. The results show a tendency in the variability of the PMOL, which fit those orientations formed by the diagonals of the viewing window (in this case, a landscape rectangle). This tendency was modulated in C1, C3, C4, but not in C2. So, except in C2, two different frames were shown in the response frame: the inner (trapezoidal) frame and the outer (rectangular) frame. This could account for the absence of such 'diagonal effect'. In order to test this hypothesis we carried on Experiment 2.

In summary, our results show two patterns of results. One pattern related to the C2 and C4, where observers reached same PMOL but a difference in response time. Another pattern related to C1 and C3, where PMOL was modulated by inclination, and RT was similar and lower than for C4. This pattern of results allow us thinking that observers have to perform more than one transformation for solving some of the tasks probed in this experiment direct and inverse transformations (related to direct (C1) and inverse (C2, C4) perspective tasks). Also three kinds of processes were implied: encoding of the end points, rotating them in a mental transformation and responses them in a frontal or inclined plane.

This way, our results suggest, first, some of the proposed tasks needed to apply just one spatial transformation (C1, C2, C4) whereas other needed applying two (C3) and, second, the tasks implied two processes: one related with encoding of the stimulus in memory and the other related with motor performance of the response. The study allowed us to dissociate perception (encoding) and response (motor) and shows PMOL variation is more likely derived from the motor performance than from the encoding of the stimulus.

In experiment 2 we aimed to verify how changes in the global figure shape of the surface contour (or the aspect-ratio, in orthogonal surfaces), modulates observer's PMOL. As a result we found a bias in the so-called "carpentered-world effect". Thus, we showed that the angles subtended by the diagonals seem to be used by observers as useful references in order to match the orientation for correcting the distortion caused by apparent inclination. The shape of the contour and the viewing window attracted their responses towards the cardinal axes and an implicit oblique axis. This means that responses were biased to the oblique effect. An oblique bias in the responses could be expected for orthogonal frames (squared, portrait and landscape rectangle). PMOL is higher at cardinal orientations, but it also was enhanced at those orientations fitting the diagonals. None-orthogonal frames (circle and like-star) lead to a better mean PMOL (Daini, Wenderoth & Smith, 2003). In this case, observers used the bisectors of the cardinal axis of the none-orthogonal contour-frames (circle and star-like) in order to match orientation with highest precision.

In short, for the new four conditions of the Experiment 2 just orientation was a modulation factor. This result confirms that when the observer should respond in a frontal plane there is no modulation in PMOL derived from the presentation stimulus inclination. Results derived from the new four conditions shown more similarity between the circle and star shape frames than between landscape and portrait frames.

Thus, differences between direct and inverse perspective that we found provide insights into the 'grammar of vision' (Kanizsa, 1980). If one imagined the pictorial depth cues as a sign system, then our study would contribute to a better understanding of the semiotic of perspective. The semiotic should establish the rules according to which the visual world is constructed in their spatial parameters. The understanding of these rules has a theoretical interest, e.g. for understanding the role of pictorial depth cues in depth perception and a practical one, e.g. for people that use visual expression to communicate ideas and information.

Conclusion

To estimate line orientation of drawings on inclined surfaces, first, observers must solve an inverse perspective problem, which implies to translate a 2D image to a 3D representation (as if it they were projected on the frontoparallel plane), a spatial transformation that involve some decrease in PMOL. After this encoding they are able to transform oriented lines drawn on whatever inclined surfaces to other inclined surface. These results show clearly that the brain uses at least two spatial transformations related to direct and inverse perspective. But also, the contour and the global shape of the frame can bias the responses towards the cardinal axes and an implicit oblique axis.

Acknowledgments

This research was supported by grants to Hans Supèr (PSI 2010-18139 & SGR2009-308) and to José Antonio Aznar-Casanova (PSI2012-35194) from the Spanish Ministry of Economy and Competitiveness (MECOM). MSK is funded by the Ramon and Cajal program from the Spanish Government, and the national grant DPI2010-21513.

References

Appelle, S. (1972). Perception and discrimination as a function of orientation: The “oblique effect” in man and animals. *Psychological Bulletin*, *78*, 266-278.

Blakemore, C. & Campbell, F. W. (1969). On the existence of neurons in the human visual system selectively sensitive to the orientation and size of retinal images. *The Journal of Physiology*, *203*, 237-260.

Blakemore, C. & Sutton, P. (1969). Size adaptation: A new after-effect. *Science, N. Y. 166*, 245-247.

Borra, T., Hooge, I. T. C. & Verstraten F. A. J. (2007). The use of optimal object information in fronto-parallel orientation discrimination. *Vision Research, 47*(26), 3307-3314.

Campbell, F. W. & Kulikowski, J. J. (1966). Orientational selectivity of the human visual system. *Journal of Physioogy, 187*(2), 437-445.

Campbell, F. W. & Robson, J. G. (1968). Application of Fourier analysis to the visibility of gratings. *Journal of Physiology* (London), *197*, 551-566.

Carpenter, R. H. & Blakemore, C. (1973). Interactions between orientations in human vision. *Experimental Brain Research, 26*, 287-303.

Daini, R., Wenderoth, P. & Smith, S. (2003). Visual orientation illusions: Global mechanisms involved in hierarchical effects and frames of reference. *Perception & Psychophysics, 65*(5), 770-778.

Dakin, S. C., Williams, C. B. & Hess, R. F. (1999). The interaction of first- and second-order cues to orientation. *Vision Research 39*, 2867-2884.

De Valois R. L., Yund E. W. & Hepler, N. (1982). The orientation and direction selectivity of cells in macaque visual cortex. *Vision Research, 22*, 531-544.

Ellis, S. R., Smith, S., Grunwald, A. & McGreevy, M. W. (1991). Direction judgment error in computer generated displays and actual scenes. Book chapter in "Pictorial communication in virtual and real environments." Ed. S. R. Ellis (London: Taylor and Francis), 504-526.

Foley J. M. (1980). Binocular distance perception. *Psychological Review, 87*(5), 411-434.

Foley, J. M., Ribeiro-Filho, N. P. & Da Silva, J. A. (2004) Visual perception of extent and the geometry of visual space. *Vision Research, 44*(2), 147-156.

Gilinsky, A. (1951). Perceived size and distance in visual space. *Psychological Review, 58*, 460-482.

Greene, E. (1993). Angular induction is modulated by the orientation of the test segment, but not its length. *Perception & Psychophysics, 54*, 640-648.

Greene, E. & Frawley, W. (2001) Evaluating models of collinearity judgment for reliability and scale. *Perception, 30*, 543-558.

Howard, I. P. (1982). *Human Visual Orientation*. Chichester, Sussex: John Wiley.

Hubel, D. H. & Wiesel, T. N. (1959). Receptive fields of single neurones in the cat's striate cortex. *The Journal of Physiology, 148*(3), 574–591.

Hubel, D. H. & Wiesel, T. N. (1962). Receptive fields, binocular interaction and functional architecture in the cat's visual cortex. *The Journal of Physiology, 160*(1), 106–154.

Hubel, D. H. & Wiesel, T. N. (1968). Receptive fields and functional architecture of monkey striate cortex. *Journal of Physiology, 195*, 215-243.

Kanizsa, G. (1980). *Grammatica del Vedere. Saggi su Percezione e Gestalt*. Bologna (Italy): Il mulino.

Keil, M. S. & Cristóbal, G. (2000) Separating the chaff from the wheat: possible origins of the oblique effect. *Journal of the Optical Society of America A, 17*, 697-710.

Li, B., Peterson, M. R. & Freeman, R. D. (2003). Oblique effect: A neural basis in the visual cortex. *Journal of Neurophysiology, 90*, 204-217.

Loomis, J. M. & Philbeck, J. W. (1999). Is the anisotropy of perceived 3-D shape invariant across scale? *Perception & Psychophysics, 61*, 397-402.

Meng, X. & Qian, N. (2005). The oblique effect depends on perceived, rather than psysical, orientation and direction *Vision Research*, *45*(27), 3402-3413.

Morgan, M. J. & Baldassi, S. (1997) How the human visual system encodes the orientation of a texture and why it makes mistakes? *Current Biology*, *7*, 999-1002.

Nundy, S., Lotto, B., Coppola, D., Shimpi, A. & Purves, D. (2000). Why are angles misperceived? *Proceedings of the National Academy of Sciences of the USA*, *97*(10), 5592-5597.

Predebon J. (1994). Illusion of length in acute and obtuse angle figures. *Perceptual & Motor Skills*, *78*(1), 259-264.

Saunders, J. A. & Backus, B. T. (2006). The accuracy and reliability of perceived depth from linear perspective as a function of image size. *Journal of Vision*, *6*(9), 933-954.

Saunders, J. A. & Backus, B. T. (2007). Both parallelism and orthogonality are used to perceive 3D slant of rectangles from 2D images. *Journal of Vision*, *7*(6), 1-11.

Saunders, J. A. & Knill, D. A. (2001). Perception of 3D surface orientation from skew symmetry. *Vision Research*, *41*(24), 3163-3183.

Segall, M., Campbell, D. & Herskovits, M. J. (1966). *The Influence of Culture on Visual Perception.* New York: The Bobbs-Merrill Company.

Shepard, R. N. & Metzler, J. (1971). Mental rotation of three-dimensional objects. *Science*, *191*, 701-703.

Tharp, G. K. & Ellis, S. R. (1990). The effects of training on errors of perceived direction in perspective displays NASA TM 102792, NASA Ames Research Center, Moffett Field CA.

Wagner, M. (1985). The metric of visual space. *Perception and Psychophysics*, *38*, 483-495.

Wagner, M. (2006). *The Geometries of Visual Space*. Lawrence Erlbaum Associates, Inc., Publishers New Jersey.

Wenderoth, P., Parkinson, A. & White, D. (1979). A comparision of visual tilt illusions measured by the techniques of vertical setting, parallel matching, and dot alignment. *Perception*, *8*(1), 47-57.

Westheimer G. (1984). Sensitivity for vertical retinal image differences. *Nature*, *307*(5952), 632-634.

Westheimer, G. (2003). The distribution of preferred orientations in the peripheral visual field. *Vision Research*, *43*, 53–57.

Xu, X., Collins, C. E., Khaytin, I, Kaas, J. H. & Casagrande, V. A. (2006). Unequal representation of cardinal vs. oblique orientations in the middle temporal visual area. *Proceedings of the National Academy of Sciences of the USA*, *103*(46), 17490-17495.

In: Advances in Visual Perception Research
Editor: Thomas Heinen

ISBN: 978-1-63482-455-2
© 2015 Nova Science Publishers, Inc.

Chapter 10

The Error-Correction Process – A Heuristic Concept

Damian Jeraj[1,2,*]***, Linda Hennig***[1] ***and Thomas Heinen***[1]
[1]University of Hildesheim, Germany
[2]German Sport University Cologne, Germany

Abstract

In sport and training situations, augmented feedback is commonly used to improve the performance of athletes. Especially in sports such as artistic gymnastics, figure skating or trampoline gymnastics, coaches use augmented feedback procedures to guide athletes' attention with the aim of highlighting particular movement errors that occurred in the performance of sport-specific skills. Prior to the generation of a particular feedback the coach (visually) observes and perceives a skill, compares the skill performance at hand with a particular target performance, and detects one or more particular errors as well as their causes. Since the mentioned process highly relies on information from coaches' visual perception system, factors influencing the visual perception of (sport-specific) skills are likely to influence the error correction process. It is argued, that in particular (a) visual perspective, (b) visual experience, (c) motor experience, (d) coach-athlete interaction, (e) methodical knowledge and (f) biomechanical knowledge influence the error correction process in sports. Evidence on the factors just mentioned is summarized and discussed. Conclusions are drawn and implications for future work are given.

Keywords: feedback factors, coach, sport, gymnastics

* Corresponding author; CeLeB, University of Hildesheim, Universitätsplatz 1, 31141 Hildesheim, Germany. Email: damian.jeraj@uni-hildesheim.de.

Introduction

In sport and training situations, augmented feedback is commonly used to improve the performance of one or several athletes (Arkaev & Suchilin, 2004; Schmidt & Lee, 2011). Other aims of augmented feedback are guiding the attention of an athlete, highlighting specific aspects of a movement or naming errors and their solutions, especially in technical oriented sports like trampoline gymnastics, figure skating or artistic gymnastics (Arkaev & Suchilin, 2004; Shiavon, Heinen, Coelho Bortoleto, Nunomura, & de Toledo, 2014). Particularly with regard to demonstrated movements in competitions, the significance of qualitative feedback given in training situations is evident. The more accurate the demonstration of the technique of a particular skill, the higher the score of the judges and finally the ranking. It is obvious that correct feedback during training situations is essential for the athlete to perform as effectively as possible. A main question that remains, however, is where are the possibilities to influence or adjust this process, and what factors can improve the feedback as a result of the error-correction process?

In order to enlighten the error-correction process, first, let us take a closer look at a specific example: Imagine a gymnastics competition where a female athlete is presenting a routine on the balance beam and you (as a coach) are standing a few metres away observing the situation. You know that the next element that she will present is a cartwheel (see Figure 1 for an illustration). At the starting point, everything looks fine and she begins performing the cartwheel. She moves from her feet over her two hands to her first foot but then, she can barely put her second foot on the balance beam and afterwards she falls down. Physically, she looks fine, but she made a small error, resulting in a low score for her routine. What would your advice for her be, if you were the person able to guide her in order to avoid such an error in the future? First, you will probably try to understand what happened and start to analyze the information you perceived during the situation. As you are not alone in the gymnasium and the volume level is high, you most likely have to rely on visual information only. You compare the target movement in your head with the actual movement information. If this information matches, the movement should have been performed without errors. However, at some point during the actual movement execution, shortly before her second foot touches the balance beam, a slight angle in her hip catches your attention. The angle in her hip does not match your target movement. Could this be the reason for the mistake? If so, you might think about mechanical links between this impression and the mistake. Is it possible that such a hip angle can produce a fall from the beam? Or is it more likely that the gymnast just did not produce enough kinetic energy, which in turn forced her to fall? This is a crucial factor in your analysis, as it would shape the feedback you will give her in the training process. You are not sure if there exist more reasons for such a fall, but in each case, you will adapt your feedback to help her avoiding such mistakes in the future.

The Error-Correction Process

In a more general regard, let us look at the steps of such an information process (Jeraj, Veit, Heinen, & Raab, in press): The coach (1) observes the movement, (2) perceives the movement, (3) does an actual–target comparison, (4) detects the (movement) error(s),

(5) detects the cause(s) of the (movement) error(s), and (6) gives feedback to one or more athletes (see Figure 2).

In the first two steps of the above-mentioned process (observation and perception of the movement) the coach does not only see the movement but he also may use auditory information or even tactile information when for example using manual guidance. The dominant information source that is used may be situation-dependent. Nevertheless, all perceived information leads to a judgment of the movement. The key points of the performed movement are compared with the target movement (Bless, Fiedler, & Strack, 2004; Plessner & Haar, 2006). As an expert, the coach knows the rules and technical regularities of the observed movement allowing for a direct comparison of the actual and the target movement. In the next steps, the coach tries to detect the error in the performance and its probable cause, based on further knowledge, such as mechanical principles. This clearly distinguishes the current error-correction process from a pure judgment process. Finally, the coach provides feedback to the athlete to focus the athlete's attention on the steps within the movement prior to the error, or just provides positive reinforcement of the movement if it was already correct.

The process just described should be seen as an idealization of the error-correction-process in sports. In some cases and depending on the coach, the athlete, and the situation, certain steps may be skipped, such as when a coach does not care about errors and their causes, and instead directly generates feedback. And it should also be remarked that this process is time discrete, meaning that steps within the process could be repeated during an observed movement. Furthermore, it is also possible that the perception of the movement influences the steps of the process and vice versa; the perceived information of the movement leads to a specific processing and the processing leads to a specific perception.

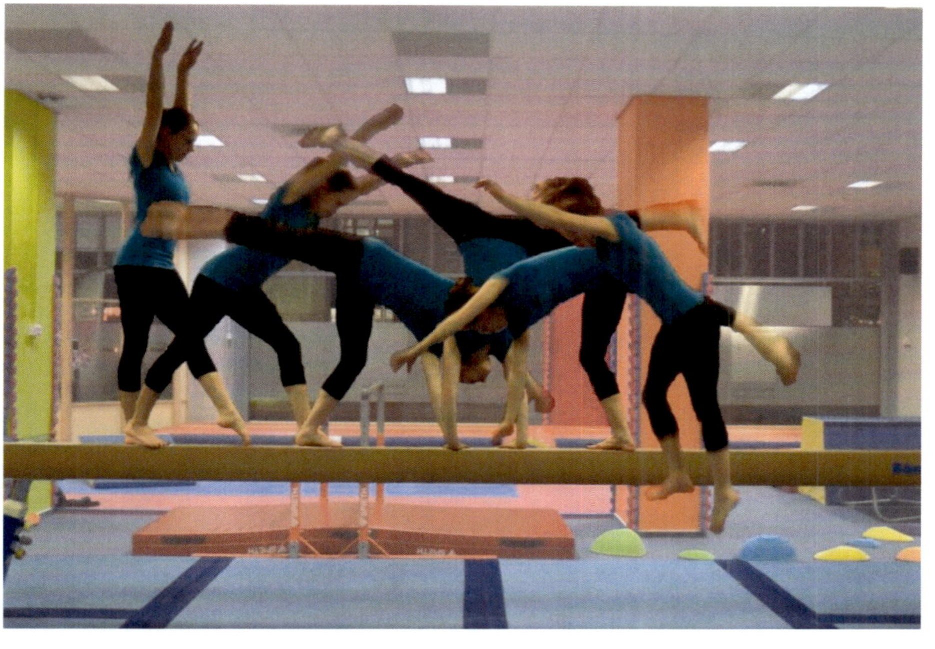

Figure 1. The movement example used within this manuscript: A female gymnast performs a cartwheel on the balance beam. The illustration highlights the coaches' point of view, which is orthogonal to the movement plane. The gymnast's movement direction is from left to right.

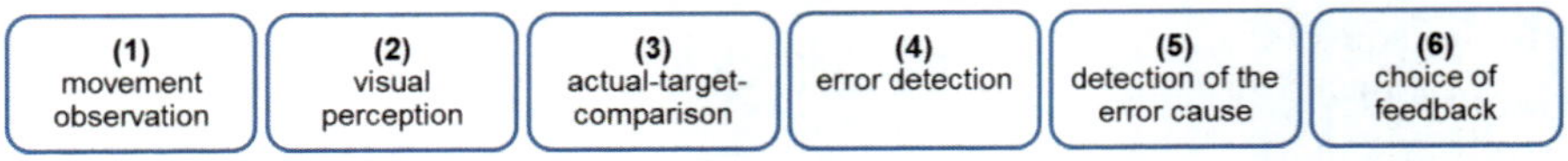

Figure 2. Illustration of the different steps of an idealized error-correction process in sport on the basis of the observation of a coach.

Following this thought, the observation situation could have an impact on the error-correction process, in a way that different tasks lead to different feedback. The coach's performance observation may differ when judging a competition performance in contrast to watching a training session, consequently changing the given feedback. The simple difference of the situation might change the aims and could also change the gaze behavior of a coach.

Literature so far, is not conclusive as to the specific factors influencing or changing error-correction processes in coaches. Hancock and Ste-Marie (2013) asked for instance thirty referees to observe ice hockey videos and judge whether the video showed a penalty or not. The referees were divided a priori into two groups with different levels (*n = 15 higher-level* and *n = 15 lower-level ice hockey referees*). During the decision task, the participants were equipped with an eye-tracking measurement device and the decision accuracy as well as the decision sensitivity was analyzed. Results revealed significantly higher accuracy and sensitivity decision of the higher-level referees. Interestingly, however, gaze behavior did not differentiate between the two expertise levels. Although there is a general remark that one can show differences in the gaze behavior from persons with different expertise levels (Gegenfurtner, Lethinen, & Säljö, 2011). Hancock and Ste-Marie (2013) concluded that higher-level referees exhibit more effective information processing as compared to lower-level referees. This could go along with indifferences in gaze behaviour between the two experimental groups because the decision process in their study could elapse on a higher cognitive level. In contrast, one can also assume that higher-level and lower-level referees do not differ in gaze behavior because they had the same very specific task (Cohen & Ebbesen, 1979). In other words, it could be possible that this specific task leads to the same gaze behavior because the variability of this behavior is constrained by the task. In order to enlighten this point, future research could address this issue by analyzing gaze behavior in different tasks during the same video clip.

Feedback Factors

Besides such a likely influence of the task during the error-correction process, one could assume that there are more factors, which could influence the error-correction process. This in turn leads to an influence on feedback, because feedback is usually given to the athlete at the end of the aforementioned process. Based on Bless, Fiedler, and Strack's concept of a judgment process, each step of this information process is susceptible to error(s) or changes (Bless, Fiedler, & Strack, 2004; Plessner & Haar, 2006). As mentioned above, the similarity of an error-correction process and a judgment process leads to the assumption that some of the biases stated in the literature could be transferred to the error-correction process (Jeraj, Veit, Heinen, & Raab, in press). These biases refer to the following aspects: (a) visual perspective, (b) visual experience, (c) motor experience, (d) coach-athlete interaction, (e) methodical knowledge, and (f) biomechanical knowledge. In the next few paragraphs, empiricial evidence on the aspects just mentioned is highlighted and their implications for the error-correction process in sports are discussed.

Visual Perspective

For example, two studies investigated the influence of the point of view on the accuracy of observed gymnastic elements (Dallas, Mavidis, & Chairopoulou, 2011; Plessner & Schallies, 2005). In the study of Plessner and Schallies (2005), $n = 40$ judges and $n = 40$ laypeople were asked to evaluate photographs of the gymnastic element *cross on rings*, which were taken from different point of views. All participants had to generate a value of the angle between the arms of each gymnast on each photograph and the horizontal axis. The authors found that both groups were influenced by their point of view, albeit the experienced judges were significantly less influenced than the laypeople. The further away from the orthogonal point of view the higher the error rate of the perceived angle was. Dallas, Mavidis, and Chairopoulou (2011) chose a similar approach. $N = 16$ judges scored photographs of the gymnastic element *inverted cross on rings*, which were taken from different perspectives. All participants had to evaluate the angle between the arms of each photograph and the horizontal axis in a similar way like in the previous study, resulting in three error deviation ranges. The authors stated that judge's score was influenced by their point of view and by the presented angles. In sum, one can assume that an orthogonal view on a movement is not sufficient enough, since different aspects of a movement were perceived in different ways. The two mentioned studies only used photographs for the judgment processes. Transferred to a real setting and assuming that aspects and angles a coach wants to regard changes during the movement observation, this leads to the conclusion that the perspective a coach should take is not clear.

Returning to our example from the beginning, your original point of view is that you are on the side of the balance beam, meaning orthogonal to the movement direction and orthogonal to the movement plane. Let us imagine that you would have the possibility to watch the cartwheel from different points of view. Thus, perhaps standing at the end of the balance beam, it would be easier to perceive the lower and upper extremities of the gymnast during the cartwheel performance and to perceive if this movement is demonstrated in a straight plane. Additionally, you would be able to perceive if your gymnast bends at the hip, which as you earlier identified as the main error leading to the fall. However it would be harder to perceive if your gymnast touches the balance beam at the optimal points because the gymnast themselves hide the grasps with their following touches making the distances of these touching points harder to estimate. These examples, clearly illustrate that a different point of view can lead to a different analysis of the movement, hence leading to different feedback.

Visual Experience

Another study addressed the influence of visual experience on a judging process (Heinen, Vinken, & Velentzas, 2012). They asked 23 judges with visual experience and 23 laypeople with motor experience to rate video clips of a handspring on vault. All judges reported that they cannot perform a handspring on vault but all of them have approximately 8 years of (visual) experience in judging gymnastics. All laypeople were able to perform a handspring on vault but none of them had (visual) experience in judging gymnastics. The results showed a significant difference in the rating, i.e. judges tended to rate the movements about one point higher than the laypeople, even though the overall pattern of results showed similar ratings in both groups. In addition, the authors analyzed if there was a relation between the participant's scores and either to time-discrete kinematic parameters or to form-aspects of the handspring. They concluded that specific visual experience is closely connected to time-discrete parameters. An argument for the influence of visual experience might lie in the experience of watching a large number of specific gymnastics movements. A further possible explanation could be that the visual experience leads to specific visual gaze behavior, i.e. longer fixation on relevant areas in combination with fewer fixation points, which might lead to a better extraction of time-discrete information (Heinen, Vinken, & Velentzas, 2012; Page, 2009). Taken together both explanations, it seems likely that visual experience affects the error-correction process.

Returning to the balance beam example, imagine that you would have the possibility to watch thousands of cartwheels from different gymnasts. This would most likely change your ideal cartwheel target. This, in effect, allows for a better comparison between the perceived and the ideal cartwheel, as you have a better identification of key points and classifications of the observed movement. In the end, again, expertise of visual experience might enable you to provide your athlete(s) with better feedback.

Motor Experience

The influence of motor experience of a judgment process was addressed in a study of Pizzera (2012). She investigated the role of a specific motor experience in gymnastics for judging an element on the balance beam. She asked $N = 58$ gymnastics judges to rate video clips of the named gymnastic skill. She divided the judges into two groups, with and without motor experience of this specific gymnastic element. Her results show that a specific motor experience leads to a better judging performance and she assumes that these specific experiences are used to identify and categorize specific movements. Furthermore, Pizzera shows with a review that field of embodied cognition (motor experience and visual experience) should be implemented in order to understand how expertise is built and how this influences judgments like during an error-correction process (Pizzera, in press). Pizzera and Raab (2012) realized an intervention study where they induced motor and visual experience of $N = 40$ participants. Participants either had to learn fake fouls during training or to watch those training sessions. Afterwards, the authors reported a slight effect on decision-making performance (accuracy and reaction time) in posttest and retention test, but a more stable performance of the motor group. One can assume according to those mentioned studies (Heinen, Vinken, & Velentzas, 2012; Pizzera, 2012; Pizzera, in press; Pizzera & Raab, 2012) that it seems to be clear that motor experience influences the error-correction process. But it is still unclear how specific the motor experience has to be in order to show a specific effect.

Regarding the example from the beginning, let us imagine that you would have the possibility to perform thousands cartwheels by your own. This would maybe change your ideal target cartwheel in your brain and you are better in a comparison of the perceived and the target cartwheel because you know better to identify the key points and to classify the observed movement with your target movement. The effect would be that you are able to give a more helpful feedback than when you don't have such a motor experience.

Coach-Athlete Interaction

The research field of a coach-athlete interaction is already widely investigated. For example, the behavior of coaching and its effects are shown, as well as influences on motivational aspects (Din & Paskevich, 2013; Mageau & Vallerand, 2003) but as far as the current state tells, only little is known about influences of the coach-athlete interaction. Especially in regard to error-correction situations, this point reaches a higher importance. Subsequent studies investigating situations from an athlete's point of view and from a coach's point of view, show that the pictures of coaches and athletes differ (Lorimer & Jowett, 2011; Macqueta & Stanton, 2014). A similar mechanism based on such made interactions could lead to a positive or a negative influence for an error-correction situation or even medalists (Jowett & Cockerill, 2003). More specifically, two directions of the influence are possible: If the coach pays specific attention to parts of the athlete's movement, he or she does this because he or she anticipates a movement error based on the past interactions between coach and athlete. This could be very helpful to ensure that this error is well perceivable and with such an approach the feedback could be addressed effectively in relation to this specific error. But as a second result the coach could be insensitive for further errors or further movement aspects, which would lead to a more appropriate feedback.

Returning to the example from the beginning, let us imagine that you remember very well that your gymnast performed within her learning process of the cartwheel several trials where she did a little error in the middle part of the cartwheel resulting in a complete fall (like in Fig. 1) and you know that this error is caused during her hand support, which is the reason that your attention is focused to the estimated hand touch on the balance beam. But when you focus her hands you can't perceive very well other aspects of the movement for the same time. It would be hard to perceive if she is performing the cartwheel still in a straight manner. It is hard to say from a scientific point of view how you should focus your attention in order to perceive most of the possible errors, one possibility is to focus a central point in order to perceive a greater attention breadth (Hüttermann, Memmert, Simonas, & Bock, 2013). But one can assume that a different gaze behavior could lead to a different error-correction as mentioned above, and here, this is based on the past interaction of coach and athlete.

Methodical Knowledge

Relating to an error-correction situation, one can easily differentiate between methodical and biomechanical knowledge (see next section). Methodical knowledge comprises the details, approaches and principles, which build the learning steps for a specific movement or interaction. The authors Cloes, Premuzak, and Pieron (1995) stated that it is necessary to have a similar knowledge level (when comparing feedback of two judges) to give appropriate feedback to the athlete(s). They used an intervention pre-posttest design to investigate effects of a video feedback training (Cloes, Denève, & Piéron, 1995). As a result the participants of the treatment group ($n = 10$) reached a higher level of specific knowledge and identified more errors than the participants of the control group ($n = 8$). This shows that the influence of knowledge is present and important during a judgment or error-correction process. Transferred to the methodical knowledge, it seems plausible to assume that a higher knowledge level of methodical aspects helps to provide effective and appropriate feedback.

Regarding the example from the beginning, let us imagine that you would have the possibility to train again with your athlete for a while and your aim is to avoid the presented error. You are pretty sure that she made this error because she was afraid to fall down. This would change your feedback totally in comparison to when she would not be afraid because you know that you have to use a different approach to help your gymnast that she can avoid such a fall. And based on the different solving strategy, you should adapt also the feedback.

Biomechanical Knowledge

The influence of biomechanical knowledge is also based on the study of Cloes, Premuzak, and Pieron (1995). In comparison to the methodical knowledge, a biomechanical knowledge especially in gymnastics is important because here, forecasts of the angle-time histories for the movement and the physical understanding of the movement function is present for almost all training and competition situations (Irwin, Williams, & Kerwin, 2014). Transferred to the error-correction process, the relation between biomechanics, type of error, and visible error is strong (Hughes & Hodges, 2008). One can assume that for a correct identification and categorization, a coach needs also this biomechanical knowledge to provide adequate feedback to the athlete(s).

Drawing back the attention to the example from the beginning, again, let us imagine that you would have the possibility to train again with your athlete for a while and your aim is to avoid the presented error. You are pretty sure that she made this error because she produced too less angular momentum in the first phase, which later led to the complete fall down. Having this error cause in mind would change your feedback totally in comparison to the assumption that the error cause would be a curved movement direction. Based on the correct error cause you would adapt your feedback and either you are going to train the first phase of the movement or to train a straight movement direction. Here, we can see clearly the impact of different identified error causes.

Conclusion and Implications for Future Work

Regarding the feedback factors above and their influence on an error-correction process, it should be remarked that this heuristic concept gives an overview about the known relations. One can assume that there are more factors, which influence this process. In addition, these factors are probably also interrelated with each other, meaning that just for an example a higher methodoical knowledge could be based on a higher visual experience or a higher expertise level as well. But this error-correction process concept could be a starting point for future work within this research field and has the aim to build the base for identifying essential factors, which could be individually manipulated and should be considered during coaches' education programs. Overall, according to observations of coaching experts there are no precise and always working rules, which would be helpful to provide effective movement feedback to the athlete(s). Two coaches can use different approaches and use different feedback but their athlete could reach the same performance level. This approach is based on the weak scientific knowledge, which often also leads to a *trial and error* approach. The future work should focus on the particular steps or particular factors in order to examine this process and to provide clear results with explicit implications for the applied field.

Acknowledgment

We want to thank Juliane Veit for her voluntary participating in demonstrating a cartwheel on the balance beam.

References

Arkaev, L. & Suchilin, N. (2004). *How to Create Champions*. Oxford: Meyer & Meyer Sports.

Bless, H., Fiedler, K. & Strack, F. (2004). *Social Cognition: How Individuals Construct Social Reality*. New York: Psychology Press.

Cloes, M., Denève, A. & Piéron, M. (1995). Interindividual Variability of Teachers' Feedback: Study in Simulated Teaching Conditions. *European Physical Education Review*, *1*(1), 83-93.

Cloes, M., Premuzak, J. & Pieron, M. (1995). Effectiveness of a Video Training Program Used to Improve Error Identification and Feedback Processes. *International Journal of Physical Education*, *32*(3), 4-10.

Cohen, C. & Ebbesen, E. (1979). Observational Goals and Schema Activation: A Theoretical Framework for Behavior Perception. *Journal of Experimental Social Psychology*, *15*(4), 305-329.

Dallas, G., Mavidis, A. & Chairopoulou, C. (2011). Influence of Angle of View on Judges' Evaluations of Inverted Cross in Men's Rings. *Perceptual and Motor Skills*, *112*(1), 109-121.

Din, C. & Paskevich, D. (2013). An Integrated Research Model of Olympic Podium Performance. *International Journal of Sports Science and Coaching*, *8*(2), 431-444.

Gegenfurtner, A., Lethinen, E. & Säljö, R. (2011). Expertise Differences in the Comprehension of Visualizations: A Meta-analysis of Eye-tracking Research in Professional Domains. *Educational Psychology Review*, *23*(4), 523-552.

Hancock, D. J. & Ste-Marie, D. M. (2013). Gaze Behaviors and Decision Making Accuracy of Higher- and Lower-Level Ice Hockey Referees. *Psychology of Sport and Exercise*, *14*(1), 66-71.

Heinen, T., Vinken, P. M. & Velentzas, K. (2012). Judging Performance in Gymnastics: A Matter of Motor or Visual Experience? *Science of Gymnastics*, *4*(1), 63-72.

Hughes, M. & Hodges, I. M. (2008). *The Essentials of Performance Analysis.* London: Routledge.

Hüttermann, S., Memmert, D., Simonas, D. J. & Bock, O. (2013). Fixation Strategy Influences the Ability to Focus Attention on Two Spatially Separate Objects. *PLoS ONE, 8*(6), p. e65673.

Irwin, G., Williams, G. K. & Kerwin, D. G. (2014). Gymnastics Coaching and Science: Biomechanics Perspectives. In L. M. Shiavon, T. Heinen, M. A. Coelho Bortoleto, M. Nunomura, & E. de Toledo, *High Performance Gymnastics* (163-175). Hildesheim: Arête Verlag.

Jeraj, D., Veit, J., Heinen, T. & Raab, M. (in press). How Do Gymnastics Coaches Provide Movement Feedback in Gymnastics? *International Journal of Sport Science and Coaching.*

Jowett, S. & Cockerill, I. M. (2003). Olympic Medallists' Perspective of the Athlete–Coach Relationship. *Psychology of Sport and Exercise, 4*(4), 313-331.

Lorimer, R. & Jowett, S. (2011). Empathic Accuracy, Shared Cognitive Focus, and the Assumptions of Similarity Made by Coaches and Athletes. *International Journal of Sport Psychology, 42*(1), 40-54.

Macqueta, A.-C. & Stanton, N. A. (2014). Do the Coach and Athlete Have the Same "Picture" of the Situation? Distributed Situation Awareness in an Elite Sport Context. *Applied Ergonomics, 45*(3), 724-733.

Mageau, G. A. & Vallerand, R. J. (2003). The Coach-Athlete Relationship: A Motivational Model. *Journal of Sports Sciences, 21*(11), 883-904.

Page, J. L. (2009). The Development and Effectiveness of Perceptual Training Programme for Coaches and Judges in Gymnastics. (Unpublished doctoral dissertation). University of Liverpool, United Kingdom. Retrieved from http://chesterrep.openrepository.com/ cdr/bitstream/10034/118015/41/ jennifer%20page. pdf

Pizzera, A. (2012). Gymnastic Judges Benefit From Their Own Motor Experience as Gymnasts. *Research Quarterly for Exercise and Sport, 43*(4), 603-607.

Pizzera, A. (in press). The Role of Embodied Cognition in Sports Officiating. *Movement & Sport Science - Science & Motricité.*

Pizzera, A. & Raab, M. (2012). Does Motor or Visual Experience Enhance the Detection of Deceptive Movements in Football? *International Journal of Sports Science and Coaching, 7*(2), 269-284.

Plessner, H. & Haar, T. (2006). Sports Performance Judgments from a Social Cognitive Perspective. *Psychology of Sport and Exercise, 7*(6), 555-575.

Plessner, H. & Schallies, E. (2005). Judging the Cross on Rings: A Matter of Achieving Shape Constancy. *Applied Cognitive Psychology, 19*(9), 1145-1156.

Schmidt, R. A. & Lee, T. D. (2011). *Motor control and learning. A behavioral emphasis* (5th ed.). Champaign, IL: Human Kinetics.

Shiavon, L. M., Heinen, T., Coelho Bortoleto, M. A., Nunomura, M. & de Toledo, E. (2014). *High Performance Gymnastics.* Hildesheim: Arête Verlag.

In: Advances in Visual Perception Research
Editor: Thomas Heinen

ISBN: 978-1-63482-455-2
© 2015 Nova Science Publishers, Inc.

Chapter 11

Visual Perceptual Learning in Cytopathology

Andrew Evered*[*], *Darren Walker, Andrew Watt and Nick Perham

Department of Applied Psychology, Cardiff School of Health Sciences,
Cardiff Metropolitan University, Wales, UK

Abstract

Cytopathology (cytology) involves the microscopic examination of cells for the diagnosis of diseases such as cancer. Little is known about how the perceptual abilities of cytologists develop, which is the focus of research described in this chapter. The acquisition of visual skills in cytology may involve two strategies. Analytical strategies require trainees to base diagnostic decisions on exhaustive feature lists, a process that is inefficient. Non-analytical pattern recognition strategies are rarely encouraged, even though this approach is characteristic of expert diagnostic behaviour. Experiment 1 evaluated the role of non-analytical learning (*perceptual learning*) in cytopathology as an efficient alternative to analytical training. Participants' diagnostic accuracy improved significantly following both training regimens ($p < .001$) but the degree of improvement was not statistically different between the two groups ($p > .05$). Speed of response to test images was generally faster under non-analytical than under analytical conditions. Experiment 2 replicated the results of experiment 1, confirming the effectiveness of perceptual learning in cytology, but went further by investigating image difficulty and diagnostic category as independent variables. Diagnostic accuracy improved for participants who were trained on normal/abnormal image pairs in which at least one member of the pair was easy to interpret ($p < .05$). Training was not effective when images pairs were of the same diagnostic category or when both members of the pair were difficult to interpret ($p > .05$). These studies make an important contribution to the development of perceptual learning modules in cytology.

[*] Department of Biomedical Science, Cardiff School of Healthcare Science, Cardiff Metropolitan University, Llandaff Campus, 200 Western Ave, Cardiff, South Glamorgan CF5 2YB. Email: aevered@cardiffmet.ac.uk

Keywords: cytopathology, perceptual learning, visual perception, categorical perception

Introduction

What Is Cytology?

Cytology was pioneered by 20th century healthcare practitioners who realised the potential clinical benefits of visually examining suitably prepared body fluids under a microscope for signs of certain diseases (Papanicolaou & Traut, 1941; Koss, 1961; Grunze & Spriggs, 1983). The types of disease that can be investigated in this way are many and varied and include one of the most prevalent and lethal of those known to mankind: cancer. It is estimated that at least one in three people will develop some form of cancer during their lifetime and that the disease claims as many as 7.4 million lives each year across the globe (WHO, 2009). Cancer, or neoplasia, is a genetic disease that manifests at the cellular level as characteristic changes in the shape, size, texture, and density of cell nuclei (Figure 1; Evered, 2011; Vogelstein & Kinzler, 1998).

Cytology As a Medical Image Perception Problem

An image of cells viewed through a microscope is a type of medical image. Like all medical images, cell images are not self-explanatory; they have to be perceived and understood.

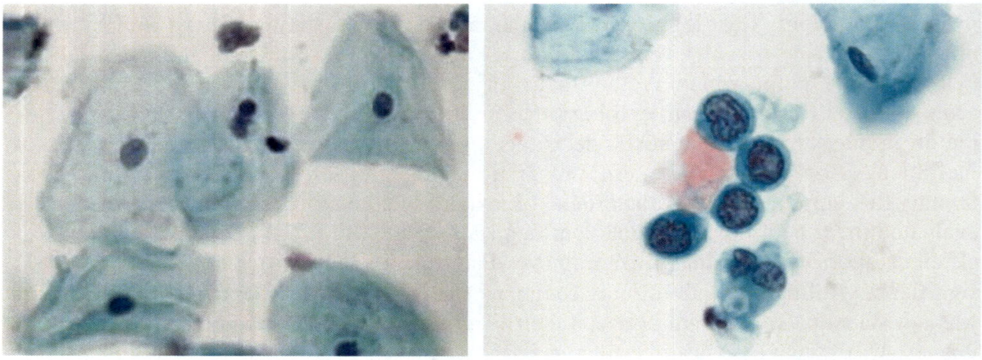

Normal cells from a human cervix. Each cell contains a relatively small, oval-shaped nucleus with a finely granular texture and a smooth outline.

At the centre of the image are four neoplastic cells from a human cervix. The nucleus of each cell is intensely stained, has an irregular outline, is coarsely granular and is disproportionately enlarged.

Figure 1. Examples of normal (left) and neoplastic cells (right).

Discovering cells that are suspicious but not diagnostic of neoplasia is not at all uncommon, and the task for the cytologist is to make a decision whether the cells are normal or neoplastic. If the cytologist reports them as normal and he is wrong, the patient might ultimately die because of delays in treatment. On the other hand, if the cells are normal and the cytologist reports neoplasia, the patient may suffer needless anxiety and undergo further unnecessary tests.

The cytologist must make a diagnostic decision, and when that decision deviates from the ground truth (i.e. the true health status of the patient) then we say that a diagnostic error has occurred. When errors occur in medical image perception tasks, the clinical consequences can be dire.

If we are to find solutions to the problem we must first elucidate the mechanisms by which cytologists acquire and maintain their visual perception skills, and we must discover the underlying causes of perceptual failure.

Cervical Cytology As a Model System for Studying Medical Image Perception

Cervical cytology has been chosen as a model system for studying medical image perception in this chapter for several reasons. First, as the primary means of screening women for precancer of the cervix, cervical cytology as an image perception problem has never been addressed empirically.

Second, cervical cytology provides a rich and abundant source of complex images from which meaningful perception experiments can be devised. Finally, the visual characteristics of normal cells and neoplastic cells lie on an ill-defined morphological spectrum (Figure 2; Frost, 1986), making cervical cytology an ideal candidate for medical image perception studies.

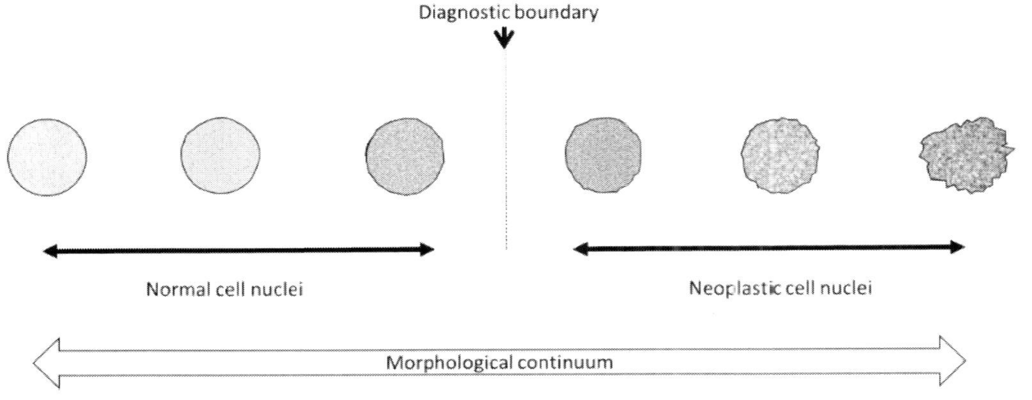

Figure 2. The morphological spectrum of normal and neoplastic cells.

How Do Cytologists Develop Their Pattern Recognition Skills?

Cytologists must learn how to visually discriminate cells that might appear very similar but have different neoplastic potential. How do these skills develop and how can this knowledge inform the design of cytology training and skill maintenance programmes? The nature of cytology expertise is poorly researched and is the focus of the experiments described below.

Experiment 1: Analytical vs. Non-Analytical Learning in Cytology

Background

Making a cytological diagnosis of neoplasia can be broken down into three separate but interdependent problems: visual search for a cellular abnormality, the recognition of one or more cells as "abnormal" in appearance, and a final decision as to whether any cells are sufficiently atypical to warrant further investigation of the patient. Cutting across each facet is the question of how cytologists develop their visual and cognitive skills with training and practice. This question is important because visual recognition and classification of abnormal cells is a subjective and error-prone task, even among highly skilled cytologists (Mitchell & Medley, 1995; Stoler & Schiffman, 2001). Surprisingly little is known about the nature of the visual learning process in cytology, which hinders the development of evidence-based training programmes (Evered, 2005).

As a fundamental contributor to human expertise, perceptual learning is rarely addressed in the cytology literature or in traditional cytology training programmes. We can start by defining perceptual learning in cytology as *experience-induced enhancements in the ability of learners to discriminate normal from neoplastic cells.* Cytology training usually involves the exhaustive application of morphological feature lists and diagnostic rules, all of which must be carefully and systematically considered before arriving at a diagnosis (City and Guilds, 2007; NHSCSP, 1995). The reasons for this highly analytical strategy are unclear but probably result from a desire to instil in students a consistent diagnostic approach and to prevent premature closure and other cognitive biases, such as anchoring, base rate neglect, expectancy and overconfidence, to name but a few (Pohl, 2004). Research in fields other than cytology indicates that perceptual learning techniques, which emphasise non-analytical strategies, can be an effective form of discrimination training. Such strategies often involve nothing more than visual exposure to a sufficient number of exemplars to induce a learning effect. Perceptual learning modules have been developed for subjects as diverse as mathematics (Kellman, Massey, & Son, 2010), aircraft pilot training (Kellman & Kaiser, 1994), surgery (Guerlain, 2004), and are of proven value in speech and language therapy (Merzenich, Jenkins, Johnstone et al., 1996). It seems curious why such a tactic is not usually considered in cytology training programmes, which, with their emphasis on the development of visual interpretation skills, would seem to be an ideal candidate for such an approach.

Although it is convenient to divide visual learning strategies into analytical and non-analytical processes, in reality they are probably not mutually exclusive and may both contribute to learning (Eva, 2005; Norman, Young, & Brooks, 2007; Pelaccia, Tardif, Triby, & Charlin, 2011). In a study by Ark et al. (2006), for instance, groups of non-medical novice observers were trained to diagnose a variety of cardiac disorders via electrocardiogram images using analytical or non-analytical reasoning strategies, or a combination of the two.

The results indicated that participants who were instructed to use both strategies performed significantly better than those who used either tactic alone (Ark, Brooks, & Eva, 2006). This approach was tested in the present experiment, the aim of which was to explore the effectiveness of non-analytical visual learning in cytology. It was hypothesised that novices who adopted a purely non-analytical reasoning strategy could achieve levels of diagnostic accuracy not inferior to that achieved using a purely analytical approach. To satisfy the dual process protagonists, an additional hypothesis was that novices instructed to adopt a combination of non-analytical and analytical reasoning would achieve diagnostic accuracy greater than those instructed to emphasise either tactic alone.

Procedure

Figure 3 illustrates a mixed design experiment. Training strategy served as the between group variable (two levels) and test number as the within-group variable (three levels).

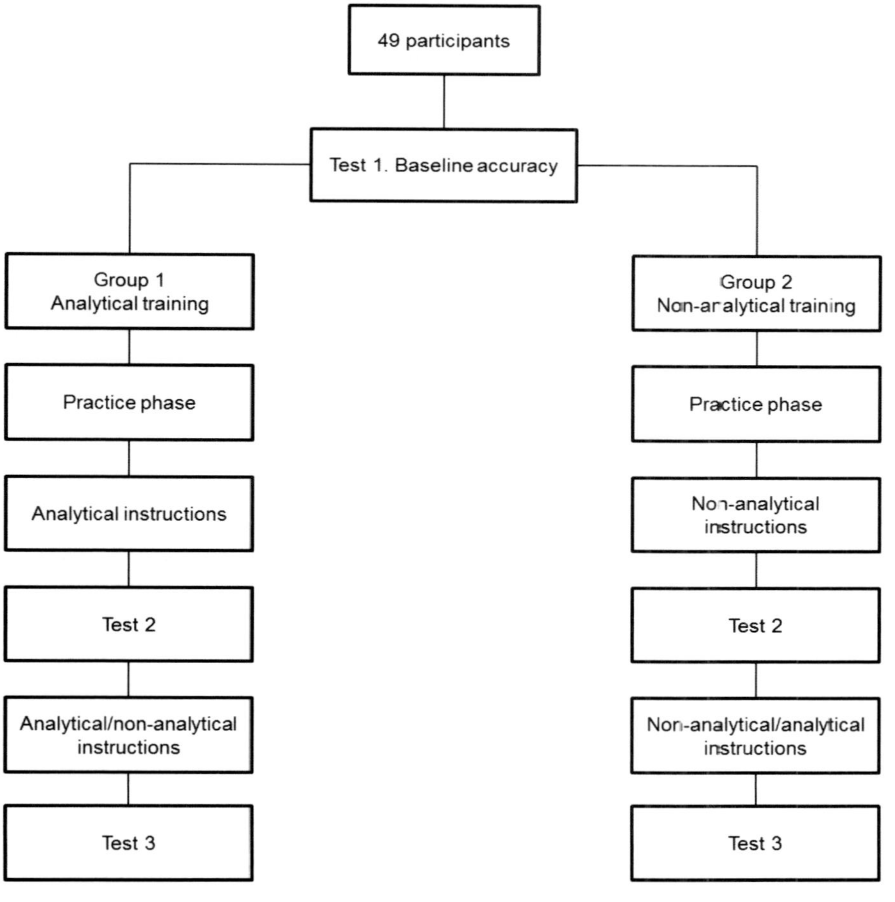

Figure 3. Diagram illustrating the design of experiment 1.

Briefly, 49 cytologically naïve participants undertook an initial cell interpretation test (test 1) to establish baseline diagnostic accuracy for untrained novice observers. The test comprised 60 cell images (30 normal and 30 abnormal) presented on a computer screen in random order via DMDX presentation software (DMDX, 2014). The ground truth diagnostic status for each image was previously established by expert consensus opinion from three trained cytologists. An example of one of the test images is shown in Figure 4.

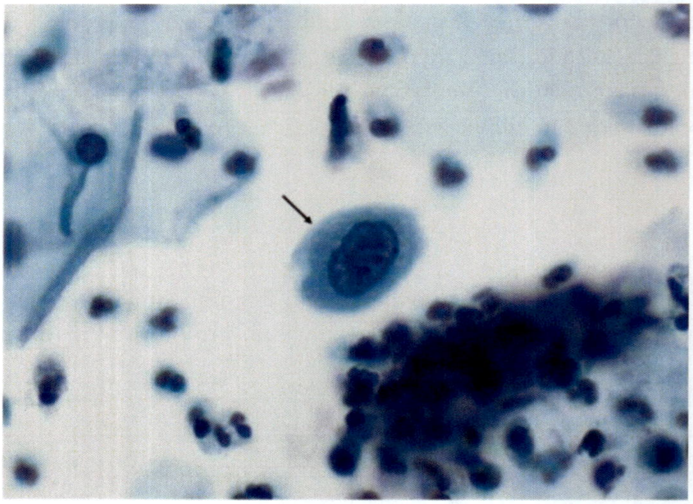

Figure 4. An example of an abnormal cell image used for testing. Participants responded "normal" or "abnormal" and provided a confidence rating on a scale of 1 (definitely normal) to 5 (definitely abnormal). The arrow indicates the relevant cell but arrows were not presented in the actual experiment.

Participants responded "normal" or "abnormal" for each test image and provided a confidence rating on a 1-to-5 ordinal scale using a computer keyboard. To test the efficiency of the decision making process, the software automatically recorded the time to respond to each test image.

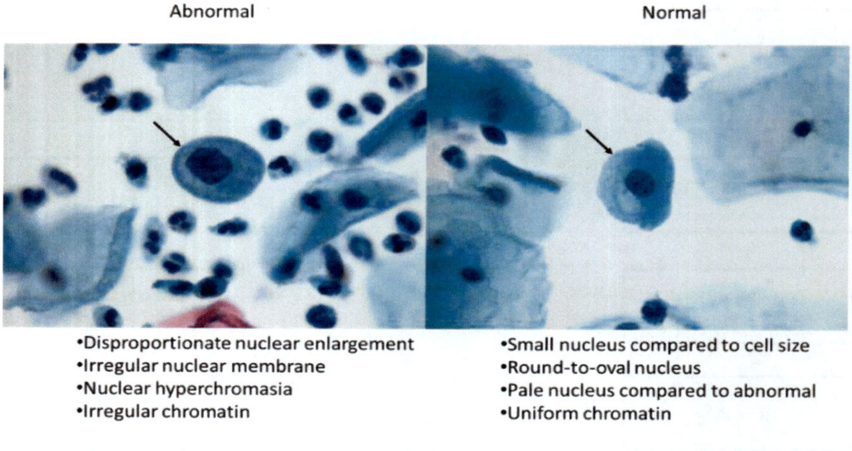

Figure 5. Example of an image-pair from the analytical training set. Cells of interest were positioned near the centre of each image. The arrows indicate the relevant cells but these were not presented in the actual experiment. To direct participants' gaze to the correct cell, each image was preceded by a visual cue.

Participants were then randomly allocated to receive either analytical training (group 1; 24 participants) or non-analytical training (group 2; 25 participants). Participants who received analytical training were taught the morphological features of normal and abnormal cells by a trained cytologist and shown 20 pairs of images on a computer screen. Each image pair comprised one normal and one abnormal cell and images were annotated with the relevant diagnostic features (see Table 1). Participants were also given a typed list of features for future reference and a full explanation of the relevant cytological terminology was provided (see Figure 5). All images were preceded by a visual cue to direct participants' gaze to the correct cell. The trainer answered all queries and clarified any points of uncertainty before proceeding further.

Table 1. List of abnormal cell features given to participants in the analytic training group

Feature
Irregular chromatin distribution
Irregular nuclear membrane
Disproportionate nuclear enlargement
Nuclear hyperchromasia
Abnormalities of the number, form and size of nucleoli
Multinucleation associated with any of the above.

Non-analytical training also comprised image-pairs but in this instance no tuition was provided and image annotation was restricted to the labels "normal" or "abnormal" (see Figure 6). The intention in this group was for participants to develop non-analytical pattern recognition skills without assistance from the trainer.

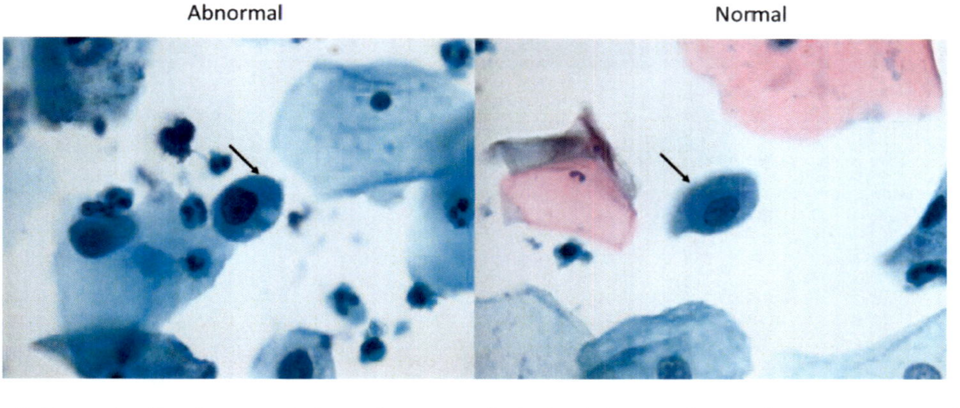

Figure 6. Example of an image-pair from the non-analytical training set. Annotations were not provided and the cells of interest were positioned near the centre of each image. The arrows indicate the relevant cells but these were not presented in the actual experiment. To direct participants' gaze to the correct cell, each image was preceded by a visual cue.

For practice, participants both groups examined a further 20 cell pairs but these were not annotated. After displaying each image, participants were instructed to make a mental note of their diagnosis and then press a computer key to see the correct answer. There was no element of performance measurement at this stage; the intention was purely to facilitate the learning process.

As in the training phase, all images were preceded by a visual cue to direct participants' gaze to the correct cell.

Following training and practice, and in preparation for test 2, participants in group 1 (the analytical training group) were instructed to base their diagnosis solely on an analysis of the cytological features observed. Participants were specifically instructed not to trust any sense of familiarity with previous images and to use only the analytical reasoning skills acquired during the training phase. Before proceeding to test 3, instructions were amended to permit participants to augment the decision making process with any non-analytical reasoning skills they may have developed during training and practice. In other words, participants were instructed to trust their sense of familiarity with previous images to amend their initial decision as necessary.

In contrast to the pre-test instructions for group 1, participants in group 2 (the non-analytical training group) were asked to provide their first impression of each image based on their similarity to images seen during training and practice. Following test 2, participants were asked to write a list of features they felt were helpful in making their diagnostic decisions. Instructions for the final test (test 3) were then modified to permit participants to augment their non-analytical reasoning strategy with their self-generated diagnostic rules and amend their initial impressions as necessary.

The dependent variables were raw error rate, area under the receiver operating characteristic (ROC) curve (AUC), *criterion* (an objective measure of observer response bias) and response time. All inferential tests were conducted using SPSS and two-sided p values of $< .05$ were considered to be statistically significant.

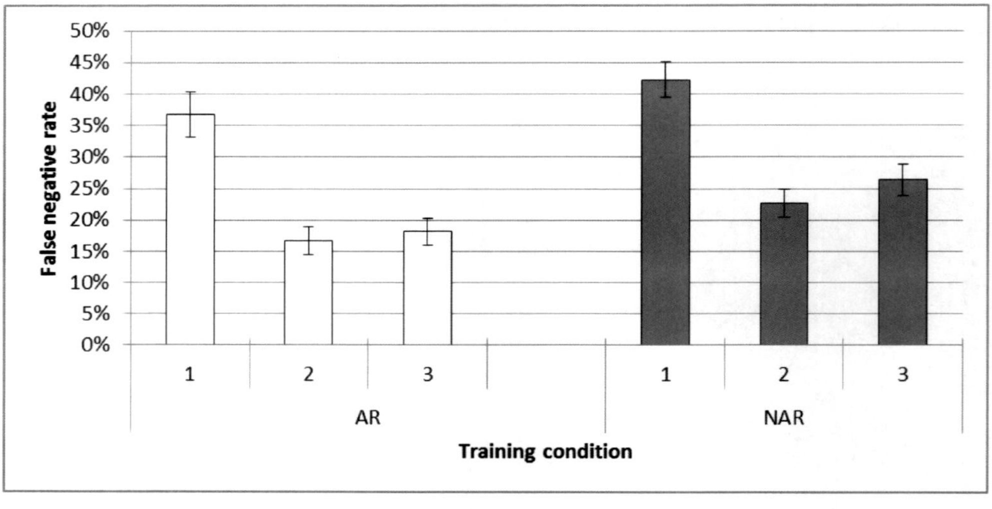

Figure 7. False negative rate as a function of training condition. Horizontal axis: tests 1, 2 and 3 under analytical reasoning (AR) and non-analytical reasoning (NAR) conditions, respectively. Error bars represent ±1 standard error of the mean.

Results

Error Rate

Pre- and post-training error rates are plotted in Figure 7 and Figure 8. The most striking changes were seen in the false negative rates. Before any training was provided (test 1) false negative rates were 36.8% and 42.3% for the analytical and non-analytical conditions, respectively.

Under both conditions, false negative rates declined dramatically to 16.7% and 22.7% following the respective training protocols (test 2). Curiously, miss errors increased to 18.2% and 26.4% in the final test, in which participants were instructed to adopt a combined analytical/non-analytical strategy.

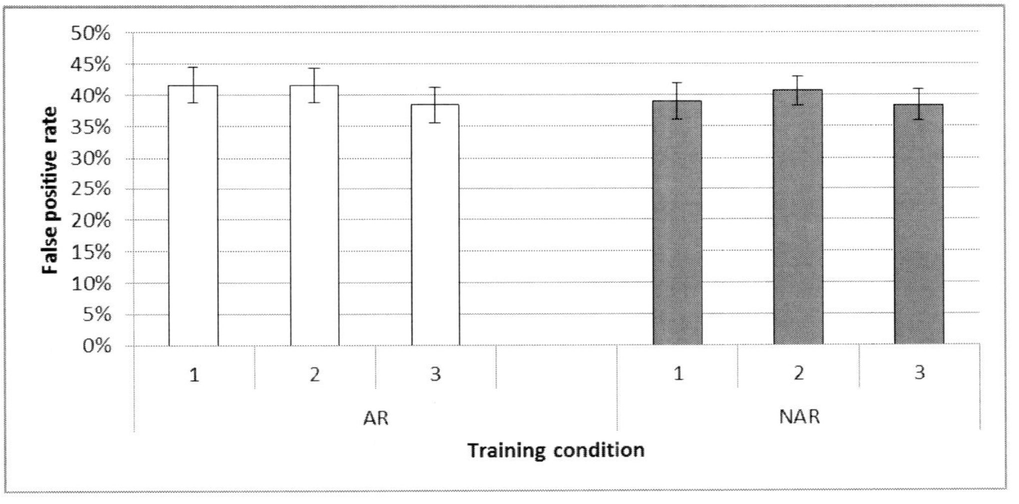

Figure 8. False positive rate as a function of training condition. Horizontal axis: tests 1, 2 and 3 under analytical reasoning (AR) and non-analytical reasoning (NAR) conditions, respectively. Error bars represent ±1 standard error of the mean.

Changes in false positive rates were less noticeable (Figure 8), dropping overall from 41.7% to 38.5% in the analytical group and from 39.1% to 38.4% in the non-analytical group.

The raw error rate data were not suitable for parametric analysis ($p < .05$, Kolmogorov-Smirnov test).

Area under the ROC Curve

Under both analytical and non-analytical conditions there was a notable increase in mean AUC between tests 1 and 2, from .603 to .744 for analytical training and from .581 to .721 for non-analytical training. For both training protocols, AUC changed only marginally between tests 2 and 3 (Figure 9).

A two-way mixed design ANOVA showed that the main effect of test number was significant ($F_{1.42,66.57} = 68.72$, $p <.001$) (Greenhouse-Geisser correction) while the main effect of training method was not significant ($F_{1,47} = 3.93$, $p = .053$). There was no significant interaction between training protocol and test number ($F_{1.42,66.57} = .51$, $p = .540$) (Greenhouse-

Geisser correction). Pairwise comparisons indicated a significant improvement in AUC between test 1 and 2 ($p < .001$) but not between test 2 and 3 ($p = .813$).

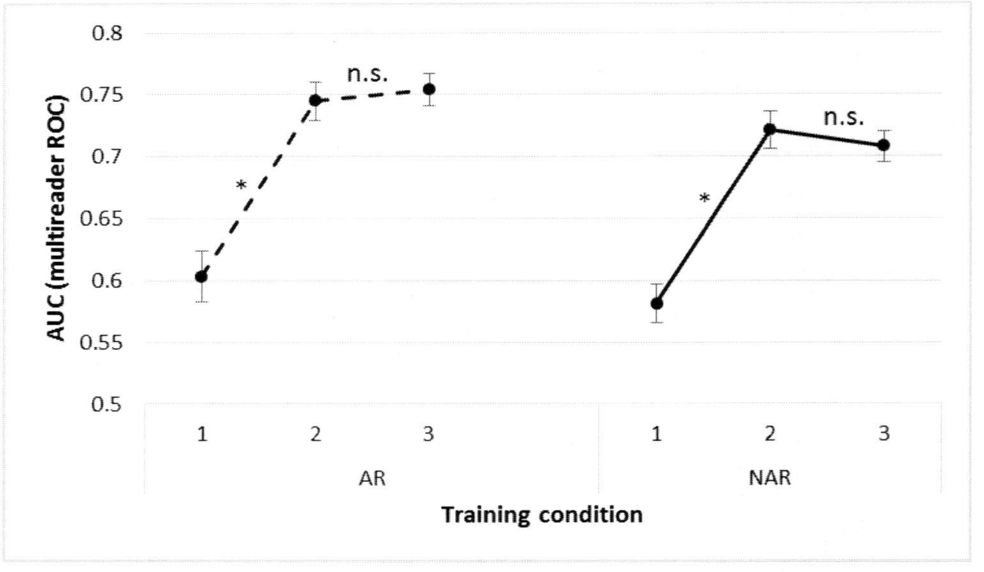

Figure 9. Multireader ROC analysis. AUC as a function of training condition. Horizontal axis: tests 1, 2 and 3 under analytical reasoning (AR) and non-analytical reasoning (NAR) conditions, respectively. Error bars represent ±1 standard error of the mean. * $p < .001$, n.s. not significant.

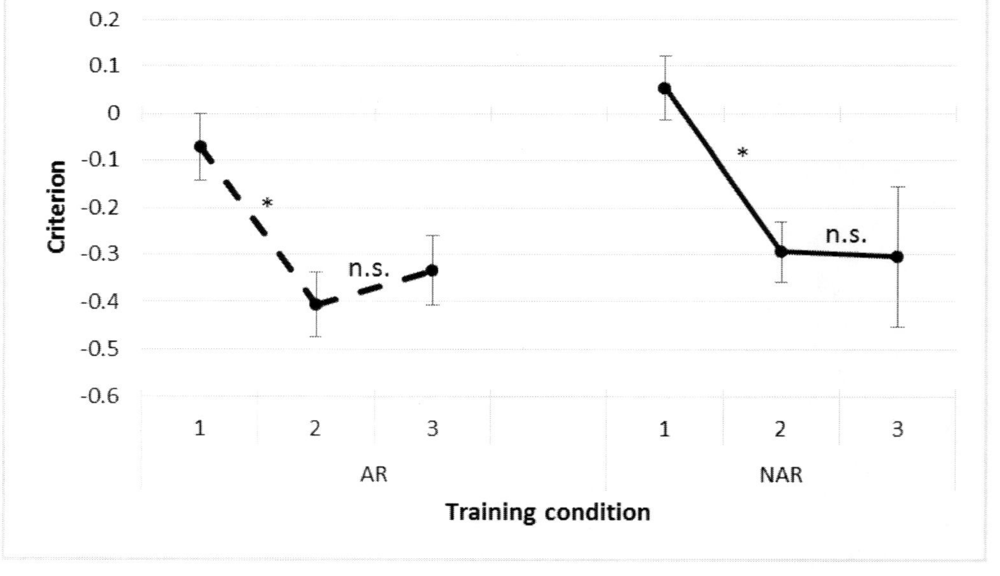

Figure 10. Changes in criterion with condition. Horizontal axis: tests 1, 2 and 3 under analytic reasoning (AR) and non-analytic reasoning (NAR) conditions, respectively. Vertical axis: criterion is devoid of units and only relative values are important. Error bars represent ±1 standard error of the mean. *$p < .001$, n.s. not significant.

Criterion

Criterion decreased markedly between tests 1 and 2 under bcth analytical and non-analytical conditions, from -.072 to -.406 for analytical training and from .053 to -.294 for non-analytical training.

This was followed by a small increase between tests 2 and 3 under analytical conditions and a small decrease under non-analytical conditions (Figure 10). The magnitude of the *criterion* shifts was similar in both groups.

A two-way mixed design ANOVA showed a significant main effect of test number ($F_{1.56,73.47} = 11.57$, $p < .001$) (Greenhouse-Geisser correction), a non-significant main effect of training method ($F_{1,47} = 1.29$, $p = .262$) and there was no significant interaction between training method and test number, $F_{1.56,73.47} = 0.16$, $p = .802$) (Greenhouse-Geisser correction). Pairwise comparisons showed that the *criterion* shifts between test 1 and test 2 were highly significant ($p < .001$), while those between test 2 and test 3 were not significant ($p = .579$).

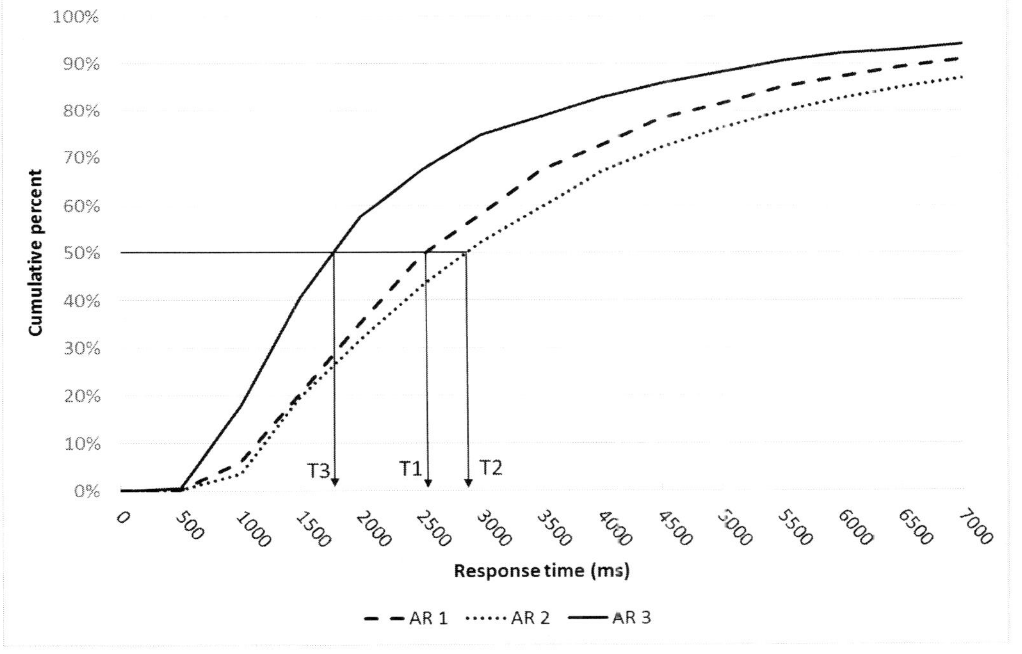

Figure 11. Cumulative distribution functions for response times in tests 1(T1), 2(T2) and 3(T3) under analytical (AR) conditions.

Response time

In the analytical training group the median time for participants to respond "normal" or "abnormal" to each image increased from 2523ms to 2887ms between tests 1 and 2 (Fehler! Verweisquelle konnte nicht gefunden werden. and Figure 12). Response times in the non-analytical group were notably lower than the analytical group for the first two tests (2114ms and 1899ms respectively). However, response times essentially equalised by the final test (1744ms and 1886ms for the analytical and non-analytical groups, respectively).

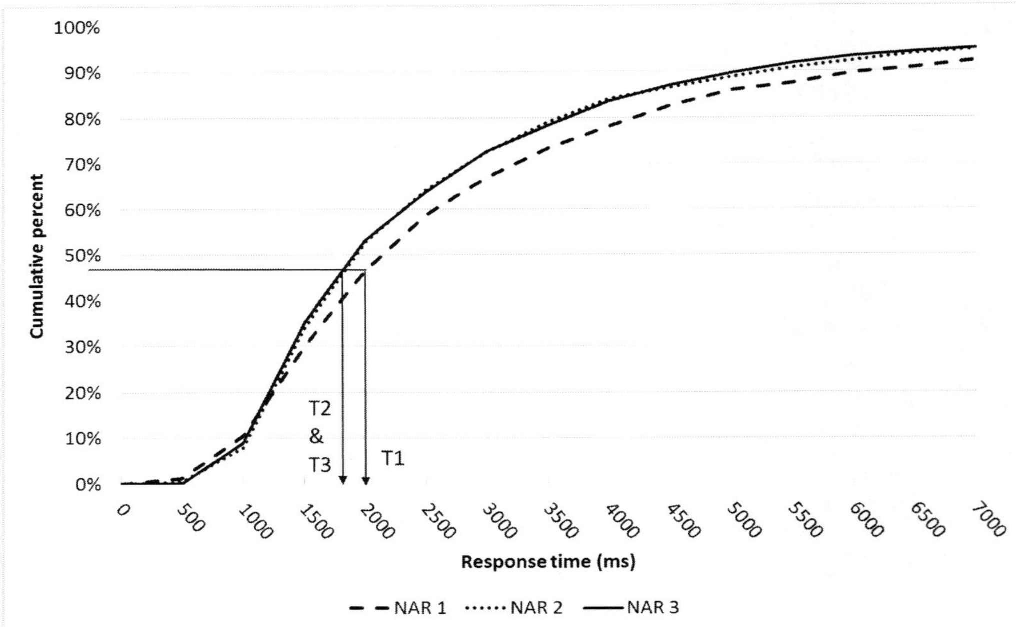

Figure 12. Cumulative distribution functions for response times in tests 1 (T1), 2(T2) and 3(T3) under non-analytical (NAR) conditions.

Response time data deviated significantly from normality ($p < .001$, Kolmogorov-Smirnov test), rendering standard parametric statistical testing problematic. Several types of data transformation and filtering, including inverse transformation, square root, logarithms and removal of potentially spurious response times, failed to correct the non-Gaussian data ($p < .001$, Kolmogorov-Smirnov test). More advanced analytical methods based on hierarchical modelling of whole response time distributions are available but these are mathematically complex, difficult to interpret and not widely employed in cognitive psychology research (Leber, Lechak, & Tower-Richardi, 2013; Rouder, Speckman, Sun, & Jiang, 2005; Whelan, 2008). The significance of the response time data in this experiment must therefore remain speculative.

Features of Abnormal Cells Generated by Participants in the Non-Analytical Training Group

Table 2 summarises the features that participants in the non-analytical group claimed were helpful in identifying abnormal cells, together with the frequency with which they were quoted. Although written in layman's terms, the morphological descriptions are surprisingly similar to the standard list of features provided by the trainer to the analytical training group.

Discussion

The experiment showed that perceptual (non-analytical) learning is comparable to traditional analytical approaches to cytology training, in terms of its contribution to the development of visual interpretation skills in novice observers. The training phase of the non-analytical arm of the experiment involved presenting participants with randomly selected pairs of normal and abnormal cell images without providing diagnostic features lists or any other form of tutor-led training.

Table 2. Features of abnormal cells generated by participants in the non-analytical training group

Features	Total number of occasionsfeature was quoted as 'helpful'.
"Dark nucleus"	15
"Irregularly shaped nucleus"	14
"Large nucleus"	11
"Irregular cell shape"	10
"Spots / blotches / rough texture in nucleus"	7
"Disproportionate nucleus / small cytoplasm"	6
"Joining of cells"	5
"More than one nucleus"	4
"Large cell"	4
"Dark cytoplasm"	4
"Nucleus sometimes lighter than cytoplasm"	2
"Splitting of nucleus"	1
"Spots in cytoplasm"	1
"Pale cytoplasm"	1

The improved performance took the form of a decline in false negatives without any noticeable increases in false positives. The increase in AUC and decrease in *criterion* between tests 1 and 2 are consistent with improvements in the ability of participants to discriminate between normal and abnormal cells and a corresponding shift to a more liberal threshold for reporting images as abnormal. This pattern of results is not entirely unexpected. When participants become aware of the features of abnormal cells, discrimination should improve alongside a greater readiness to report cellular abnormalities. The non-significant *criterion* shift between test 2 and 3 indicated a stabilisation of decision threshold as participants became increasingly confident in their diagnostic abilities.

What is perhaps more surprising is that improvements in diagnostic performance did not require intensive rule-based training, thus supporting the hypothesis that a non-analytical reasoning strategy can achieve levels of diagnostic accuracy equal to that achieved using a purely analytical approach. Moreover, the response time data suggest that non-analytical strategies are more efficient than rule-based training. This finding is encouraging because rule-based training in cytology is time-consuming and labour intensive. Given the noninferior performance of non-analytical strategies, their incorporation into cytology training and skill maintenance programmes might be of tremendous benefit to cytology services and could shorten training times considerably. In the UK for instance, non-medical trainees are mandated to attend an intensive four-week introductory course followed by two years of closely supervised screening of a minimum of 5000 cytology slides (City and Guilds, 2007; NHSCSP, 1995). Although it is difficult to estimate the full costs of this labour-intensive activity for the whole of the UK cervical screening programme, they are no doubt considerable. While no cytologist would argue against the need for thorough preparation of cytology trainees, any evidence-based strategy that offers the potential for reducing training times whilst achieving the same outcome should be taken very seriously.

The deterioration in diagnostic performance between tests 2 and 3 under the non-analytical training conditions, although not statistically significant, is worthy of discussion. Other researchers have noted an improved performance when observers are instructed to combine analytical and non-analytical reasoning strategies (Ark, Brooks, & Eva, 2006), but participants in both training groups showed a marginal decline in AUC in the final test. The hypothesis that a combined non-analytical/analytical reasoning strategy can achieve diagnostic accuracy greater than that employing either method alone is therefore not supported. Participant boredom and/or fatigue could have contributed to the decline in performance during the final test, but an alternative explanation is the possibility that participants were confused by the instructions given just prior to the test. It is acknowledged that the meaning and validity of an instruction to "combine" analytical and non-analytical reasoning might not have been entirely clear to participants, and in any case practitioners are unlikely to consciously do this in practice. Such explanations must of course remain speculative until further studies of this nature are undertaken.

While the focus of the experiment was on diagnostic accuracy, the opportunity was taken to gather response time data to gauge the efficiency of each training modality. Although the interpretation and meaning of response times is uncertain, several investigators propose that short response times (generally less than one second), at least among experts, indicate rapid non-analytical cognitive processing (Norman et al., 2007; Kundel, Nodine, Conant, & Weinstein, 2007). The results of this study support the notion that novices can also respond very quickly to complex visual scenes, with generally quicker response times noted under non-analytical reasoning conditions than under analytical conditions. Importantly, the fast response times did not appear to be at the expense of diagnostic accuracy.

The results generally support a long history of theories generated mainly in the cognitive psychology and radiology literature that put rapid visual perceptual processing at the heart of expert performance and how it develops (Ahissar & Hochstein, 2004; Lesgold, Rubinson, Feltovic et al., 1988; Mackworth & Morandi, 1967; Neisser, 1967). The data fit well with such theories and for the first time it has been demonstrated that cytopathology has much in common with radiology with regard to visual learning. Furthermore, the experiment has shown that the ability of novices to assess, rapidly and accurately, complex cytology images appears to develop very early in the learning process. Indeed, the list of morphological criteria generated spontaneously by naive observers in this experiment was surprisingly similar to those appearing in cytology textbooks and atlases. The similarities between the standard criteria listed in Table 1 and those produced by naive participants in Table 2 are readily apparent. This experiment has clearly demonstrated that inexperienced observers were able to generate diagnostic criteria without assistance from an expert trainer and with minimal exposure to cytology images, a finding that has important implications for cytology training programmes.

Experiment 2: Further Development of the Non-Analytical Learning Paradigm

Background

This experiment developed the perceptual learning theme further by exploring whether exposure to paired cell images of different levels of interpretive difficulty influences the acquisition of cytopathology image interpretation skills. Training on stimuli at different levels of discrimination difficulty is an interesting concept that has been investigated by several researchers, but with mixed results (Fahle, 2005; Garcia, Kuai, & Kourtzi, 2013; Liu & Weinshall, 2000; Sagi, 2011; Wright & Zhang, 2009). An additional aim was to investigate the relative importance of pairing images from different diagnostic categories (i.e. normal vs. abnormal cells) compared with same-category image pairs (i.e. normal cell pairs and abnormal cell pairs).

A closer examination of perceptual learning theory is required to understand the basis for the experiment. Dating back at least to Gibson and Gibson's seminal paper on the subject, (Gibson & Gibson, 1955) the idea that perceptual learning takes place at a "low level" of cortical information processing has prevailed.

In other words, simple visual stimuli such as object orientation, edges, contrast and brightness are selected and processed in the primary visual cortex and learning takes place at this level. An alternate view is that perceptual learning occurs at a "high level" of processing in a way that permits the recognition of objects as coherent wholes rather than by their component parts (Mollon & Danilova, 1996). Contemporary theorists contend that the low vs. high level argument is too simplistic to explain the wide variety of perceptual learning phenomena observed empirically.

Today, cognitive scientists are more inclined to propose a unified theory of perceptual learning, in which learning occurs at a number of different levels of processing, with "higher" levels playing a role in adjusting the processing at "lower" levels (Kellman & Garrigan, 2009). The key concept is that of a "salience hierarchy" in which obvious features are learned first followed by less salient features that require more effort and an extended period of learning.

In these terms, the goal of perceptual learning is to increase the salience of features that were previously not noticeable. Perhaps the best known multilevel model of perceptual learning is Reverse Hierarchy Theory (RHT), which asserts that perceptual learning is a top-down guided process (Ahissar & Hochstein, 2004).

In simple terms, object recognition is said to occur at a high level (i.e. rapidly and holistically) wherever possible, but when these processes do not suffice, learning occurs at increasingly lower levels, sometimes at the level of basic visual stimuli such as line orientations and the edges of objects. In a cytological context, RHT is represented diagrammatically in Figure 13.

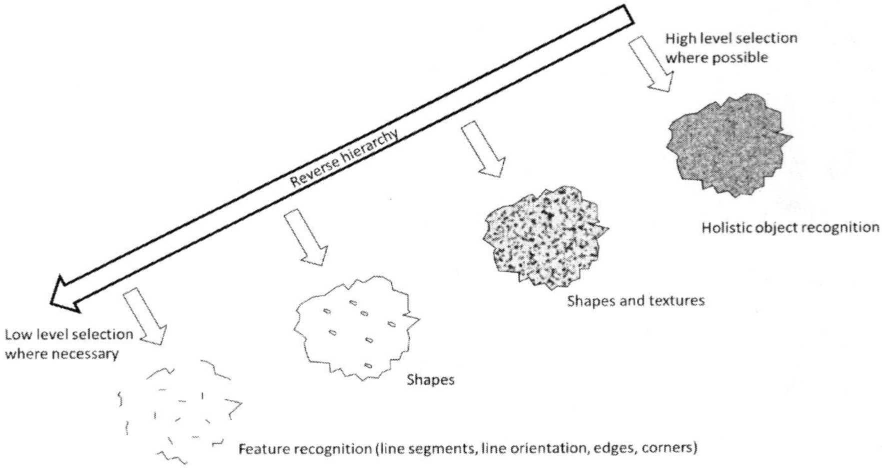

Figure 13. A cytological interpretation of Reverse Hierarchy Theory. Each shape represents a cell nucleus.

Cytopathology can be envisaged as a visual discrimination task, analogous to discrimination tasks encountered elsewhere in the perception literature, such as the vernier alignment task (Astle, Li, Webb et al., 2013), motion discrimination (Matthews & Welch, 1997), discrimination of spatial frequencies (Fiorentini & Berardi, 1980) and texture discrimination (Karni & Sagi, 1991). The main difference between cytopathology images and the relatively simple stimuli used in many visual perception studies is that cell images are rich multidimensional stimuli.

To illustrate the visual discrimination task in cytopathology, consider Figure 14, which is an elaborated version of Figure 2. Each shape represents the nucleus of a cell and the challenge for the trainee cytologist is to learn how to discriminate normal from neoplastic cells.

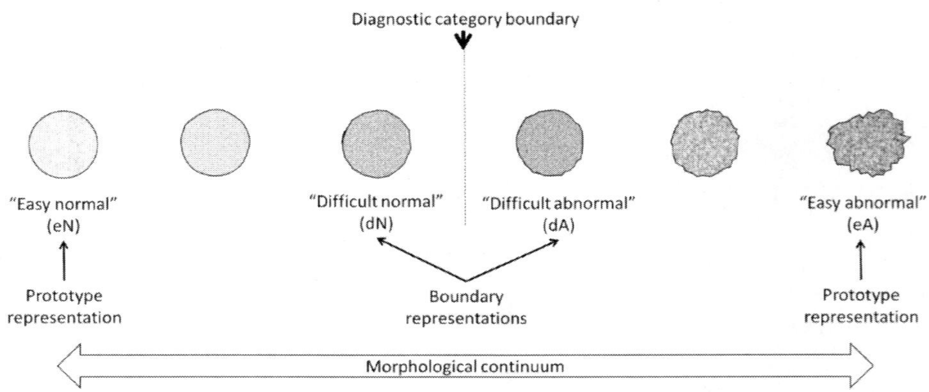

Figure 14. A simple diagrammatic representation of the visual discrimination task in cytopathology. Each shape represents the nucleus of a cell. For notation, the upper case letters N and A are used to indicate the diagnostic categories "normal" and "abnormal" whilst the level of interpretive difficulty ("easy" or "difficult") is represented by the lower case letters "e" and "a", respectively. This latter concept is explained more fully in the main text.

Information derived from chromatin texture, the shape and size of nuclei, the intensity of staining and nuclear size must be carefully integrated to yield consistently accurate results. The task can be difficult because the morphological continuum between definite normality (far left) and definite abnormality (far right) can lead to uncertainties in the location of the boundary between the two diagnostic categories. In the present experiment, cell images were either "normal" (N) or "abnormal" (A), and "easy" (e) or "difficult" (d) to interpret. While the terms "normal" and "abnormal" are readily understood, the concept of *interpretive difficulty* requires brief elaboration. The ease with which visual stimuli are discerned is best described in signal detection terms. Put simply, "easy" visual discriminations are those in which the signal-to-noise ratio is high and differences are said to "pop out" of the visual scene, whereas "difficult" tasks have a lower signal-to-noise ratio, involve finer discriminations and demand greater cognitive effort (Ahissar & Hochstein, 1996, 1997, 2004).

For the present experiment, we start with the idea that presenting images in pairs will affect the visual learning process in naïve participants, a premise that is supported by the results of the previous experiment (Evered, Walker, Watt, & Perham, 2013) and by other investigators (Dwyer, Mundy, & Honey, 2011; Mundy, Honey, & Dwyer, 2007, 2009). Suppose also that the paired images are presented to naive observers using the non-analytical paradigm, as described in the previous experiment and by others (Evered et al., 2013; Nodine & Mello-Thoms, 2010; Norman et al., 2007).

Image pairs may be drawn from the same diagnostic category (i.e. N paired with N or A paired with A) or from the opposite category (i.e. N paired with A). With two levels of interpretive difficulty (e and d) there are 10 possible image pair combinations, the following six of which were of potential interest: Difficult normal paired with difficult abnormal (dN/dA); difficult normal paired with easy abnormal (dN/eA); easy normal paired with difficult abnormal (eN/dA); easy normal paired with easy abnormal (eN/eA); easy normal paired with difficult normal (eN/dN), and; easy abnormal paired with difficult abnormal (eA/dA).

The remaining four combinations (eAeA, dAdA, eNeN and dNdN) were not evaluated because each of these image-pairs occupies the same location on the morphological continuum shown in Figure 14, and successful perceptual learning most plausibly requires examination of dissimilar stimuli (Gibson & Gibson, 1955).

Accepting that the primary purpose of cytopathology is to discriminate neoplastic from normal cells (i.e. it is a category discrimination task), we must also consider the notion of *categorical perception*, which describes the way in which humans perceptually exaggerate the differences between objects that belong to different categories whilst de-emphasising the differences between objects that lie in the same category (Goldstone & Hendrickson, 2010). In cytopathology, we can think of categorical perception as the ability to discriminate between normal and abnormal cells while perceptually de-emphasising the morphological variation seen among cells in the same diagnostic category.

The extent to which categorical perception is learned rather than innate is not clear (Pastore, 1987), but there is some evidence that the skills improve with practice, at least for auditory stimuli (Lane, 1964; Logan, Lively, & Pisoni, 1991). If the same is true of visual stimuli, there are two models that can be drawn upon in order to operationalize the learning process in cytopathology. The first approach might be termed "easy training", which, as its name suggests, would involve the presentation of images that are typical of the diagnostic category they represent. So, eN/eA image pairs would be the purest form of easy training in cytopathology, an example of which is shown in Figure 15.

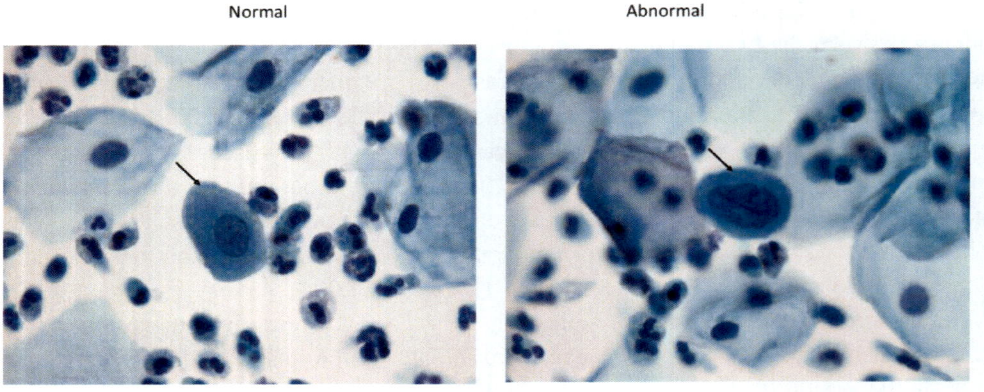

Figure 15. An example of an "easy" image pair (eN/eA). The cells in the centre of each image are easily distinguished from each other because of the highly salient differences in nuclear size, texture, shape and staining intensity. The arrows indicate the relevant cells but these were not presented in the actual experiment. Each image was preceded by a visual cue to direct participants' gaze to the correct cell.

We might also consider "difficult training", in which observers examine a number of paired images that lie at the morphological boundary of normality (i.e. dN/dA pairs). Although normal and abnormal cells can be difficult to discriminate for different reasons, the key concept is the low salience of the features to be discriminated. For instance, a normal cell might have an unusually large nucleus, or an abnormal nucleus might have an unusually bland texture. Figure 16 shows an example of a dN/dA image pair.

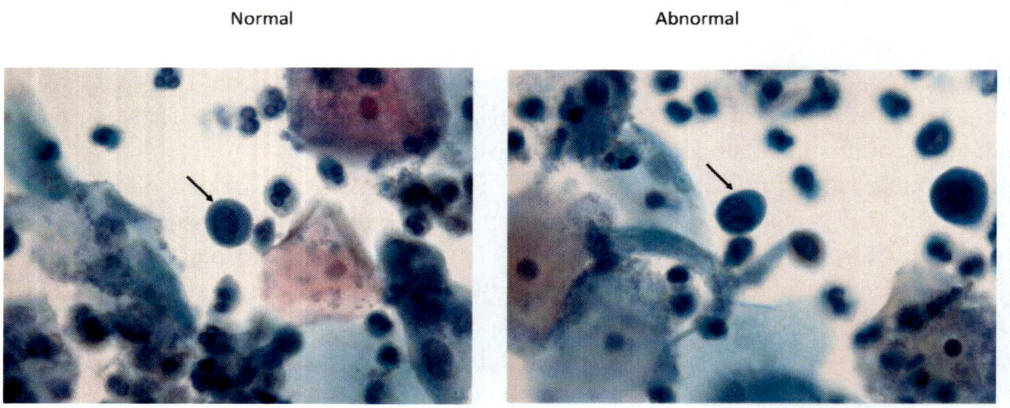

Figure 16. An example of a "difficult" image pair (dN/dA). In the centre of the image on the left is a normal cell with a nucleus that is relatively large but is uniform in texture and has a smooth border. It is strikingly similar to the abnormal cell in the centre of the image on the right, in which the irregularity of nuclear texture and outline are subtle. The arrows indicate the relevant cells but these were not presented in the actual experiment. Each image was preceded by a visual cue to direct participants' gaze to the correct cell.

Of course it is possible to experiment with any one or a mixture of the possible image pair combinations described above, including paired easy/difficult images (i.e. eN/dA and dN/eA); there is evidence that both difficult and easy training can be effective (Acker, Pastore, & Hall, 1995; McFadden & Callaway, 1999; Kuhl & Miller, 1975). However, categorical perception theory intuitively suggests that training on paired images drawn from the same diagnostic category, regardless of difficulty level, (i.e. eN/dN or eA/dA) would not be very effective, simply because observers might require exposure to objects from different diagnostic categories if they are to learn to distinguish them. In purely practical terms we would like to know which of the paired image combinations leads to the best outcome, in terms of speed of learning and diagnostic performance.

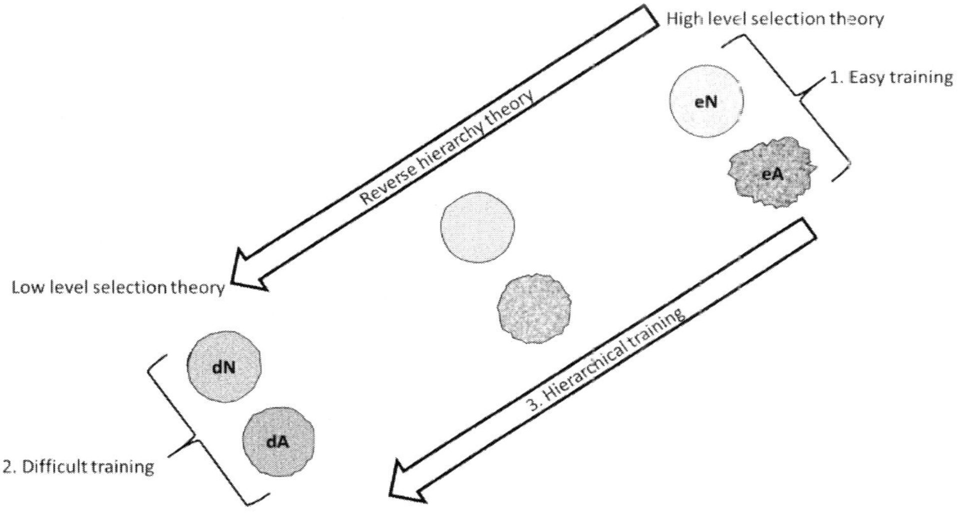

Figure 17. Three possible approaches to perceptual training in cytopathology and their theoretical underpinnings. 1: Easy training exposes participants to prototypical examples of paired normal and abnormal cells (eN/eA). 2: With difficult training, participants are presented with paired images of normal and abnormal cells that lie on the morphological boundary of diagnostic categories (dN/dA). 3: Hierarchical training involves the use of paired images of graded difficulty, from easy to difficult. The shapes in the figure represent cell nuclei.

The theories described above make specific predictions about visual learning in cytopathology. If learning occurs at the highest level of processing, i.e. at the level of whole "objects" such as cells and cell groups, then perceptual training using images of easy normal (eN) and abnormal (eA) cells should improve cytologists' discrimination skills. On the other hand, if learning is predominantly low level then we might expect training on difficult images that lie on diagnostic category boundaries to be more effective (i.e. dN/dA). If however, learning occurs by selecting the most appropriate level of processing for the task in hand, as asserted by RHT, then presenting participants with cell images of graded difficulty, from easy prototypical cases to difficult images that lie on the diagnostic boundary, would be the most effective approach. These predictions are summarised in Figure 17.

An experiment was designed to test the two competing theories of high level and low level perceptual selection in the context of cytopathology education and training. The effectiveness of hierarchical training using stimuli of graded difficulty is supported by recent empirical evidence (Kadar & Ben-Shahar, 2012), but was not explored here.

Procedure

The procedure is shown in Figure 18.

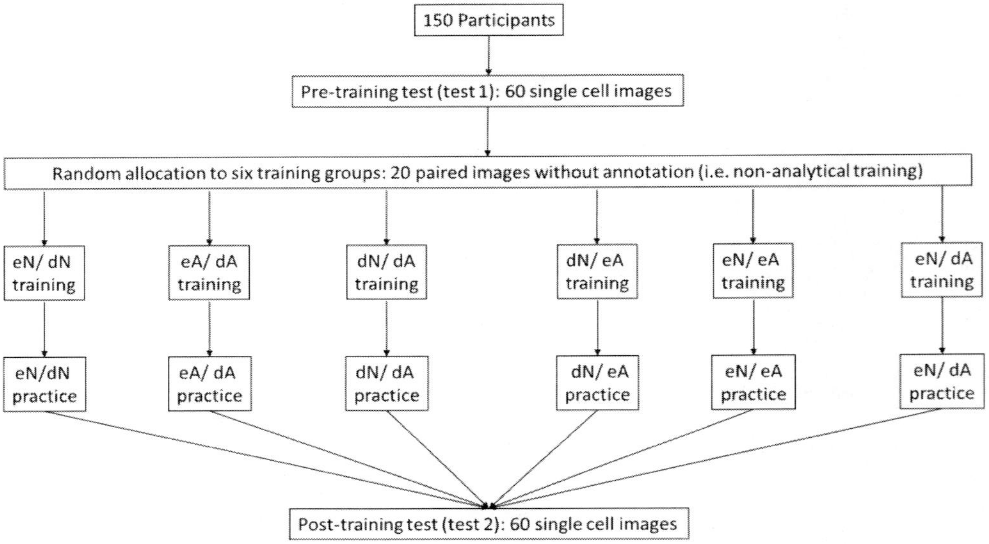

Figure 18. Diagram illustrating the design of experiment 2.

Briefly, 150 participants (none of whom participated in experiment 1) undertook an initial pre-training image interpretation test (test 1) identical to that used in experiment 1. Participants were then randomly divided into six equally sized groups and trained according to one of the following non-analytical training protocols.

1. Difficult normal paired with difficult abnormal (dN/dA)
2. Difficult normal paired with easy abnormal (dN/eA)
3. Easy normal paired with difficult abnormal (eN/dA)
4. Easy normal paired with easy abnormal (eN/eA)
5. Easy normal paired with difficult normal (eN/dN)
6. Easy abnormal paired with difficult abnormal (eA/dA)

Every effort was made to ensure that judgments regarding image difficulty were consistent with the way in which they would be perceived by new cytology trainees and, although subjective, were based on the lead author's experience as a cytology trainer. To provide additional reassurance, all images were corroborated by two independent cytology experts, each with over 20 years' experience in cytology education and training. The expert consensus opinion of normal, abnormal, easy and difficult provided the ground truth status for each image. Following a practice phase, each group was subjected to a post-training test (test

2) as previously described. Training protocol served as the between group independent variable and test position (pre-training vs. post-training) as the repeated measures independent variable, giving a 6x2 factorial design. The dependent variables were raw error rate, AUC, *criterion.*

Results

Extending the non-analytical learning paradigm of experiment 1, experiment 2 showed that while some easy/difficult and normal/abnormal image pair combinations promoted learning, others did not. Figure 19 shows that three of the six training strategies, namely dN/eA, eN/eA and eN/dA training, enhanced learning, but eN/dN, eA/dA and dN/dA were less effective.

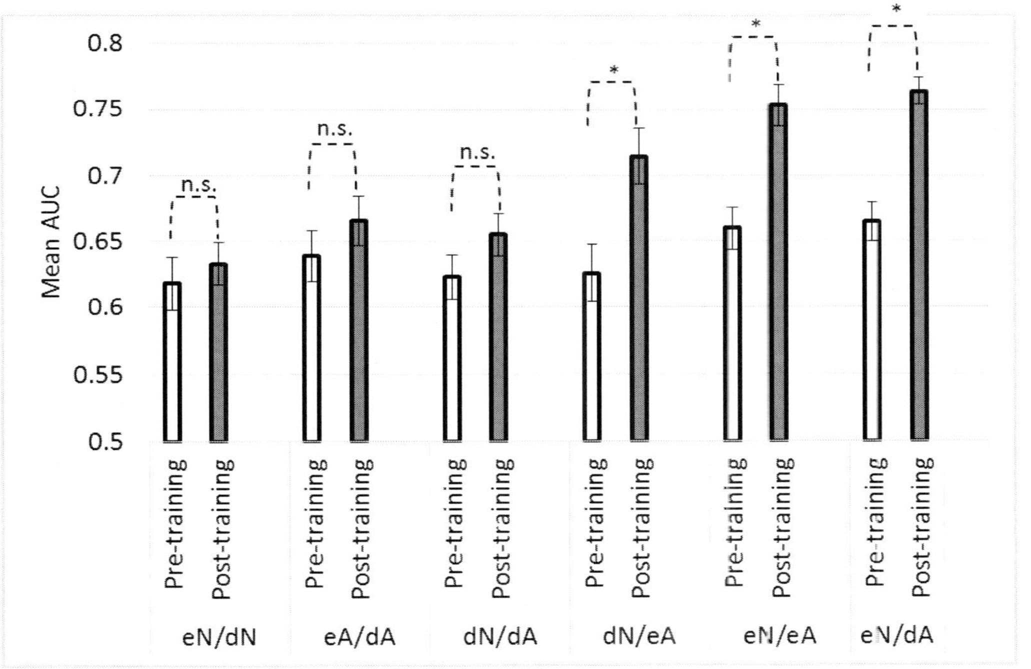

Figure 19. Bar chart showing changes in AUC for each non-analytical training protocol. Error bars represent ±1 standard error of the mean. $*p < .05$, n.s. not significant.

A one-way ANOVA provided reassurance that the variation noted in pre-training test performance between groups was random rather than systematic ($F_{6,168} = 2.03$, $p = .064$). A two-way mixed design ANOVA revealed a significant main effect of training strategy ($F_{5,144} = 6.35$, $p = .001$), a significant main effect of test number ($F_{1,144} = 51.21$, $p = .001$) and a significant interaction between training strategy and test number ($F_{5,144} = 3.55$, $p = .005$). Pairwise comparisons showed interesting differences between training protocols. The key finding was a significantly improved performance following dN/eA, eN/eA and eN/dA training ($p < .05$). The error rates shown in Figure 20 and Figure 21 also show interesting group differences. Except for the eN/dN and eA/dA protocols, in which participants were trained using only normal or only abnormal image pairs, training resulted in some reduction in false negatives with little discernible increase in false positive rates, thereby replicating the results of experiment 1.

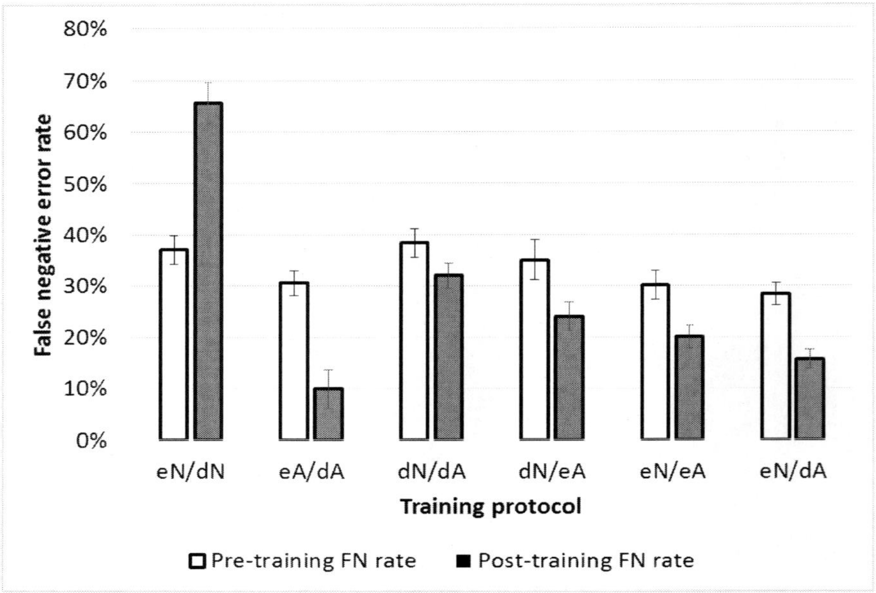

Figure 20. False negative (FN) error rates by training condition. Error bars represent ±1 standard error of the mean.

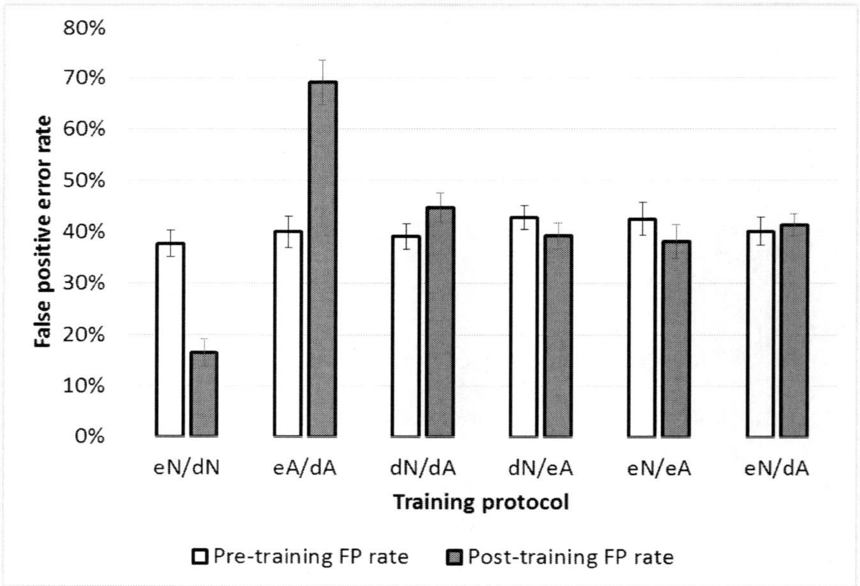

Figure 21. False positive (FP) error rates by training condition. Error bars represent ±1 standard error of the mean.

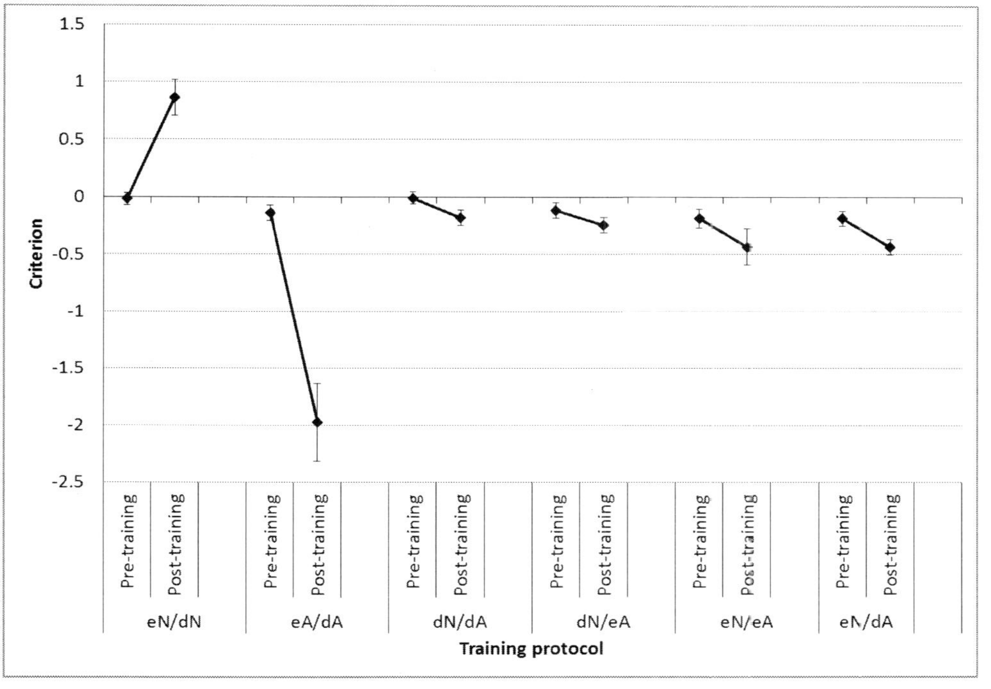

Figure 22. Pre- and post-training diagnostic thresholds. Criterion is an objective measure of observer response bias and is derived from true positive and false positive rates. Low values indicate low thresholds for reporting a positive result and high values indicate high thresholds. Error bars represent ±1 standard error of the mean.

However, the extent to which the observed changes in raw error rates may be due to *criterion* shifts should be carefully noted. Figure 22 clearly shows such a shift for all training scenarios, but is most noticeable for the eN/dN and eA/dA strategies.

Note the large shift to a higher threshold for the eN/dN group and an even greater downward shift for the eA/dA group, indicating that the dramatic changes in false negative and false positive rates observed for these two groups can be largely explained by *criterion* shifts. The changes in *criterion* noted for the remaining groups were more modest, but all were in a downward direction, indicating a greater willingness to report an abnormal following any training protocol that involved exposure to abnormal cell images.

Discussion

The purpose of experiment 2 was to extend the perceptual learning model developed in experiment 1 by testing the extent to which six non-analytical training strategies, involving untutored exposure of naïve participants to selected pairs of cell images, enhanced image interpretation skills.

Experiment 2 replicated the finding in experiment 1 that naive observers appear to develop cell discrimination skills very early during the learning process (Evered, Walker, Watt, & Perham, 2014). Of greater interest in this experiment were the differences between pre- and post-training diagnostic performance across the six training groups and these are described in the sections below.

Training on Images from the Same Diagnostic Category (eN/dN and eA/dA) Is Ineffective

Training on image pairs from the same diagnostic category was not as effective as cross-category training, regardless of the level of interpretive difficulty. Intuitively and theoretically, this finding was not entirely unexpected. Reductions in false negative rates following eA/dA training were matched by an increase in false positive rate of equal magnitude.

The large downward *criterion* shift for this group amply illustrates the dependence of error rate data on the diagnostic thresholds adopted by observers, and in terms of perceptual learning the results for this group of participants should be interpreted with caution.

Likewise, the decrease in false positive rates following eN/dN training should not be interpreted as perceptual learning because they are accompanied by a corresponding increase in false negative rates and a large increase in *criterion*. A change in observer response bias as a result of training is therefore the most likely explanation for the observed results in these two groups.

Training on Difficult Images from Different Diagnostic Categories (dN/dA) Is Ineffective

This is a key result, and one that has great relevance for the design of perceptual learning modules in cytopathology.

Specifically, when participants were trained on difficult image pairs that straddle the diagnostic boundary, diagnostic performance did not improve. It would appear that training on such restricted stimuli did not transfer to test conditions, a finding that contravenes low level selection theory (Sagi, 2011).

This phenomenon has been noted by others (Aberg & Herzog, 2009; Adini, Wilkonsky, Haspel, Tsodyks, & Sgi, 2004; Evered, Walker, Watt, & Perham, 2014; Yu, Klein, & Levi, 2004) and is referred to as perceptual "over-fitting" (Sagi, 2011). Educators should therefore be cautious about incorporating boundary images when developing perceptual learning modules for cytopathology.

Training on Easy Images (eN/eA) and Mixed Easy/Difficult Images (eN/dA and dN/eA) from Different Diagnostic Categories Is Effective

Training on paired images from different diagnostic categories in which at least one member of the image pair was easy to interpret was the key feature of these three strategies. A valuable finding was the significant improvement in diagnostic performance in all three conditions. It appears that cross-boundary easy training prevents the over-fitting that occurs with difficult training. The benefits of mixed easy/difficult training have been reported by others (Liu, Zu, & Dosher, 2012).

Experiment 2 clearly demonstrated the benefits of learning on some types of image pair combinations over others. Specifically, training on dN/eA, eN/eA and eN/dA image pairs was more effective than eN/dN, eA/dA and dN/dA combinations (Evered, Walker, Watt, & Perham, 2014).

General Discussion and Conclusion

Taken together, the results of both experiments provided convincing evidence that a structured approach to perceptual learning in cytopathology can result in discrimination performance that is equally effective and more efficient than analytical training. Furthermore, the skills acquired during perceptual learning on normal/abnormal image pairs, in which at least one member of the image pair is easy to interpret, appears to transfer to categorisation tasks involving more difficult images. The findings are consistent with a theory of high level selection, in which training involving easy tasks facilitates the learning of more difficult ones, (39) (60) and is in concordance with other studies that have demonstrated this effect (Ahissar & Hochstein, 1997; Liu, 1999; Liu & Weinshall, 2000; Rubin, Nakayama, & Shapley, 1997).

Interestingly, some studies have shown that perceptual learning that starts with difficult items can also be effective. For example, in an experiment involving a difficult perceptual categorization task, one group of participants began with easy training examples and then moved to more difficult examples, in a second condition the order was reversed, and in a third condition participants saw examples in a random order. Participants who began with the most difficult items performed much better than participants in the other two conditions (Liu, 1999). In another study, sequential groups of participants were trained to classify stimuli that previous groups had found difficult. In all experiments, classification accuracy was greatest in the later groups, thus suggesting that learning might be more effective when training begins with the most difficult items and concludes with the easiest (Lee, MacGregor, Bavelas et al., 1988). Notwithstanding the previous paragraph, the phenomenon of *transfer along a continuum*, in which training is most effective when it begins with easy conditions and moves gradually to more difficult conditions, is well established. The phenomenon was first reported by Pavlov and later confirmed in other behavioural experiments with humans and non-human animals (Baker & Osgood, 1954; Haberlandt, 1971; Lawrence, 1952; Mackintosh, 1965, 1970; Sutherland, Mackintosh, & Mackintosh, 1963; Walker, Younglim, & Bitterman, 1990; Williams, 1968).

Reverse Hierarchy Theory provides a plausible neuronal-cortical explanation for these observations. In its simplest form, RHT proposes that perceptual learning proceeds along a cortical hierarchy in which the learning of easy conditions guides the learning of hard ones (Ahissar & Hochstein, 1996). Of particular interest in applied fields such as cytology is the consistent finding that the effectiveness of learning is highly sensitive to the choice of the first few training trials rather than the total amount of practice. Similar results in the domain of cytology training would provide a firm foundation for the development of short but effective training programmes.

By demonstrating that training strategies incorporating easy cell images enhance diagnostic performance beyond that achieved when only difficult images are used, and that such training does not require explicit tuition, these experiments have advanced our understanding of the visual learning process in cytopathology.

Important clues have been gleaned for the development of perceptual learning modules that might be usefully integrated into existing cytology training programmes. Non-analytical learning strategies are worthy of further exploration as an innovative technique that could expedite the acquisition of diagnostic expertise in cytology, a skill that purportedly takes several years to master.

References

Acker, B.E., Pastore, R.E., & Hall, M.D. (1995). Within-category discrimination of musical chords: perceptual magnet or anchor? *Perception & Psychophysics, 57*, 863-874.

Aberg, K.C., & Herzog, M.H. (2009). Interleaving bisection stimuli – randomly or in sequence – does not disrupt perceptual learning, it just makes it more difficult. *Vision Research, 49*, 2591-2598.

Adini, Y., Wilkonsky, A., Haspel, R., Tsodyks, M., & Sagi, D. (2004). Perceptual learning in contrast discrimination: the effect of contrast uncertainty. *Journal of Vision, 4*, 993-1005.

Ahissar, M., & Hochstein, S. (1996). Learning pop-out detection: specificities to stimulus characteristics. *Vision Research, 36*, 3487-3500.

Ahissar, M., & Hochstein, S. (1997). Task difficulty and the specificity of perceptual learning. *Nature, 387*, 401-406.

Ahissar, M., & Hochstein, S. (2004). The reverse hierarchy theory of visual perceptual learning. *Trends in Cognitive Science, 8*, 457-464.

Ark, T.K., Brooks, L.R., & Eva, K.W. (2006). Giving learners the best of both worlds: do clinical teachers need to guard against teaching pattern recognition to novices? *Academic Medicine, 81*, 405-409.

Astle, A.T., Li, R.W., Webb, B.S., Levi, D.M., & McGraw, P.V. (2013). A Weber-like law for perceptual learning. *Scientific Reports, 3*, 1158.

Baker, R.A., & Osgood, S.W. (1954). Discrimination transfer along a pitch continuum. *Journal of Experimental Psychology, 48*(4), 241-246.

City and Guilds (2007). *Level 3 Diploma in Cervical Cytology* (Cervical Cytology 3166). Retrieved from http://www.cityandguilds.com/qualifications-and-apprenticeships/health-and-social-care/health/3166-cervical-cytology#tab=documents.

Dwyer, D.M., Mundy, M.E., & Honey, R.C. (2011). The role of stimulus comparison in human perceptual learning: effects of distractor placement. *Journal of Experimental Psychology Animal Behavior Processes, 37*(3), 300-307.

Eva, K.W. (2005). What every teacher needs to know about clinical reasoning. *Medical Education, 39*, 98-106.

Evered, A (2005). What can cytologists learn from 25 years of investigations in visual search? *British Journal of Biomedical Science, 62*(4), 182-192.

Evered, A. (2011). Abnormal cervical cytology. In B. Shambayati (Ed.), *Fundamentals of biomedical Science – cytopathology* (pp. 108-136). London: Oxford University Press.

Evered, A., Walker, D., Watt, A., & Perham, N. (2013). To what extent does non-analytic reasoning contribute to visual learning in cytopathology? *Cancer Cytopathology, 121*(6), 329-338.

Evered, A., Walker, D., Watt, A., & Perham, N. (2014). Untutored discrimination training on paired cell images influences visual learning in cytopathology. *Cancer Cytopathology, 122*(3), 200-210.

Fahle, M. (2005), Perceptual learning: specificity versus generalization. *Current Opinion in Neurobiology, 15*(2), 154-160.

Fiorentini, A., & Berardi, N. (1980). Perceptual learning specific for orientation and spatial frequency. *Nature, 287*, 43-44.

Frost, J.K. (1986). *The cell in health and disease: an evaluation of cellular morphologic expression of biologic behavior.* 2nd edn. New York : Karger.

Garcia, A., Kuai, S.G., & Kourtzi, Z (2013). Differences in the time course of learning for hard compared to easy training. Frontiers in Psychology, 4, 110.

Gibson, J.J., & Gibson, E.J. (1955). Perceptual learning; differentiation or enrichment? *Psychological Review, 62*(1), 32-41.

Goldstone, R.L., & Hendrickson, A.T. (2010). Categorical perception. *WIREs Cognitive Science, 1*, 69-78.

Grunze, H., & Spriggs, A.I. (1983). *History of clinical cytology: a selection of documents*, 2nd edn. Darmstadt : Ernst Giebler.

Guerlain, S. (2004). Improving surgical pattern recognition through repetitive viewing of video clips. *IEEE Transactions on Systems Man and Cybernetics – Part A Systems and Humans, 34,* 699-707.

Haberlandt K. (1971). Transfer along a continuum in classical conditioning. *Learning & Motivation, 2*(2), 164-172.

Karni, A., & Sagi, D. (1991). Where practice makes perfect in texture discrimination: evidence from primary visual cortex plasticity. *Proceedings of the National Academy of Sciences, 88*, 4966-4970.

Kadar, I., & Ben-Shahar, O. (2012). A perceptual paradigm and psychophysical evidence for hierarchy in scene gist processing. *Journal of Vision, 12*(13), 1-17.

Kellman, P.J., Massey, C.M., & Son, J.Y. (2010). Perceptual learning modules in mathematics: enhancing students' pattern recognition, structure extraction, and fluency. *Topics in Cognitive Science, 2*, 285-305.

Kellman, P.J., & Kaiser, M.K. (1994). Perceptual learning modules in flight training. *Human Factors and Ergonomics Society Annual Meeting Proceedings, 38*, 1183-1187.

Kellman, P.J., & Garrigan, P. (2009). Perceptual learning and human expertise. *Physics of Life Reviews, 6*(2), 53-84.

Koss, L.G. (1961). *Diagnostic cytology and its histopathologic bases*, 1st edn. Philadelphia: JB Lippicott.

Kuhl, P.K., & Miller, J.D. (1975). Speech perception by the chinchilla: voice-voiceless distinction in alveolar plosive consonants. *Science, 190*, 69-72.

Kundel, H.L., Nodine, C.F., Conant, E.F., & Weinstein, S.P. (2007). Holistic component of image perception in mammogram interpretation. *Radiology, 242*, 396-402.

Lane H. (1964). Motor theory of speech perception: a critical review. *Psychological Review, 72*, 275-309.

Lawrence, D.H. (1952). The transfer of a discrimination along a continuum. *Journal of Comparative and Physiological Psychology, 45*(6), 511-516.

Leber, A.B., Lechak, J.R., & Tower-Richardi, S.M. (2013). What do fast response times tell us about attentional control? *Journal of Vision, 13*(3), 31.

Lee, E.S., MacGregor, J.N., Bavelas, A., Mirlin, L., Lam, N., & Morrison, I. (1988). The effects of error transformations on classification performance. *Journal of Experimental Psychology: Learning, Memory, and Cognition, 14*, 66-74.

Lesgold, A., Rubinson, H., Feltovich, P., Glaser, R., Klopfer, D., & Wang, Y. (1988). Expertise in a complex skill: diagnosing x-ray pictures. In R. Glaser, M.T.H. Chi, & M.J. Farr (Eds.), *The nature of expertise* (pp. 311-342). Hillsdale: Erlbaum.

Liu Z. (1999). Perceptual learning in motion discrimination that generalizes across motion directions. *Proceedings of the National Academy of Science, 96*, 14085-14087.

Liu, J., Lu, Z.L., & Dosher, B.A. (2012). Mixed training at high and low accuracy levels leads to perceptual learning without feedback. *Vision Research, 61*, 15-24.

Liu, Z., & Weinshall, D. (2000). Mechanisms of generalization in perceptual learning. *Vision Research, 40*(1), 97-109.

Logan, J.S., Lively, S.E., & Pisoni, D.B. (1991). Training Japanese listeners to identify /r/ and /l: a first report. *The Journal of the Acoustic Society of America, 89*, 874-886.

Mackworth, N.H., & Morandi, A.J. (1967). The gaze selects informative details within pictures. *Perception & Psychophysics, 2*, 547-552.

Mackintosh, N.J. (1965). Selective attention in animal discrimination learning. *Psychological Bulletin, 62*(2), 124-150.

Mackintosh, N.J., & Little, L. (1970). An analysis of transfer along a continuum. *Canadian Journal of Psychology, 24*(5), 362-369.

Matthews, N., & Welch, L. (1997). Velocity-dependent improvements in single-dot direction discrimination. *Perception & Psychophysics, 59*, 60-72.

McFadden, D., & Callaway, N.L. (1999). Better discrimination of small changes in commonly encountered than in less commonly encountered auditory stimuli. *Journal of Experimental Psychology, 25*, 543-560.

Merzenich, M.M., Jenkins, W.M., Johnstone, P., Schreiner, C., Miller, S., & Tallal, P. (1996). Temporal processing deficits of language impaired children ameliorated by training. *Science, 271*(5245), 77-81.

Mitchell, H., & Medley, G. (1995). Differences between Papanicolaou smears with correct and incorrect diagnoses. *Cytopathology, 6*(6), 368-375.

Mollon, J.D., & Danilova, M.V. (1996). Three remarks on perceptual learning. *Spatial Vision, 10*(1), 51-58.

Mundy, M.E., Honey, R.C., & Dwyer, D.M. (2007). Simultaneous presentation of similar stimuli produces perceptual learning in human picture processing. *Journal of Experimental Psychology: Animal Behavior Processes, 33*(2), 124-138.

Mundy, M.E., Honey, R.C., & Dwyer, D.M. (2009). Superior discrimination between similar stimuli after simultaneous exposure. *Quarterly Journal of Experimental Psychology, 62*(1), 18-25.

Neisser, U. (1967). *Cognitive Psychology.* Englewood Cliffs NJ: Prentice-Hall, Inc.

NHS Cancer Screening Programmes (1995). Qualifications and training for non-medical laboratory staff. NHSCSP Publication No 12. Sheffield.

Nodine, C., & Mello-Thoms, C. (2010). The role of expertise in radiologic image interpretation. In E. Samei, & E. Krupinski (Eds.), *The handbook of medical image perception and techniques* (pp. 139-156). New York: Cambridge University Press.

Norman, G., Young, M., & Brooks, L. (2007). Non-analytic models of clinical reasoning: the role of experience. *Medical Education, 41*(12), 1140-1145.

Papanicolaou, G.N., & Traut, H.N. (1941). The diagnostic value of vaginal smears in carcinoma of the uterus. *American Journal of Obstetrics and Gynecology, 42*, 193-205.

Pastore, R.E. (1987). Categorical perception: some psychophysical models. In *Categorical perception* (pp. 29-52). Cambridge: Cambridge University Press.

Pelaccia, T., Tardif, J., Triby, E., & Charlin, B. (2011). An analysis of clinical reasoning through a recent and comprehensive approach: the dual-process theory. *Medical Education Online.* doi: 10.3402/meo.v16i0.5890.

Pohl, F. (2004). *Cognitive illusions: a handbook on fallacies and biases in thinking, judgement and memory.* Hove: Psychology Press.

Rouder, J.N., Lu, J., Speckman, P., Sun, D., & Jiang, Y. (2005). A hierarchical model for estimating response time distributions. *Psychonomic Bulletin & Review, 12*(2), 195-223.

Rubin, N., Nakayama, K., & Shapley, R. (1997). Abrupt learning and retinal size specificity in illusory contour perception. *Current Biology, 7*, 461-467.

Sagi, D. (2011). Perceptual learning in vision research. *Vision Research, 51*(13),1552-1566.

Stoler, M.H., & Schiffman, M. (2001). Interobserver reproducibility of cervical cytologic and histological interpretations: realistic estimates from the ASCUS-LSIL Triage Study. *JAMA, 285*(11), 1500-1505.

Sutherland, N.S., Mackintosh, N.J., & Mackintosh, J. (1963). Simultaneous discrimination training of octopus and transfer of discrimination along a continuum. *Journal of Comparative and Physiological Psychology, 56*(1), 150-156.

University of Arizona. DMDX display software (2014). Retrieved from http://www.u.arizona.edu/~kforster/dmdx/dmdx.htm.

Vogelstein, B., & Kinzler, K.W. (1998) (Eds.). *The Genetic Basis of Human Cancer.* New York: McGraw-Hill.

Whelan, R. (2008). Effective analysis of reaction time data. *Psychological Review, 58*, 475-482.

Wright, B.A., & Zhang, Y. (2009). A review of the generalization of auditory learning. *Philosophical Transactions of the Royal Society. B Biological Sciences, 364*(1515), 301-311.

Walker, M.M., Younglim, L., & Bitterman, M.E. (1990). Transfer along a continuum in the discriminative learning of honeybees (Apis mellifera). *Journal of Comparative Psychology, 104*(1), 66-70.

Williams, D.I. (1968). Transfer along a continuum in the pigeon. *Journal of Comparative and Physiological Psychology, 65*(2), 369-371.

World Health Organization (2009). *Cancer Fact Sheet No 297.* Retrieved from http://www.who.int/mediacentre/factsheets/fs297/en/index.html.

Yu, C., Klein, S.A., & Levi, D.M. (2004). Perceptual learning in contrast discrimination and the (minimal) role of context. *Journal of Vision, 4*, 169-182.

In: Advances in Visual Perception Research
Editor: Thomas Heinen ISBN: 978-1-63482-455-2
© 2015 Nova Science Publishers, Inc.

Chapter 12

Visuomotor Behavior in Computer-Simulated Display

Hirofumi Ida [*]
Department of Sports and Health Management,
Jobu University, Japan

Abstract

Our world never seems to stop computerization. Thus, we must work effectively with computer displays in our daily lives. This is often the case for experimental participants who are instructed to respond to computer-generated visual stimuli. This chapter reviews the literature on human visuomotor behaviors, for which computer-simulated displays, such as virtual reality, served as a tool of stimulus presentation. At the beginning a brief technical overview is provided, followed by arguments on the findings derived from the investivgations of several representative perceptual motor tasks. In studies on posture control, immersive and interactive visual environments are useful to examine the balance response to an apparent motion in the visual scene, known as optical flow. With regard to interceptive action, various types of environments have been utilized depending on tasks, although stereoscopic displays seem to be a technique of choice. For biological motion perception, computer-generated graphical characters can be an alternative to the simple traditional model called point-light display. Some recent topics are also provided, in which computer-simulated displays are effectively utilized to address longstanding scientific problems. At the end of the review, the results from comparisons between simulation and reality are presented in order to highlight the specific effect of computer-generated stimuli on the viewer's response. Researchers should thoroughly recognize the advantages and disadvantages of a computer-simulated display, and at times, may need to consider whether the visual stimuli on the screen evoke valid visuomotor responses that meet the purpose of their study.

[*] 634-1, Toyazuka-Machi, Isesaki, Gunma 372-8588, Japan. Email: hiroida@me.com

Keywords: Visuomotor control, Perception-Action coupling, Posture control, Interception, Biological motion, Virtual reality, Stimulus perturbation, Simulation versus reality

Introduction

Visuomotor Control

Seeing is an act and doing is another act—this notation more or less holds true in the history of vision science. That is to say, studies on visual systems have taken a separated trail from those on motor systems in classical physiology and psychology (Goodale, 1998). An ideological barrier for theorization does exist explicitly and implicitly between these two systems. This can be seen, for example, in the famous textbook "Principles of Neural Science" (Kandel, Schwartz, Jessell, Siegelbaum, & Hudspeth, 2012), which has two separate chapters for "Perception" and "Movement". This dualistic thinking, however, might no longer make sense, at least for modern researchers who attempt to explore systematic understandings of perceptual motor control. Acquisition of dynamic and fine motor skills, or motor learning, is the lawful operation that strengthens the coordination between perception and action (Newell, 1991). More specifically, visual input works hand-in-hand with motor output to achieve a purposeful action. The term 'visuomotor control' encompasses both of these processes, and is now widely accepted.

In advance of understanding how computer-simulated displays affect the visuomotor behavior of the observers, we need general knowledge about the characteristics of human perceptual and motor processing in a normal environment (Figure 1). First, visual perception can be defined as a process in the sensory system to recognize and interpret the optical information of visible light from the surrounding environment. On the other hand, motor control is a process in the motor system to generate muscle activations and to purposefully coordinate the movements of the body segments. The traditional model describes the sensory system as first integrating the external and internal information, and thereafter the motor system activates a set of muscles at an adequate level and ratio, as required. This 'one-way' diagram from perception to motion, however, is being replaced with a 'two-way' or 'multi-way' model. Such an interactive nature in perceptual motor control is well conceptualized by the term 'perception-action coupling', which represents that the nervous system has intrinsically intertwined processing functions for perception and action (Sperry, 1952). More recently, the idea is passed down to 'common coding theory', which claims perceptual representations and motor representations share a common code for processing (Prinz, 1997; Schutz-Bosbach & Prinz, 2007).

In the case of vision and motion, this concept can be called 'visuomotor coupling'. Besides, the term 'visually guided action' is often used to collectively represent the motor tasks that are carried out under vision-based control, e.g., steering, intercepting, and avoiding (Fajen, 2005; Gibson, 1958). Although various types of control laws have been proposed, it is commonly recognized that different tasks involve different available information, require different strategy, and are well explained by different models. That is to say, they are strongly task dependent. However, several theories are traditionally and frequently drawn as a basement hypothesis. 'Optical flow', which is the pattern of apparent motion in a visual scene, is regarded as one of the dominant control variables for postural control (Gibson, 1958). 'Tau (τ)', which is expressed as the inverse of the relative expansion rate of an approaching object on the retina, is referred as an optical invariant to control locomotive movements or interceptive actions (Lee, 1976). Provided that a person is in a communicative environment, another specific perceptual function of human (and most likely other animals), namely 'biological motion perception', should be taken into account where appropriate (Johansson, 1973).

For decades, brain functions related to visuomotor control have been investigated in detail using vertebrate animals (Livingstone & Hubel, 1988). From the inspections of hamster's behaviors after brain ablation, it was first postulated that there would be two visual processing systems for spatial localization and for object identification (Schneider, 1969). And later, from monkey studies, dorsal stream and ventral stream were distinguished as processing pathways for localization and for identification, respectively (Ungerleider, 1982). These findings are sophisticatedly reconceptualized as a 'two-streams hypothesis', which separates the visual processing system into a 'where' system (or 'how' system) to localize, and a 'what' system to identify (Goodale & Milner, 1992).

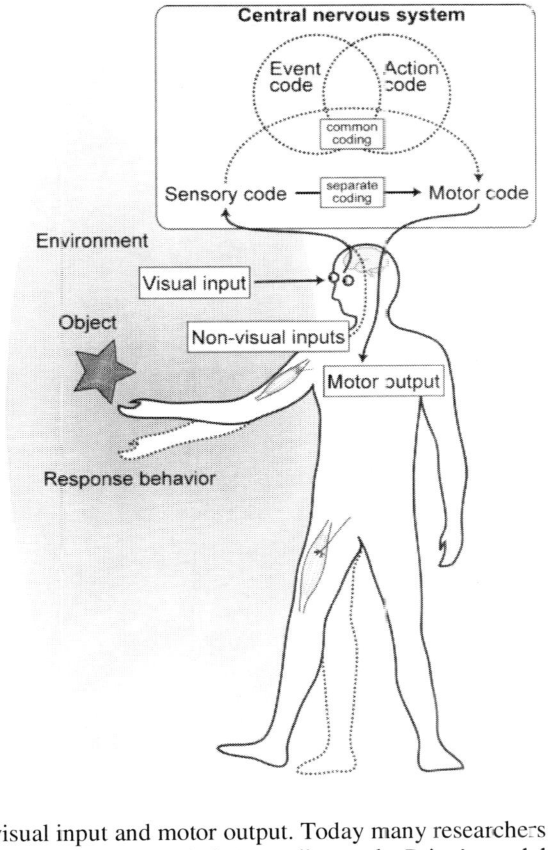

Figure 1. Processing of visual input and motor output. Today many researchers support the notion that perception and action are functionally coupled. According to the Prinz's model (1997), for example, perceived information and motor planning share the same representation (common coding), while many traditional models assume that the sensory information is serially translated into motor commands (separate coding).

The dorsal stream, which begins with the primary visual cortex (V1) in the occipital lobe, passes through visual area V2 and V5 (MT), and terminates in the parietal lobe, and works as the 'where' system. On the other hand, the ventral stream that serves as a 'what' system travels from V1, through visual area V2 and V4, and to the temporal lobe. In particular, the dorsal stream is considered to play a central role in visually guided actions due to its speeded processing nature. The two-streams hypothesis, however, may be an oversimplified schematic of information processing; hence, arguments over this notion are still in progress. In addition to the stream of neural processing, the brain areas activated are of interest in studies on perceptual motor control. Some studies addressed the visuomotor function through brain imaging, such as functional magnetic resonance imaging (fMRI) and positron emission tomography (PET). This approach enables the examination from the aspect of neural function.

Computer-Simulated Display

By the way, our modern life is surrounded by a huge number of computers. Those who work with a personal computer (PC), smartphone, or tablet computer would be conscious that they actually use a computer system, but in other situations they may be unconscious of using a computer, particularly when the devices are controlled by embedded systems, e.g., elevators, air conditioners, and washing machines. As is often the case, the existence of a computer is recognized when we see the visual display, or monitor, connected to the computer. It can be also said that our life is surrounded by computer visual displays. We can talk with friends face to face online, play tennis in a video game, watch digital three-dimensional (3D) movies, and occasionally experience a computer-simulated imaginary world in a museum. Although vision science has concentrated on exploring basic visual functions and mechanisms to date, for modern people, the performance for displayed computer images is of increasing importance. The visuomotor control in response to computer-simulated displays would be categorized into applied vision science, and thus have practical significance to develop our vision-related skills in real life. This may lead to a paradigm shift in future vision science.

Computer monitors, however, are not newcomers in the field of vision science. Traditionally, cathode ray tube (CRT) monitors have been widely used for presenting visual stimuli, and recently liquid crystal display (LCD) monitors and other display monitors are increasingly in use. In this chapter, the author does not go into detail on the property (specifications and compatibility) of these computer monitors, instead the effect of computer-simulated display on visuomotor control will be the main issue of concern. The term computer-simulated display here comprehensively denotes the presentation techniques that computationally and artificially mimic a real-world event, happening, phenomenon, scenario, action, and other scenes. Hence, the following discussions will deal specifically with the viewers' responses to reality-based contexts of simulated environment, while responses to simple visual stimuli, e.g., flash light, cue signal, and position indicator, is out of scope no matter if these stimuli are displayed in computer monitors. Additionally, the techniques in computer-simulated display do not merely mean computer-based visualization, such as computer graphics (CG) and virtual reality (VR), but also computational simulation such as mathematical manipulation and numerical perturbation. Although some display equipment may be constructed to involve other sensory displays such as acoustic and haptic devices, the visuomotor response to computer-simulated visual display is the main topic of this chapter.

While enthusiastic discussions on visuomotor function have been ongoing for a century or more, studies on perceptual motor behaviors in computer-simulated displays emerged only in the past few decades. After the birth of computer-generated imagery techniques in the 1950s and the 1960s, and the commercial success in the 1970s and later, taking a few decades, computer-simulated displays became rapidly popular as a technique for visual stimuli presentation in the 2000s. The technique offers some advantages that traditional experimental settings in laboratory did not have. First, it facilitates researchers to bring in realistic scenes and contexts to their laboratories under computer-based control, although it is more or less an approximation of the real world. Therefore further realistic, naturalistic, interactive, and complicated visumotor tasks became more available than ever. This is figuratively shown in the evolution process of the table tennis simulator (Figure 2), from the early video game 'PONG' (Atari Inc., CA, USA) in the 1970s, to a virtual simulator in the 1990s (Todorov, Shadmehr, & Bizzi, 1997), and to the more advanced environment 'V-Pong' in the 2000s (Brunnett, Rusdorf, & Lorenz, 2006).

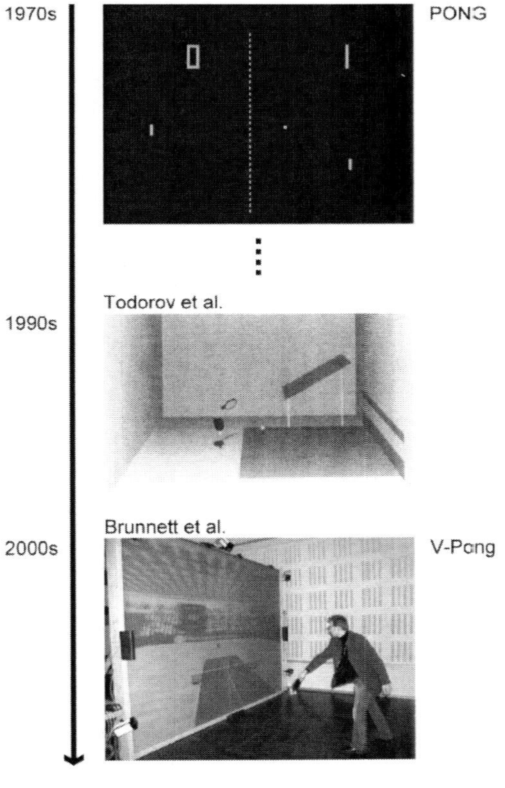

Figure 2. History of table tennis simulator. 'PONG' (Atari Inc.) was first released in 1970s as video game, and after decades interval, a virtual table tennis simulator was used in a motor learning study (Todorov et al., 1997). More recently further sophisticated simulator 'V-Pong' successfully realized a large field of view, higher fidelity, and faster interaction (Brunnett et al., 2006). Reproduced with permission from the publishers.

Second, contrastingly, the technique also makes it possible to reconstruct unrealistic, unnatural, and unfamiliar situations. Users may virtually experience an astronaut's view of walking in space, a bug's view in the grass, and a racer's view in the Formula One. Third, the phenomenon displayed as visual stimulus can be arbitrarily and computationally simulated with numerical exactness. This is applicable for natural and unnatural environmental scenes, more specifically, both adherence and violation to physical laws can be permitted. Furthermore, thanks to the development of computer performance, researchers may conduct all the experimental preocedures even with one computer, i.e., presentation of the visual stimuli, recording of the observer's response, and possibly the synchronization of these two are all-in-one. Being inspired by longstanding topics, e.g., optical flow, outfielder problem, and biological motion perception, some studies attempt to find out the answer of unsolved questions or raise a new question to be solved in the future. The computer-simulated displays possess great potential to offer good solutions for the problems that have not been approached due to practical problems such as cost, ethics, and physical impossibility.

At the same time, researchers should be aware of the disadvantages of computer-simulated displays. First of all, no matter how the technology advances in the future, it never becomes exactly the same thing to the real world. Hence, observers' actions emerged in response to a computer-simulated visual stimuli are nothing more than a simulated performance. It might be very difficult to distinguish whether or not the action was performed in a similar manner as done in the real situation. When we want to understand the characteristics of a simulated visuomotor behavior, though it may seem paradoxical, sufficient understandings for the perceptual motor control in unsimulated (natural) environments should be established beforehand. Thus, the comparative consideration between simulated and unsimulated, or virtual and real, has a critical importance. This approach strengthens the validity of the results obtained from the computer-simulated experiment, and in doing so, the causal inference derived from the findings can be generalized. The problem of 'external validity' or 'ecological validity' are fundamentally inevitable for the studies using a computer-simulated display. The validity of computer-simulated experiments should be taken into account more seriously than that of normal laboratory experiments.

Purpose

In this chapter, the author will develop an argument on human visuomotor functions, which have been revealed by using computer-simulated displays that imitate the real-world environments and objects. What did computer-simulated display techniques newly find out? How do the computer-simulated displays modulate the motor behavior of the viewers? What type of computer-simulated displays will be expected in future studies? First, the technical aspects of display techniques will be briefly overviewed.

Thereafter, the findings in various perceptual motor tasks are presented by reviewing related previous literatures, where posture control, interceptive action, and biological motion perception are the main topics to be discussed. Lastly, studies that verified the characteristics of computer-simulated displays in comparison with the realistic scene will be reviewed in order to highlight the specific effect of computer-simulated displays on visuomotor control. In addition to behavioral, psychological, physiological, and biomechanical performance data, the results from recent brain imaging will be presented where appropriate.

Technical Overview

Visual Display Device

CRT monitors have been widely used in the studies on vision and related areas. LCD monitors are believed to be inadequate for experimental use due to their poorer temporal response characteristics for a long time. Recent studies, however, gave evidence against this belief. It was reported that LCD was comparable to CRT for an attentional blink task and metacontrast masking task (Kihara, Kawahara, & Takeda, 2010), or better regarding visible persistence (Lagroix, Yanko, & Spalek, 2012) and visual search tasks (Menozzi, Lang, Näpflin, Zeller, & Krueger, 2001). In addition, the superiority of LCD was also suggested in a practical screening task for mammography (Krupinski et al., 2004). These findings provided positive impacts on using LCDs for the display of visual stimuli. Moreover, this leads to practical convenience, because CRT is now rarely offered in markets. In addition to LCD, other flat-panel displays, such as plasma display panels and organic light-emitting diodes become available (Mentley, 2002).

For the study of visuomotor behavior, other options may be considered in accordance with the intended use. For example, for a large-size screen with a projector, digital light processing (DLP) projectors have the dominant market share, and will be helpful for the presentation of a life-size scene. A head mount display (HMD) is preferred if the task requires immersion in the environment. In some cases, a binocular stereoscopic display may be chosen if the effect of depth perception is interested. Regarding the stereoscopic display, we can readily utilize commercial products called 3D projectors, 3D television, and 3D cameras. Although there are so many options available as visual displays, the selected one should match the purpose of the study.

Computer-Generated Imagery

The key technique of computer-based visualization is computer-generated imagery, which includes both static images and dynamic scene renderings. Among them, CG animation takes a central role in studies on visuomotor control. Thanks to commercial success of CG technologies in the area of entertainment, researchers of today benefit from various kinds of visualization hardware and software. Application programming interface (API) such as OpenGL (Silicon Graphics Inc., CA, USA) or DirectX (Microsoft Inc., WA, USA) are regarded as basic programming tools for the 2D or 3D rendering, and have been broadly used in studies on visual perception. More comprehensive CG software is an alternative option to create visual stimuli. Among a variety of CG modeling application programs, for example, Maya (Autodesk Inc., CA, USA), 3ds Max (Autodesk Inc., CA, USA), and Blender (Blender Foundation, Netherlands) are popular. Effective use of CG software saves time and effort in the creation of visual stimuli without learning fundamental techniques of programming and rendering. In addition, commonly-used computing and programming languages such as Matlab (MathWorks Inc., MA, USA), GNU Octave, Mathematica (Wolfram Research Inc., IL, USA), and Python (Python Software Foundation, DE, USA) are available as well (Yoonessi & Yoonessi, 2011). In psychological and physiological studies, these application languages may be coupled with some toolbox packages such as Psychtoolbox for Matlab or GNU Octave (Pelli, 1997), and Psychopy for Python (Peirce, 2007).

Virtual Reality

Higher integrated environments, known as VR, are also available for modern scientists. In spite of public interest in such a leading-edge technology, even before the realization of computer-generated imagery technology in 1950s, the serious application of VR in experimental psychology started only in the last couple of decades (Fisher, McGreevy, Humphries, & Robinett, 1987; Tarr & Warren, 2002). This is largely due to the limitations in hardware and software, and the shortage of commercial markets seem to exist as a background factor. Today, however, researchers as well as other consumers, enjoy rich VR technologies thanks to the improvement of computer power, enhancement of the peripheral products, and convenience of CG modeling software.

Most current VR systems are composed of 3D visual displays, realized by the binocular stereoscopic imaging. Some VR systems also include the acoustic and/or haptic devices that help further integrated sensory experiences. Also, immersion in the displayed environment and interaction with the presented world are also key concepts of VR. Visual immersion can be realized by HMD, which blocks the optical information from the outer world by enclosing the eyes within a light shield (Figure 3A).

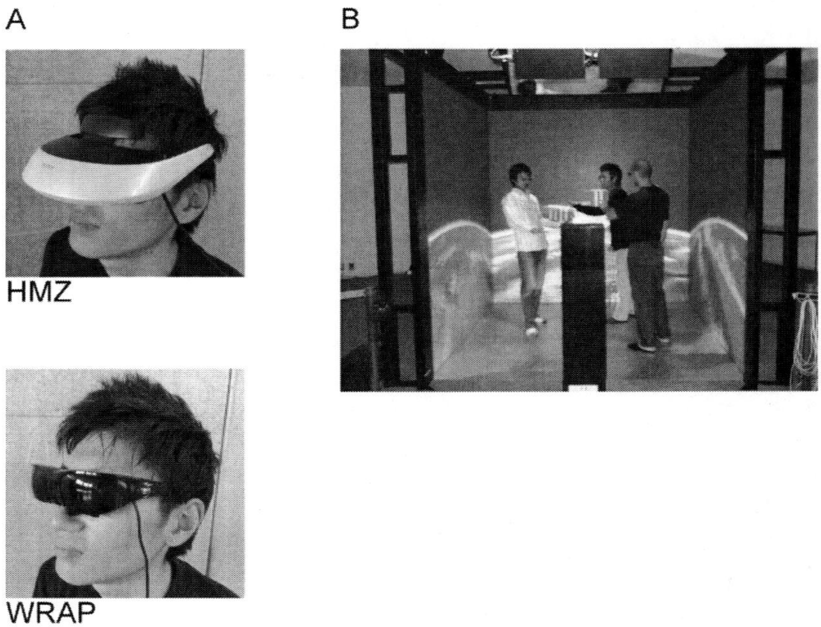

Figure 3. Head mount display (HMD, A) and CAVE (B). HMDs shown are HMZ series (Sony Inc., Japan) and WRAP series (Vuzix Inc., NY, USA). HMD enables visual immersion, while CAVE allows both visual and full-body immersion.

Nowadays, a wide variety of HMD products are available from cheap and accessible models to expensive and high-end models, depending on their functions and specifications, e.g., resolution, 3D vision, and motion tracking. CAVE (Computer Assisted Virtual Environment, Figure 3B), which has room-sized multiple cubic walls, allows the users to experience both visual and full-body immersion as they wear 3D glasses, and to walk around in the space within the screen (Cruz-Neira, Sandin, & DeFanti, 1993; Cruz-Neira, Sandin, DeFanti, Kenyon, & Hart, 1992). Interaction between the user and the environment is mediated by peripheral input devices such as keyboard and joystick, or in advanced VR systems, by embedding highly automated equipment such as motion tracking and motion capturing. Not only the effects of depth cue provided by stereoscopic display, but also those of immersion and interaction, are topics for studies on visuomotor control in VR. Although telepresence exemplified by video-conference is one of the framework concepts for VR (Lanier, 2001), this is mainly addressed from the aspect of social behavior rather than that of perceptual motor control.

While the application of VR is escalating, attention should be called to the problem of construction of a veridical 3D visual space, which is almost impossible with the current stereoscopic display technologies (Wann, Rushton, & Mon-Williams, 1995). One reason is the disruption of natural oculomotor synchronization. That is, unlike real conditions, the accommodation movement of the viewer's eye is kept on the fixed screen while the vergence movement is forced by the image offset for the binocular disparity in VR. Another reason regards perspective representation. Since the vergence movement of the eye generates a small change in the distance between the left and right eyes, it can cause a spatial bias if the displayed images are fixed, irrespective of ocular movement.

The 'sense of presence', or more simply 'presence', is the term indicating the extent to which the computer-simulated environment represents the world of concern, and used to assess how much the users feel or behave as if they are in the world presented. Hence, the sense of presence is worthy of examination not only for VR developers and video creators but also for scientists interested in perceptual behavior (Sanchez-Vives & Slater, 2005). In fact, several inventories and questionnaires for psychological tests have been developed to assess the level of presence in VR and 3D presentation (Banos et al., 2008; Witmer & Singer, 1998). The sense of presence, although it may be a product of illusionary effect, would have no small effect on the visuomotor performance in VR space.

Motion Capture System

If an experimenter needs to include a human-like performer in computer-simulated visual stimuli, a motion capture system should be one of the most powerful tools used to create the CG animation of moving character. In the studies on biological motion, although video-based motion measurement technique such as direct linear transformation method (Abdel-Aziz & Karara, 1971) is also useful, 3D auto motion capture systems appear to be gaining a larger share in the last few decades. Motion capture is fundamentally a recording procedure for the physical movements of an object, however now widely recognized as one of the core technologies for digital character animations. The most commercially successful product to date would be the retroreflective optical system, such as Vicon (Vicon Inc., NY, USA) and

MotionAnalysis (Motion Analysis Inc., CA, USA), while many other optical and non-optical systems are also supplied.

There is available literature that offers methodological tips of creating character animations and archived data of created motions (Dekeyser, Verfaillie, & Vanrie, 2002; Ma, Paterson, & Pollick, 2006; Troje, 2002; Vanrie & Verfaillie, 2004). Besides, facial biological perception is also of concern, where 3D laser scanning technology is favorable to create realistic facial expressions. It becomes possible to realize morphing (Blanz & Vetter, 1999), reflecting muscular activations (Sifakis, Neverov, & Fedkiw, 2005), and etching wrinkles (Bickel et al., 2007), based on both static facial scanning and dynamic motion capture. For studies on perceptual motor control, however, motion capture systems are often used for recording the performer's movement. Thus, the system may be employed twice in an experiment project, first in creating visual stimuli of biological motion and second in recording the reactors' motions responding to the visual stimuli. Furthermore, in some laboratories, the motion capture system is integrated with the visual display or VR equipment, as the real-time input device of the user's motion.

Manipulation of Visual Stimuli

The concept of computer-simulated display in this chapter covers computational simulation of visual stimuli with mathematical and numerical manipulation as well as the display of computer-generated images. One of the advantageous points in computer-simulated display is to present intended situations that are arbitrarily and rigorously defined by parameter settings. The numerical manipulations can be applied to all of the environmental phenomena including object motion, human movement, and background space. Generally speaking, there are two possible policies in executing a computational simulation: one is to reconstruct realistic context and another is to implement unrealistic context.

Although these approaches literally seem to seek different goals, both of them are absolutely effective in revealing the characteristics of human visuomotor control. The realistic approach allows researchers to bring the quasi-natural and standardized contexts of an event into their laboratory, and further helps to control the experimental conditions as they want, with less time, cost, and effort. The results obtained would have relatively direct suggestions to perceptual motor behaviors in the real world. On the other hand, the unrealistic approach enables examination of human visuomotor control in response to physically impossible phenomena. The emerging response pattern, however, can clearly highlight the inherent function of human visuomotor control apart from the physical laws in nature and acquired skills adapted to the outer world.

'Dynamic simulation', which is designed to model the time-varying behavior of an environment or an object, using differential equations, is one of the realistic approaches used to generate the motion of stimulus images with adherence to the physical laws and some constraints. To create a ball flight animation on the basis of an aerodynamic formula is the typical simulation case. Needless to say, other dynamically-constrained motions such as the pendulum and spring are also applicable. If biological movement is simulated dynamically, valid anatomical constraints, e.g., motion axis and motion range at the joint, should be considered. Furthermore, if it has a multi-link structure (two or more segments linked with joints), inverse dynamics that calculate the joint forces and forward dynamics, which predict the outcome motion resulting from applied joint forces, might be very helpful. 'Averaging' would be also categorized as a realistic approach, which is used to standardize, neutralize, or generalize the visual stimuli by eliminating the individual and conditional factors. In this approach, a mass of original data must be collected in order to increase the validity as standard, and normalization may be needed prior to averaging if the original data are varied in size, amplitude, time period, and other physical quantity. Other computational manipulations, such as 'optimization' and 'regression', can be an alternative options to generate the standardized behavior of a system. In addition, some perturbation techniques may also be categorized into the realistic approach as long as the manipulation does not violate physical laws.

For the unrealistic approach, on the other hand, various types of perturbation techniques that ignore or change the laws governing the behavior of the original system are possible. There should be a concrete hypothesis if an unrealistic perturbation is applied, or the study can only tell that strange stimuli evoke a strange performance. 'Noise addition' is intended to disturb the normal visuomotor function by interfering or contaminating the original optical signal. The noise may be injected directly into the target object as random error or arranged onto the surrounding space as background masking. It should be noted, however, that some noise, such as visual white noise, is used in order to represent a background scene, not to contaminate the target signal. 'Exaggeration' is used to enhance the extent of the motion, shape, or duration of original image to emphasize specific visual information. 'Replacement' partially changes the original motion to a modified one. 'Inversion' is to turn upside down and 'scrambling' is to mix randomly, those are typically used in the studies on biological motion perception. Moreover, 'occlusion', 'deformation', and many other artificial treatments of spatiotemporal dynamics would be categorized into the unrealistic approach.

Posture Control

Overview of Posture Study

Postural control is a mechanism to maintain the body position in space for the purpose of balance and orientation that is regulated by visual, vestibular, and somatosensory information in principle (Warren, Kay, & Yilmaz, 1996; Woollacott & Shumway-Cook, 2002). Neurologically, it has been considered an automatic and reflex controlled task to arrange the mechanical structure of bones and joints with minimal attentional resources. To date, a number of studies have reported the mechanism of balance control during upright standing or some locomotion tasks, and provided evidence that vision plays an important role in the maintenance and adjustment of the posture. It has been widely recognized that optical flow, which refers to the apparent motion of visual array, causes the viewers' ego-motion without self-consciousness (Gibson, 1950; Lishman & Lee, 1973). More specifically, sinusoidal oscillation of the outer visual environment induces a coherent sinusoidal postural sway at the driving frequency. A qualitative interpretation for this phenomenon is that the visual system perceives the moving surroundings as if it resulted from the self-motion and makes the motor system generate compensatory responses. It is also evident that the lamellar optical flow projected onto the retinal periphery induces greater body sway than the radial flow in the center of the visual field (Stoffregen, 1985).

The assessment of the relation between vision and other sensations may more clearly highlight the roll of the visual system, so that the normal sway is critically disturbed when the visual information conflicts with the vestibular and proprioceptive inputs (Soechting & Berthoz, 1979). Although posture studies brought in computer-simulated display techniques comparatively earlier than other visuomotor task studies, it took a decade to begin serious application of such computerized stimuli after these pioneering studies. Since then to the present, various perturbing effectors are used, e.g., moving room (Lee & Lishman, 1975; Lishman & Lee, 1973; Stoffregen, 1985; Stoffregen, Schmuckler, & Gibson, 1987), mobile cart (Soechting & Berthoz, 1979), computer-generated textured wall (Dijkstra, Schoner, & Gielen, 1994; Dijkstra, Gielen, & Melis, 1992; Mahboobin, Loughlin, Redfern, & Sparto, 2005; van Asten, Gielen, & Denier van der Gon, 1988), or virtual tunnel (Greffou, Bertone, Hanssens, & Faubert, 2008), nevertheless the optical environment is mostly controlled by simple waveforms, such as sinusoid. Recently, however, more realistic and contextual paradigms are being addressed such as street walking, physical training, and communication benefiting from CG modeling technology.

Response to Computer-Simulated Optical Flow

For upright standing tasks, sinusoidal oscillation patterns of the visual environment (often in the anterior-posterior direction) have traditionally been used to generate optical flow on the retina after the milestone study using a 'moving room' paradigm (Lee & Lishman, 1975; Lishman & Lee, 1973). A computer-simulated visual room (walls) is often depicted using random dots, checkerboard, and bull's eye target textures. Postural responses to an oscillating virtual wall were measured under conditions in which viewers were exposed to computer-generated 2D monocular images (Dijkstra et al., 1992) and to 3D binocular stereograms (Dijkstra et al., 1994). The results of these studies showed that the body sway amplitude was approximately constant, irrespective of the assumed distance to the moving wall, while the optical expansion rate is inversely varied with the wall distance. This indicates that posture is adjusted based on the spatial dimension of the outer environment (distal information) rather than the optical flow on the retina (proximal information), and further implying the active involvement of the central nervous system in postural control.

Another study that also used sinusoidally-moving stimuli demonstrated an occasional switching of the postural sway from in-phase to anti-phase mode and vice versa, i.e., 180° phase shift, presumably depending on the viewer's perceptual interpretation of the environment (van Asten et al., 1988). A series of studies, in which somatosensory information using a light touch of the fingertip and visual information by random dot images are perturbed, revealed that multisensory information was integrated in a nonlinear fashion for the control of upright posture (Jeka, Oie, & Kiemel, 2000; Oie, Kiemel, & Jeka, 2001).

In the 2000s, full-fledged immersive and interactive VR displays rapidly spread in perceptual motor experiments, where studies on postural control were no exception. Such VR simulators help not only in reusing the moving room paradigm in a more convenient fashion, but also the simultaneous use of other sensory devices (Greffou et al., 2008; Sparto et al., 2006). This would accelerate the comprehensive understanding toward the role of the sensory systems in the adjustments of posture. A study created a unique simulated situation in which the optical flow was identical, but perceived self-motion relative to the environment (perceived relative motion) was different, by interchanging the stereoscopic images of HMD between the left and right eyes (Kelly, Loomis, & Beall, 2005). The reversed stereo condition caused greater postural instability as compared with the normal condition, suggesting that perceived relative motion alone can affect self-motion regardless of the optical flow available.

The development effect of children on vision-based balance control was also examined using an immersive screen and a moving platform (Sparto et al., 2006), HMD and tilted platform (Lee, Cherng, & Lin, 2004), and a virtual tunnel in CAVE (Greffou et al., 2008). These studies suggested that children around the age of 10 or younger are prone to rely heavily on the visual information, relative to the vestibular and proprioceptive inputs, than older children and adults.

Sensory Re-Weighting in Balance Control

In the stream of posture study, the phenomenon that relative contributions of the sensory systems change depending on the available information from the environment, known as 'sensory re-weighting hypothesis', is one of the current hot topics (Asslander & Peterka, 2014; Peterka, 2002; Peterka & Loughlin, 2004). A study using a computer-generated immersive optical flow and movable platform showed that the effect of visual perturbation diminished immediately after viewing a randomly moving scene, suggesting that the viewers decreased reliance on the unreliable visual information in controlling posture (Mahboobin et al., 2005).

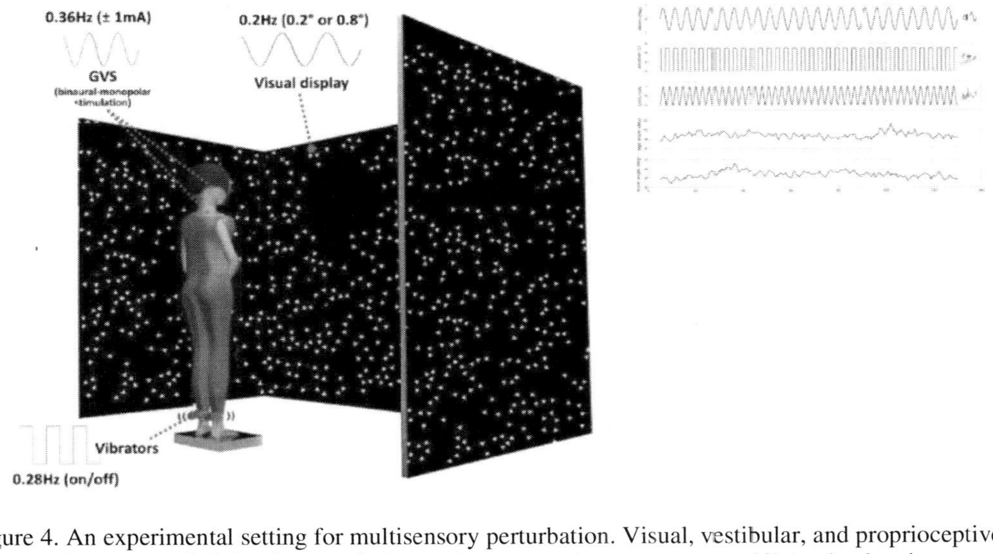

Figure 4. An experimental setting for multisensory perturbation. Visual, vestibular, and proprioceptive perturbations are applied simultaneously by random texture image on screen, bilateral galvanic vestibular stimulation, and bilateral vibration of Achilles tendons, respectively. Reproduced from Hwang et al. (2014) in accordance with the publisher's policy.

Another study using visual and light touch displays has shown that children between 4-10 years old increased the amount of re-weighting as age, indicating the developmental process of a adaptive ability (Bair, Kiemel, Jeka, & Clark, 2007). On the other hand, it has been evidenced that elderly adults have less efficient in sensory re-weighting ability from the computer-simulated display experiments of quiet standing tasks (Jeka et al., 2006) and collision avoidance tasks (Eikema, Hatzitaki, Tzovaras, & Papaxanthis, 2012). In one of the latest synthesizing experimental settings, the visual, vestibular, and proprioceptive inputs were simultaneously perturbed with a random texture on a surrounded screen, galvanic vestibular stimulation, and vibrator on the Achilles tendons, respectively (Figure 4) (Hwang, Agada, Kiemel, & Jeka, 2014). The results showed that there were intramodal visual-visual, intermodal visual-vestibular, and intermodal visual-proprioceptive re-weighting effects.

Locomotion and Other Posture-Related Tasks in Virtual Simulator

The analysis of locomotion, more specifically walk, is also longstanding theme explored not only in biomechanical studies but also in neurological studies (Warren, Kay, Zosh, Duchon, & Sahuc, 2001). Visual stimuli similar to that used to test upright stance can be applied but specific equipment that enables locomotion is needed. A study on treadmill walking in a virtual hallway suggested that the mediolateral motion was unstable and required balance control by the central nervous system from step-to-step whereas the anteroposterior component was passively stabilized through the series of falls during the step intervals (O'Connor & Kuo, 2009). Another treadmill and VR setup was used to identify the patterns of stepping parameters during passing activities through an oscillating aperture (Buekers, Montagne, de Rugy, & Laurent, 1999; Montagne, Buekers, de Rugy, Camachon, & Laurent, 2002). An electromyography study showed that the muscle activities of the lower body were correlated with the amount of foot displacement during an adaptive step of walking in both real and virtual obstacle avoidance tasks (Moraes & Patla, 2006).

A VR setting is also used in the study on heading perception during locomotion (Wann, Swapp, & Rushton, 2000). Errors in heading judgment increased with attentional load during a simulated locomotion, however, the judgment could be improved by the introduction of extra-retinal gaze information. A dynamical model in which the angular acceleration of a locomotor is a function of the angle and distance of goal and obstacle was proposed to explain the locomotors' path based on the data of VR experiment and simulation (Fajen & Warren, 2003). Subsequently the model was generalized by the results of a real-world experiment (Fink, Foo, & Warren, 2007).

Moreover, VR techniques are releasing a further new and wide variety of experimental frameworks in posture, balance, and locomotion studies. For example, postural stability in a simulated street view with rich visual scenes, such as buildings and trees (Horlings et al., 2009), balance control in a social interpersonal situation (Alatalo, Juhola, Surakka, & Tossavainen, 2009), and self-motion illusion induced by moving sounds and a photorealistic view in a simulated market place (Riecke, Väljamäe, & Schulte-Pelkum, 2009).

For clinicians, VR is expected as sensorimotor training device for neurorehabilitation. Although a number of studies have been conducted to establish the efficacy of VR rehabilitation for various clinical populations, e.g., cerebral palsy, stroke, spinal cord injury, optimal training methodology must be identified to improve real-world motor function

(Adamovich, Fluet, Tunik, & Merians, 2009; Holden, 2005). Meanwhile, it has been noticed that the immersion in VR caused motion sickness, postural instability, and behavioral delay (Akizuki et al., 2005; Horlings et al., 2009; Nishiike et al., 2013; Nyberg et al., 2006). Although there is no doubt that VR is a very powerful tool in posture study, steady and further elaboration is required to verify to what extent the simulator is effective.

Interceptive Action

Overview of Interception Study

Interception is an action to stop or change the translational motion of object or organism, including many kinds of daily activities described by various verbs, e.g., taking, seizing, halting, catching, hitting, blocking, and others. To successfully perform an interception, the effector, such as a hand, and the target, such as a ball, must be coincident both in space and in time irrespective of whether its style is capture or non-capture. There are four basic geometric configurations in regard to the relative motion of the intercepting effector and target object, i.e., pursuit, head-on, receding, and perpendicular (Tresilian, 2005). In addition, the vector summation of the perpendicular configuration and one of three other co-linear configurations makes other possible configurations, e.g., pursuit plus perpendicular. There are two major types of interceptive tasks that have been addressed in the past studies: The first one is a locomotive task in which the interceptor displaces their own body to the location where the target object will pass (Fajen & Warren, 2004; McBeath, Shaffer, & Kaiser, 1995; McLeod & Dienes, 1996; Rushton, Harris, Lloyd, & Wann, 1998).

Another one is a manual task in which the interceptor controls their hand or other end-effector without transferring the self-location (Le Runigo, Benguigui, & Bardy, 2005; Peper, Bootsma, Mestre, & Bakker, 1994; Savelsbergh, Whiting, & Bootsma, 1991; van der Kamp, Savelsbergh, & Smeets, 1997). Interception is generally classified into visually guided action as well as steering and avoidance. Although many theoretical models have been proposed to explain the pattern of visually guided action, none is commonly and universally acknowledged (Fajen, 2005). Rather, it seems suitable to stand on the notion that different tasks will involve different control strategies (Tresilian, 2005).

However, the theoretical models can be classified into two broad categories, i.e., the preprogrammed control model and the on-line control model. As far as we know, tau theory is the most influential as prototype of a preprogrammed control model, where the critical value 'tau' that initiates an action is assumed as invariant (Lee, 1976). On the other hand, the on-line control model further classified into two types, continuous control model and discrete error correction model (Tresilian, 2005). Recently, on-line models seem to be preferred rather than preprogrammed models even if the motor task discussed is rapid action.

An 'Outfielder problem', which is typically described as how a baseball fielder runs to catch a fly ball, is a longstanding topic in studies on locomotive interceptive task modeled by an on-line control theory. This was first formulated in the physical consideration as $d(\tan(\alpha))/dt$ = constant, where α is the elevation angle of the ball from the viewpoint of successful catcher (Chapman, 1968). In addition, actor and reactor match-up contexts, e.g., server and receiver in tennis, have been used to examine the expert performance that is of particular interest in the field of sports science.

Time to Contact with Computer-Generated Approaching Object

In order to successfully perform an interceptive task, one must accurately estimate the time to contact (TTC) between the intercepting effector and the approaching object. As a case of TTC perception for motion in depth, a virtual object approaching in a straight line toward the viewer's face at rest is often used as visual stimuli. In particular, how the binocular and monocular cues affect the TTC perception has been of interest to vision science. From a psychophysical study using a dichoptic experimental setting, it has been shown that estimates of TTC are more accurate when both binocular and monocular retinal image information was available than when only binocular or only monocular information is available (Gray & Regan, 1998). Regarding visuomotor control, a theoretical model for perceived TTC of an approaching object is derived from the measurement of hand closure motion during a virtual ball catch task in HMD (Rushton & Wann, 1999). First, the study made a test model that includes the binocular disparity and optical looming as information sources of motion in depth. Thereafter the model's robustness was demonstrated by predicting the catcher's response to perturbed ball trajectories.

TTC analysis can be also applied to virtual interception tasks for a moving object other than motion in depth. In manual interception tasks for the computer-generated animation of falling ball, the interceptors systematically time their motor responses on the assumption of gravity effect (gravitational free-fall), even when the simulated falling ball did not actually accelerate (uniform fall) (Zago et al., 2004). Approaching ball stimuli with pendular motion is used to compare the catching performance in real and VR settings (Dessing, Peper, & Beek, 2004). TTC judgment is a matter of importance in daily behavior such as avoidance of a collision accident. For example, the road crossing behavior of a pedestrian was examined in VR, and simulated approaching vehicles in the traffic flow (Simpson, Johnston, & Richardson, 2003). The results showed that younger children were prone to unsafe crossing behavior as compared with older counterparts. Gaze analyses during virtual driving tasks have suggested that visual strategies for TTC judgment are characterized by the saccadic eye movement between the approaching vehicle and the road ahead (van Loon, Khashawi, & Underwood, 2010).

Outfielder Problem in Virtual Simulator

The Chapman model ($d(\tan(\alpha))/dt$ = constant), later called an optic acceleration cancellation (OAC) model, was a seed of the subsequent theories known as linear optical trajectory (LOT) model (McBeath et al., 1995), control of optical velocity (COV) model (Marken, 2001), and generalized optic acceleration cancellation (GOAC) model (McLeod, Reed, & Dienes, 2006). The first VR study that addressed the outfielder problem was conducted using a CAVE system (Zaal & Michaels, 2003). The results suggested that the patterns of $d(\tan(\alpha))/dt$ can be a cue for judging whether the ball will land behind or in front of the catcher. In addition, the catching performance was higher when the catchers intercepted the approaching virtual ball with their forehead (47%) than with a hand-held wand (9%). Since the original Chapman model is expressed using eye gaze angle (α), such a head interception task might be better than the manual one because the contact point (forehead) is closer to the eyes than hand.

The outfielder problem was also addressed by investigating the locomotion pattern of soccer players who attempted to head an approaching ball in HMD (Figure 5) (McLeod, Reed, Gilson, & Glennerster, 2008). In this study the approaching pattern of the virtual ball was perturbed in mid-flight from the normal quasi-parabolic path to an abnormal linear one in order to manipulate the modality of changing d(tan(α))/dt (Figure 5A). The results were in line with the notion that the locomotion of interceptors is controlled in an on-line manner, and more specifically, supported the GOAC theory but rejected the LOT theory. This conclusion was further confirmed by another HMD study that used a similar perturbation for the ball flight pattern (from parabolic to linear) and measured the running path of baseball fielder (Fink, Foo, & Warren, 2009). It is noteworthy that this study was conducted in a relatively wide space (12 × 12 m) as compared with the former soccer heading study (3.5 × 3.5 m).

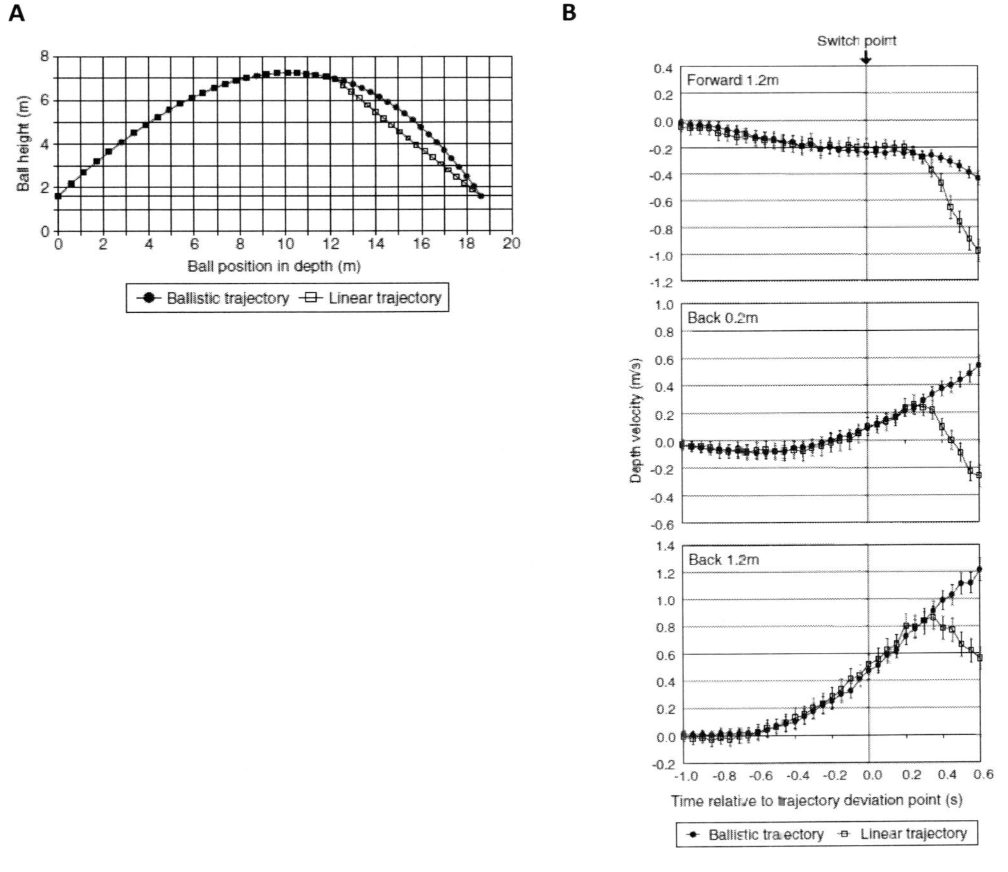

Figure 5. Perturbation of the ball flight trajectory displayed as visual stimuli (A) and resulting alteration of catcher's velocity (B) in a virtual outfielder task. Reproduced from McLeod et al. (2008) with permission from the publisher.

Interception in Simulated Sporting Context

High-demanding interceptive activities, typically seen in competitive match-up play, have been also addressed by using computer-simulated displays. Skilled versus less skilled comparisons are often accompanied with this paradigm in order to clarify the effect of expertise. A batting simulator that displayed a pitched ball and monitored the bat motion was used to investigate the spatiotemporal swing accuracy of college baseball players (Gray, 2002). The results showed that the randomness of the ball speed from pitch to pitch caused large errors in bat swing. In addition, it was also shown that the batters benefit from the information of pitch count, pitch history, and ball rotation to execute the swing. Later, by using a modified version of this simulator including a virtual field and CG humanoid pitcher, it was evident that expert batters are more accurate than less skilled counterparts in the outcome prediction where the batted ball will land, and less vulnerable to hindsight bias after feedback (Gray, Beilock, & Carr, 2007). Another integrative virtual batting simulator, which enables immersive and stereoscopic display and measurement of batters' motor response, was constructed to investigate the effect of perception-action coupling in batting behavior (Ranganathan & Carlton, 2007). The results indicated that the skilled batters attuned their stepping patterns to the pitcher's kinematics whereas their swing duration was related to the ball speed.

Goalkeepers' judgment ability toward a curved free kick was examined in a virtual stadium created through 3D modeling, where the ball flight pattern was determined with an aerodynamic model including gravity, drag, and Magnus–Robins lift forces (Craig, Berton, Rao, Fernandez, & Bootsma, 2006). The results clearly demonstrated that the laterally bended ball caused goalkeepers' erroneous predictions about the entering point. The follow-up modeling study reported that goalkeepers' movements were explained by the ball's current heading direction (position and velocity) but not by the lateral acceleration and thus resulted in the erroneously biased movement opposite to the desirable direction (Dessing & Craig, 2010). A series of these studies provided the practical evidence that curved free kicks are often chosen in soccer games.

More recently, gaze analysis during racquetball strokes simulated in HMD is providing an insight into the visual strategy in making an interception of bouncing ball with handheld gear (Diaz, Cooper, Rothkopf, & Hayhoe, 2013). This study revealed a typical gaze pattern that a large saccade occurred 150–200 ms prior to the ball bounce and followed by a fixation across the bounce. Today, such match-up interceptive behaviors are addressed in various sporting situations, e.g., thrower and goalkeeper in handball (Bideau et al., 2004), defender and attacker in rugby (Watson et al., 2011), and successive rally in table tennis (Brunnett et al., 2006).

Biological Motion Perception

Overview of Biological Motion Study

It is widely recognized that our brain has a unique visual mechanism in the detection of biped or quadruped motions, known as biological motion perception. Research on this topic originates pioneering literature that demonstrates our interpolative perceptual ability, more specifically, only a few dots depicting some body landmarks (e.g., joints) can give a compelling impression of a human walker when the dots started moving (Johansson, 1973). Dot-made stimuli like this were later called point-light display (PLD) and became commonly used in subsequent studies. Early studies demonstrated that PLD could convey the information of the sex of walkers (Kozlowski & Cutting, 1977) and identity of friends (Cutting & Kozlowski, 1977). And later, it was evident that higher-level mental states such as intention (Runeson & Frykholm, 1983) and emotions (Pollick, Paterson, Bruderlin, & Sanford, 2001) can be transmitted via PLD as well.

Brain imaging studies identified that the superior temporal sulcus (STS) is characteristically activated when observers perceive the PLD animation as biological motion (Bonda, Petrides, Ostry, & Evans, 1996; Howard et al., 1996; Vaina, Solomon, Chowdhury, Sinha, & Belliveau, 2001). In addition, it was also reported that other brain areas such as the occipital and fusiform face areas (Grossman & Blake, 2002) and premotor cortex (Saygin, Wilson, Hagler, Bates, & Sereno, 2004) selectively responded to biological motion.

To create PLD animation of human action, motion analysis techniques that output the coordinate data of body landmarks are very advantageous. The digitized motion data can be used for visual stimuli as is, and moreover, such digital data are also convenient when manipulating the stimuli by the procedures of noise addition, inverting, scrambling, occlusion, and others. Furthermore, it is possible to do more complicated manipulations such as dynamic simulation and mathematical perturbation and to do more advanced rendering such as polygon-based CG characterization.

Although biological motion is often discussed from the aspect of its perceptual effect, it surely has considerable effects on the motor generation of the observer. In particular, the acquisition of motor skill is intimately tied to observational learning and imitative learning in which the action of a demonstrator serves as the model of the learner's movements.

It should be noted that, in a broader sense, the concept of biological motion perception contains the recognition ability of facial expression. Anatomically speaking, facial expression is created by activating mimetic muscles inserted on the face skins, whereas bodily motion is generated by activating skeletal muscles attached to the adjacent bones. Partly because of such intrinsic differences in the types of motion generation, perceptual effects of face and body are often discussed separately in biological motion studies.

Graphic-Rich Model for Biological Motion Stimuli

The biological motion study started with a PLD model, but thereafter, some researchers introduced other graphical models, e.g., stick-figures, silhouette, and polygon characters. Motion capture systems facilitate the use of these models in combination with CG rendering techniques. An advantage of using a graphically rich model is that measured perceptual responses have, to some extent, direct relevance to natural performance when seeing the motion of a living creature, at least better than viewing PLD. Since the captured digital motion data can be output as any PLD and other CG characters, a direct comparison of perceptual effects is possible among these models on the identical actions (Dekeyser et al., 2002). Furthermore, if archived motion data are freely available like an open source library, various motion stimuli can be readily and commonly shared across the world and over the ages (Ma et al., 2006; Vanrie & Verfaillie, 2004). For face recognition study, 3D laser scanning plus motion capturing is helpful in rapidly creating the shape of the face and arbitrary manipulating the configurations and patterns in expression (Hill & Johnston, 2001; Vetter & Troje, 1997).

An early study reported that a polygon model evoked more accurate responses than a corresponding stick-figure model in the discrimination of running motion pattern (Hodgins, O'Brien, & Tumblin, 1998). However a contradictory finding, that the stick-figure is better than the polygon, has also been shown in tennis serve discrimination tasks (Ida, Fukuhara, & Ishii, 2012). Furthermore, it was demonstrated that handball goalkeepers adopted a different defending motor strategy when responding to a PLD thrower than when doing it to stick-figures and silhouettes (Vignais et al., 2009). The discrepancies in these findings seem to be partly attributable to the difference of the visual simuli and tasks. Nevertheless, these studies agree at the point that the types of humanoid models displayed critically affect observers' perceptual and motor performance.

A brain imaging study showed that a simplified polygon walker with four cylinder limbs selectively activated the cortical area sensitive to biological motion (STS) as well as a more human-like polygon character, whereas the motion of the disjointed cylinder limbs and grandfather clock did not trigger this type of activation (Pelphrey et al., 2003). Among various biological motion studies using computer-simulated display, one of the most advanced application cases might be a fully-computerized learning system through motor imitation. A real-time VR dance training system was implemented by integrating a HMD and optical motion capture device, and it was reported that this system successfully improved the dancing skill of learners (Chan, Leung, Tang, & Komura, 2011).

Computational Manipulation of Motion Stimuli

PLD model has been subjected to computer simulations and numerical perturbations in accordance with study hypotheses. The simplicity of the PLD component, i.e., dot, enhances the ease of manipulation, even though the biological motion itself is generally taken as having very complicated information. Conventionally upside-down inverted models and/or phase scrambled models have been frequently used as control stimuli because they can critically impair the normal perceptual processing for an intact model while preserving the quantity of visual information. In addition, background masking with mass dots, removal of specified dots, spatiotemporal occlusion of individual dots, and many other treatments are readily possible if only a modest computer system is available.

On the other hand, fairly complicated manipulation with mathematical calculation is occasionally required to create intended biological motion stimuli. As an 'averaging' approach, forty walkers' motions were analyzed with principal component analysis and summarized into an averaged PLD walker where body size, dynamic pattern, and structural configuration were normalized where appropriate (Troje, 2002). This technique is very advantageous for the purpose of eliminating the undesired bias arising from individual traits, and further, makes it possible to synthesize new motion patterns on the arbitrary parametric setting. A similar approach has been taken to identify anticipatory information embedded in the dynamic context of tennis shots (Huys, Smeeton, Hodges, Beek, & Williams, 2008) and soccer kicks (Diaz, Fajen, & Phillips, 2012).

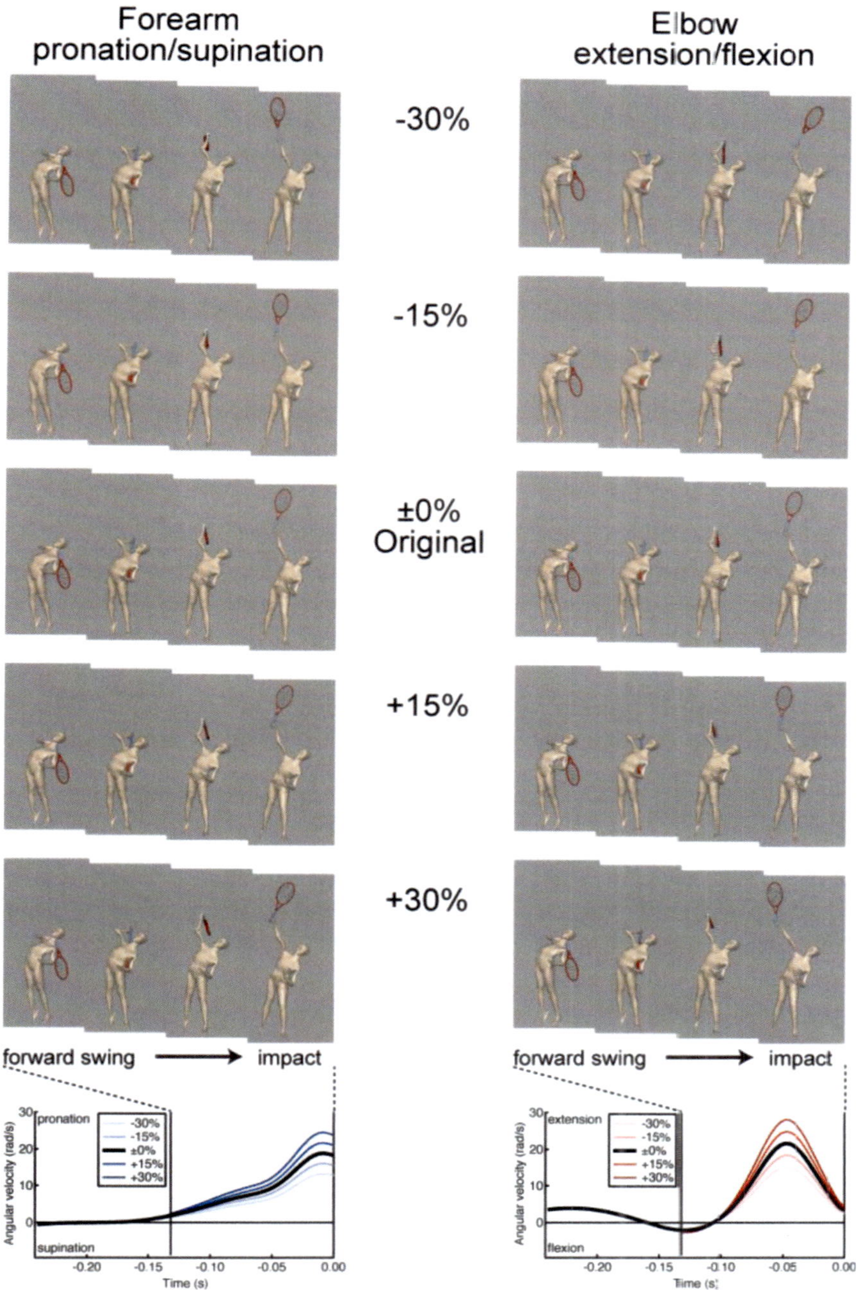

Figure 6. Computational perturbation of racket-swing pattern and CG display using humanoid model for tennis serve. Forearm pronation/supination (left) and elbow extension/flexion (right) were perturbed during the forward swing phase by proportionally modulating the joint angular velocity of the original serve motion.

More complicated models, such as polygon humanoid characters and face expressions can be computationally manipulated as well. By using a polygon character, it was shown that a spatial exaggeration of tennis serve motion enhanced the discrimination accuracy of the shot styles (Pollick, Fidopiastis, & Braden, 2001). In addition, another exaggeration manipulation was proved to heighten the impression of the intensity of 30-PLD facial emotions (Pollick, Hill, Calder, & Paterson, 2003).

It should be noted that exaggeration techniques are likely to induce unperformable movements for real-world humans if the algorithm excluded biomechanical considerations. Thus, toward the understandings of actual perceptual motor skills, manipulations must be designed without violating anatomical constraints. The perturbations that magnified the torso rotation angle or shoulder joint torque of a polygon runner (Hodgins et al., 1998) and that modulated the joint angular velocity of a polygon tennis server (Figure 6) (Ida, Fukuhara, Kusubori, & Ishii, 2011; Ida, Fukuhara, Sawada, & Ishii, 2011) would be of significance in a practical sense, because the perturbed motions could be deemed to be performable actions.

Expert Recognition in Action Observation

Expertise in specific domains has to do with not only developing motor skills of one's own motion but also acquiring perceptual skills to read anyone else's motion. This can be referred to as high-demand biological motion perception in which visual information must be processed under heavy time pressure. Numerous studies have demonstrated the superiority of skilled players compared to less skilled counterparts in information pick-up ability from the observed action. Recently it became evident that professional performers activate their brains in a distinctly different manner than untrained non-professional people when observing other's action of the performers' expertise play (Aglioti, Cesari, Romani, & Urgesi, 2008; Calvo-Merino, Glaser, Grèzes, Passingham, & Haggard, 2005).

In making a predictive judgment under a competitive situation, it is said that skilled players can effectively benefit from multiple information sources distributed across the opponent's body in addition to deterministic information at the end-effector. For example, by using temporal and spatial occlusion techniques on PLD, it has been shown that world-class badminton players are able to extract anticipation cues from the opponent's lower body, let alone from the racket (Abernethy & Zawi, 2007). Other computational manipulation techniques such as reduction of dynamic structure, neutralization, and interchanging were applied to displayed actions to draw more clear insights into the effect of expertise on extracting localized information (Huys et al., 2009; Huys et al., 2008; Williams, Huys, Cañal-Bruland, & Hagemann, 2009).

Besides, PLD techniques are further applicable to yield knowledge about various aspects of the relationship between expertise and observation ability. For example, even within professional dancers, female performers were sensitive to subtle differences in PLD exemplars in comparison with male counterparts (Calvo-Merino, Ehrenberg, Leung, & Haggard, 2010). In an observational learning of cricket bowling, a PLD that represents intra-limb relative motion of the isolated bowling arm (shoulder, elbow, wrist, and knuckle) was able to improve the observers' movement coordination more than another PLD for inter-limb relative motions of right and left wrists (Breslin, Hodges, Williams, Kremer, & Curran, 2006). Skilled drummers' brain activity was reduced when the motion of a PLD drummer was simultaneously and meaningfully matched with sound (Petrini et al., 2011). VR settings integrated with motion analysis are increasingly being introduced in order to reveal the expertise effect of sports players when they observe an opponent's action, and execute a motion reaction accordingly (Bideau et al., 2010; Ranganathan & Carlton, 2007).

Computer-Simulated Display Versus Real Scene

Implications of Environmental Comparison

Computer-simulated displays have so many advantageous points, especially in controlling the experimental conditions, and will become much more popular in the future. Researchers as users, however, should always keep in mind that what a computer-simulation presents is intrinsically different from the real thing (of course the computer-display itself is real), even if they elaborated the simulation with their best effort. Normal humans in the real world understand the layout of their surrounding space through a number of monocular sources (occlusion, perspective, relative size, familiar size, accommodation, texture gradient, and others) and binocular sources (retinal disparity and convergence), although any computer-simulated display would not be able to coherently present all these cues (Cutting, 1997). Thus, verifications to what extent the simulated environment in a laboratory setting evokes natural behaviors in a real situation would be required if need arises (Figure 7) (Ho, Gray, & Spence, 2014).

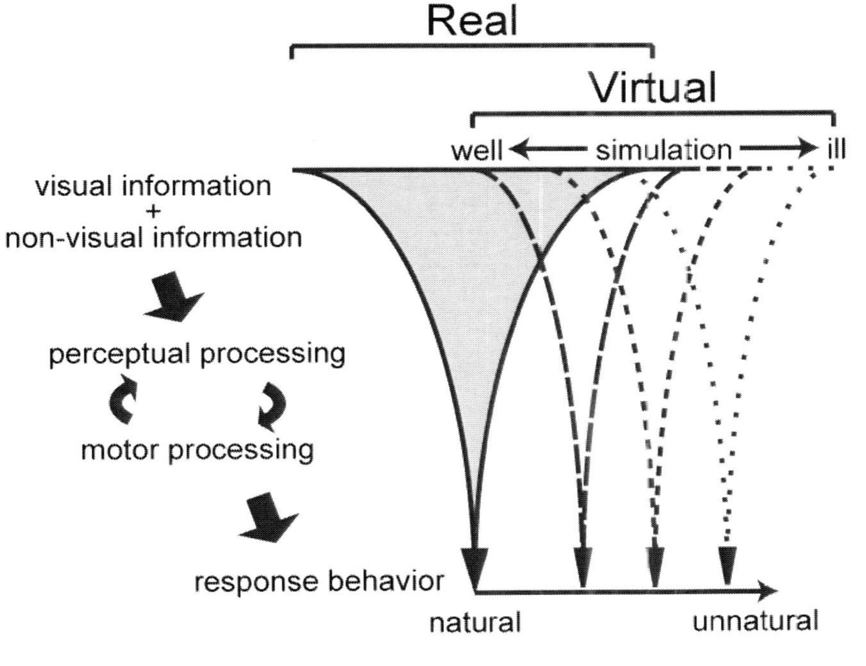

Figure 7. Schematic of simulation quality and resulting action. If a virtual environment suitably simulated the real world and matched the purpose of the test, the response action is expected to be closer to natural behavior.

One of the most straightforward approaches to this end is comparing the behaviors between computer-simulated and real (or photorealistic in some cases) environments. It is reported that virtual and real interactive experiences were comparable with one another in recalling the spatial layout of objects in a room whereas both of them induced inferior recall performance than static observation of the room through a peephole (Arthur, Hancock, & Chrysler, 1997). At brain activation level, however, virtual and real environments provide different effects in spatial learning (Mellet et al., 2010). The distance in VR generally tends to be underestimated, whereas it can be improved or overestimated depending on the tasks and conditions (Bingham, Bradley, Bailey, & Vinner, 2001; Grechkin, Nguyen, Plumert, Cremer, & Kearney, 2010; Plumert, Kearney, Cremer, & Recker, 2005). Although the conclusions about the perceptual similarity (dissimilarity) between virtual and real environments vary from study to study, a number of studies on rehabilitation and sports training have confirmed significant effects of skill acquisition in VR, which are transferable to the real world (Holden, 2005; Kemeny & Panerai, 2003; Miles, Pop, Watt, Lawrence, & John, 2012; Rose, Brooks, & Rizzo, 2005). In this regard, however, we should be always careful about thoughtless use of VR.

Comparisons between Virtual and Real Visuomotor Tasks

It is not as simple as it seems to compare the perceptual motor effects of VR with those in the real world. The first problem is to what extent researchers build up the quality of VR closer to reality, where they have to make decisions about what is replicated, what is ignored, and what is approximated. The selection of simulated events should be determined depending on study hypothesis, and fidelity of VR has a critical impact on the validity of the study. In addition, VR holds some inherent technical limitations in the field of view, spatial and temporal resolution, physical modeling, image quality, time delay, and availability of peripheral devices. Thus, even if differences between virtual and real environments were detected, the results cannot simply be attributed to the factors of experimental treatments. Even the technical problems of VR systems are concurrent and intertwined. Nevertheless, the comparisons between virtual and real are not meaningless.

Locomotors in VR wearing HMD walked slower, took a more deviated path, and kept a larger distance from obstacles than those in the equivalent real situation, while the shape of the paths were highly correlated between these two environments (Fink et al., 2007). In addition, a total change in lower body muscle activities significantly and positively correlated with the amount of foot displacement during a virtual adaptive locomotion task as well as during an equivalent real task (Moraes & Patla, 2006). A locomotive aperture-passing task in a VR environment (Montagne et al., 2002) was later replicated as a real-world task in another study (Cinelli & Patla, 2008). The latter study made retrospective comparisons, and demonstrated that the strategy of velocity adjustment was common between the real and virtual environments whereas the real passengers occasionally took an additional postural strategy, or shoulder rotation.

From the results of kinematic measurements during ball catching, it was shown that the hand motions were initiated later, less accurately, smoother, and aimed more directly toward the contact point in CAVE compared with the real environment. These findings suggest a disadvantageous aspect of VR as a display device for studies regarding on-line control.

Nowadays the visuomotor control when playing commercial video games can become a research paradigm in neuroscience. For example, brain activities during performing golf putts on Nintendo Wii was studied, and the results suggested that cortical activity patterns related to working memory were different between real and game plays (Baumeister, Reinecke, Cordes, Lerch, & Weiss, 2010).

Comparisons in Biological Motion Perception

In the early stage of biological motion perception study, PLD was most likely preferred because it exhibited a surprising phenomenon that a limited number of dots, which seem meaningless while remaining still, can provide a compelling impression of human movement once they start moving. Today, however, researchers in various disciplines are interested in the paradigm of biological motion and broadening the type of performer model, video, CG, robot, and living organism. In the context of comparison between computer-simulated display and reality, it would be reasonable to cast digital models including PLDs and CG characters into computer-simulation while regarding live actors and their filmed (photorealistic) images as real visual stimuli. For example, it has been demonstrated that a full-light display of bodily motion conveys more information about emotion than PLD (Atkinson, Dittrich, Gemmell, & Young, 2004). In another study, taking advantage of recent computer technology of CG character modeling, the perceptual effect was compared among the raw video, high resolution video-like, low resolution video-like, wooden mannequin, cartoon-like, and zombie-like models (McDonnell, Jörg, McHugh, Newell, & O'Sullivan, 2008). Even though the appearance of some models is likely to provide positively or negatively biased feelings, such as the cartoon is friendly but the zombie is scary, the results suggested that with few exceptions the perceived emotion was robust, independent of the character types displayed.

On the other hand, an fMRI study showed that the ventral (lateral fusiform gyrus) and lateral (STS) temporal cortices responded more strongly to video clips of photoreal human motions than to computer-generated PLDs (Beauchamp, Lee, Haxby, & Martin, 2003). Furthermore, a PET study also showed that the right posterior parietal cortex did not respond to displayed hand actions of the CG model even when a high-quality polygon model was used to render it, whereas obvious neural activity was found in this area for real hand actions in the natural environment (Perani et al., 2001). These findings seem reasonable because PLD or commonly-used polygon models have apparently different shapes, colors, and many optical properties than a real (photoreal) actor. In short, the information input to the visual system is essentially different in quantity and quality.

For perceptual activity in the sporting scenario, it was reported that skilled tennis players were able to more effectively extract anticipation cues from the opponent's stroke motion than novice counterparts in live and video displays, while this skill dependent difference was not evident when PLD was used (Shim, Carlton, Chow, & Chae, 2005). Another study on tennis demonstrated that a polygon CG character conveyed information about the future ball direction to the receiving observer but did poorly compared to a corresponding video display (Fukuhara, Ida, Kusubori, & Ishii, 2009). A recent brain imaging study on prediction in badminton suggests that cortical areas sensitive to the anticipation task are similar between PLD and video while visual areas responded differently (Wright, Bishop, Jackson, & Abernethy, 2011).

Summary and Conclusion

This chapter argued the past and present studies on visuomotor control where computer-simulated displays made significant contributions. First, the author made a brief technical overview on available hardware devices and software resources where some concepts in the computational manipulations of visual stimuli were also described. Second, arguments were presented on the findings from the visuomotor experiments using computer-simulated displays, particularly regarding posture, interception, and perception of action.

Several ongoing topics, e.g., sensory re-weighting in posture control and outfielder problem in interception, were referred to in order to illustrate the effective use of VR toward the understanding of longstanding perceptual motor problems. Finally, evidence on the validity of computer-simulated displays was provided by reviewing the studies that made comparisons between computer-generated visual stimuli and the real (realistic) scene. Although there were both positive and negative results in using VR, opinions and views from either side are significant to correctly formulate the application of computer-simulated display techniques in the future.

Now computer-generated imagery and VR are no longer mere visualization tools but almost standard techniques for presenting visual stimuli in modern vision science. Nevertheless, the arguments on the effects of these methods do not seem to be enough; still opening a simple question—does computer-simulated display correctly evoke normal visuomotor function? Traditionally revealing the perceptual motor function was the first priority and the computer-simulated display was nothing more than a convenient techniques that aided the achievement of this goal. However, such attitudes are disrupted in some cases. It would not be an exaggeration to say that some current research may begin with the availability of electronic devices and computer programs in designing an experiment where the study hypothesis is formulated afterward.

Although computer-simulated displays not only allow reconstruction of the realistic scene but they also allow injection of unrealistic perturbation, after all, the goal should be solid in terms of revealing the 'real' visuomotor function of human. Indeed, the current moment we are alive is the ultimate age of huge computerization in history. We may be facing the turning point in considering the meaning of computer-simulated displays in visuomotor research. Historically, the concept of perception-action coupling has offered us a new paradigm in vision science. How will the actual and virtual reality be coupled, and what does it bring us?

References

Abdel-Aziz, Y.I., & Karara, H.M. (1971). Direct linear transformation from comparator coordinates into object space coordinates in close-range photogrammetry. In: *Proceedings of the ASP/UI Symposium on Close-Range Photogrammetry* (pp. 1-18). Falls Church, VA, USA: American Society of Photogrammetry.

Abernethy, B., & Zawi, K. (2007). Pickup of essential kinematics underpins expert perception of movement patterns. *Journal of Motor Behavior*, *39*(5), 353-367.

Adamovich, S.V., Fluet, G.G., Tunik, E., & Merians, A. S. (2009). Sensorimotor training in virtual reality: a review. *NeuroRehabilitation*, *25*(1), 29-44.

Aglioti, S.M., Cesari, P., Romani, M., & Urgesi, C. (2008). Action anticipation and motor resonance in elite basketball players. *Nature Neuroscience*, *11*(9), 1109-1116.

Akizuki, H., Uno, A., Arai, K., Morioka, S., Ohyama, S., Nishiike, S., Tamura, K., & Takeda, N. (2005). Effects of immersion in virtual reality on postural control. *Neuroscience Letters*, *379*(1), 23-26.

Alatalo, T., Juhola, M., Surakka, V., & Tossavainen, T. (2009). Creation of virtual reality stimulus for a psychophysiological body balance measurement. *Psychology Research and Behavior Management*, *2*, 13-22.

Arthur, E.J., Hancock, P.A., & Chrysler, S.T. (1997). The perception of spatial layout in real and virtual worlds. *Ergonomics*, *40*(1), 69-77.

Asslander, L., & Peterka, R.J. (2014). Sensory reweighting dynamics in human postural control. *Journal of Neurophysiology*, *111*(9), 1852-1864.

Atkinson, A.P., Dittrich, W.H., Gemmell, A.J., & Young, A.W. (2004). Emotion perception from dynamic and static body expressions in point-light and full-light displays. *Perception*, *33*(6), 717-746.

Bair, W.N., Kiemel, T., Jeka, J.J., & Clark, J.E. (2007). Development of multisensory reweighting for posture control in children. *Experimental Brain Research*, *183*(4), 435-446.

Banos, R.M., Botella, C., Rubio, I., Quero, S., Garcia-Palacios, A., & Alcaniz, M. (2008). Presence and emotions in virtual environments: the influence of stereoscopy. *Cyberpsychology Behaviour*, *11*(1), 1-8.

Baumeister, J., Reinecke, K., Cordes, M., Lerch, C., & Weiss, M. (2010). Brain activity in goal-directed movements in a real compared to a virtual environment using the Nintendo Wii. *Neuroscience Letters*, *481*(1), 47-50.

Beauchamp, M.S., Lee, K.E., Haxby, J.V., & Martin, A. (2003). fMRI responses to video and point-light displays of moving humans and manipulable objects. *Journal of Cognitive Neuroscience*, *15*(7), 991-1001.

Bickel, B., Botsch, M., Angst, R., Matusik, W., Otaduy, M., Pfister, H., & Gross, M. (2007). Multi-scale capture of facial geometry and motion. *ACM Transactions on Graphics*, *26*(3), 33.

Bideau, B., Kulpa, R., Vignais, N., Brault, S., Multon, F., & Craig, C. (2010). Using virtual reality to analyze sports performance. *IEEE Computer Graphics and Applications*, *30*(2), 14-21.

Bideau, B., Multon, F., Kulpa, R., Fradet, L., Arnaldi, B., & Delamarche, P. (2004). Using virtual reality to analyze links between handball thrower kinematics and goalkeeper's reactions. *Neuroscience Letters*, *372*(1–2), 119-122.

Bingham, G.P., Bradley, A., Bailey, M., & Vinner, R. (2001). Accommodation, occlusion, and disparity matching are used to guide reaching: a comparison of actual versus virtual environments. *Journal of Experimental Psychology: Human Perception and Performance*, *27*(6), 1314-1334.

Blanz, V., & Vetter, T. (1999). A morphable model for the synthesis of 3D faces. In: *Proceedings of the 26th Annual Conference on Computer Graphics and Interactive Techniques* (pp. 187-194). Los Angeles, CA, USA: ACM Press/Addison-Wesley Publishing Co.

Bonda, E., Petrides, M., Ostry, D., & Evans, A. (1996). Specific involvement of human parietal systems and the amygdala in the perception of biological motion. *The Journal of Neuroscience*, *16*(11), 3737-3744.

Breslin, G., Hodges, N.J., Williams, A.M., Kremer, J., & Curran, W. (2006). A comparison of intra- and inter-limb relative motion information in modelling a novel motor skill. *Human Movement Science*, *25*(6), 753-766.

Brunnett, G., Rusdorf, S., & Lorenz, M. (2006). V-Pong: an immersive table tennis simulation. *IEEE Computer Graphics and Applications*, *26*(4), 10-13.

Buekers, M., Montagne, G., de Rugy, A., & Laurent, M. (1999). The regulation of externally paced human locomotion in virtual reality. *Neuroscience Letters*, *275*(3), 171-174.

Calvo-Merino, B., Ehrenberg, S., Leung, D., & Haggard, P. (2010). Experts see it all: configural effects in action observation. *Psychological Research*, *74*(4), 400-406.

Calvo-Merino, B., Glaser, D.E., Grèzes, J., Passingham, R.E., & Haggard, P. (2005). Action observation and acquired motor skills: an fMRI study with expert dancers. *Cerebral Cortex*, *15*(8), 1243-1249.

Chan, J.C.P., Leung, H., Tang, J.K.T., & Komura, T. (2011). A virtual reality dance training system using motion capture technology. *IEEE Transactions on Learning Technologies*, *4*(2), 187-195.

Chapman, S. (1968). Catching a baseball. *American Journal of Physics*, *36*(10), 868-870.

Cinelli, M.E., & Patla, A.E. (2008). Task-specific modulations of locomotor action parameters based on on-line visual information during collision avoidance with moving objects. *Human Movement Science*, *27*(3), 513-531.

Craig, C.M., Berton, E., Rao, G., Fernandez, L., & Bootsma, R.J. (2006). Judging where a ball will go: the case of curved free kicks in football. *Naturwissenschaften*, *93*(2), 97-101.

Cruz-Neira, C., Sandin, D.J., & DeFanti, T.A. (1993). Surround-screen projection-based virtual reality: the design and implementation of the CAVE. In: *Proceedings of the 20th Annual Conference on Computer Graphics and Interactive Techniques* (pp. 135-142). Anaheim, CA, USA: ACM.

Cruz-Neira, C., Sandin, D.J., DeFanti, T.A., Kenyon, R.V., & Hart, J.C. (1992). The CAVE: audio visual experience automatic virtual environment. *Communications of the ACM*, *35*(6), 64-72.

Cutting, J. (1997). How the eye measures reality and virtual reality. *Behavior Research Methods, Instruments, & Computers*, *29*(1), 27-36.

Cutting, J., & Kozlowski, L. (1977). Recognizing friends by their walk: gait perception without familiarity cues. *Bulletin of the Psychonomic Society*, *9*(5), 353-356.

Dekeyser, M., Verfaillie, K., & Vanrie, J. (2002). Creating stimuli for the study of biological-motion perception. *Behavior Research Methods, Instruments, & Computers*, *34*(3), 375-382.

Dessing, J.C., & Craig, C.M. (2010). Bending it like Beckham: how to visually fool the goalkeeper. *PLoS One*, *5*(10), e13161.

Dessing, J.C., Peper, C.E., & Beek, P.J. (2004). A comparison of real catching with catching using stereoscopic visual displays. *Ecological Psychology*, *16*(1), 1-21.

Diaz, G., Cooper, J., Rothkopf, C., & Hayhoe, M. (2013). Saccades to future ball location reveal memory-based prediction in a virtual-reality interception task. *Journal of Vision*, *13*(1):20, 1-14.

Diaz, G.J., Fajen, B.R., & Phillips, F. (2012). Anticipation from biological motion: the goalkeeper problem. *Journal of Experimental Psychology. Human Perception and Performance*, *38*(4), 848-864.

Dijkstra, T.M., Schoner, G., & Gielen, C.C. (1994). Temporal stability of the action-perception cycle for postural control in a moving visual environment. *Experimental Brain Research*, *97*(3), 477-486.

Dijkstra, T.M.H., Gielen, C.C.A.M., & Melis, B.J.M. (1992). Postural responses to stationary and moving scenes as a function of distance to the scene. *Human Movement Science*, *11*(1–2), 195-203.

Eikema, D.J., Hatzitaki, V., Tzovaras, D., & Papaxanthis, C. (2012). Age-dependent modulation of sensory reweighting for controlling posture in a dynamic virtual environment. *Age*, *34*(6), 1381-1392.

Fajen, B.R. (2005). Perceiving possibilities for action: on the necessity of calibration and perceptual learning for the visual guidance of action. *Perception*, *34*(6), 717-740.

Fajen, B.R., & Warren, W.H. (2003). Behavioral dynamics of steering, obstacle avoidance, and route selection. *Journal of Experimental Psychology. Human Perception and Performance*, *29*(2), 343-362.

Fajen, B.R., & Warren, W.H. (2004). Visual guidance of intercepting a moving target on foot. *Perception*, *33*(6), 689-715.

Fink, P.W., Foo, P.S., & Warren, W.H. (2007). Obstacle avoidance during walking in real and virtual environments. *ACM Transactions on Applied Perception*, *4*(1), 2.

Fink, P.W., Foo, P.S., & Warren, W.H. (2009). Catching fly balls in virtual reality: a critical test of the outfielder problem. *Journal of Vision*, *9*(13):14, 1-18.

Fisher, S.S., McGreevy, M., Humphries, J., & Robinett, W. (1987). Virtual environment display system. In: *Proceedings of the 1986 Workshop on Interactive 3D Graphics* (pp. 77-87). Chapel Hill, NC, USA: ACM.

Fukuhara, K., Ida, H., Kusubori, S., & Ishii, M. (2009). Anticipatory judgment of tennis serve: a comparison between video images and computer graphics animations. *International Journal of Sport and Health Science*, *7*, 12-22.

Gibson, J.J. (1950). *The perception of the visual world*. Oxford, England: Houghton Mifflin.

Gibson, J.J. (1958). Visually controlled locomotion and visual orientation in animals. *British Journal of Psychology*, *49*(3), 182-194.

Goodale, M.A. (1998). Visuomotor control: where does vision end and action begin? *Current Biology*, *8*(14), R489-491.

Goodale, M.A., & Milner, A.D. (1992). Separate visual pathways for perception and action. *Trends in Neurosciences*, *15*(1), 20-25.

Gray, R. (2002). Behavior of college baseball players in a virtual batting task. *Journal of Experimental Psychology: Human Perception and Performance*, *28*(5), 1131-1148.

Gray, R., Beilock, S.L., & Carr, T.H. (2007). "As soon as the bat met the ball, I knew it was gone": outcome prediction, hindsight bias, and the representation and control of action in expert and novice baseball players. *Psychonomic Bulletin & Review*, *14*(4), 669-675.

Gray, R., & Regan, D. (1998). Accuracy of estimating time to collision using binocular and monocular information. *Vision Research*, *38*(4), 499-512.

Grechkin, T.Y., Nguyen, T.D., Plumert, J.M., Cremer, J.F., & Kearney, J.K. (2010). How does presentation method and measurement protocol affect distance estimation in real and virtual environments? *ACM Transactions on Applied Perception*, *7*(4), 1-18.

Greffou, S., Bertone, A., Hanssens, J.M., & Faubert, J. (2008). Development of visually driven postural reactivity: a fully immersive virtual reality study. *Journal of Vision*, *8*(11):15, 1-10.

Grossman, E.D., & Blake, R. (2002). Brain areas active during visual perception of biological motion. *Neuron*, *35*(6), 1167-1175.

Hill, H., & Johnston, A. (2001). Categorizing sex and identity from the biological motion of faces. *Current Biology*, *11*(11), 880-885.

Ho, C., Gray, R., & Spence, C. (2014). To what extent do the findings of laboratory-based spatial attention research apply to the real-world setting of driving? *IEEE Transactions on Human-Machine Systems*, *44*(4), 524-530.

Hodgins, J.K., O'Brien, J.F., & Tumblin, J. (1998). Perception of human motion with different geometric models. *IEEE Transactions on Visualization and Computer Graphics*, *4*(4), 307-316.

Holden, M.K. (2005). Virtual environments for motor rehabilitation: review. *Cyberpsychology & Behavior*, *8*(3), 187-211; discussion 212-189.

Horlings, C.G., Carpenter, M.G., Kung, U.M., Honegger, F., Wiederhold, B., & Allum, J.H. (2009). Influence of virtual reality on postural stability during movements of quiet stance. *Neuroscience Letters*, *451*(3), 227-231.

Howard, R.J., Brammer, M., Wright, I., Woodruff, P.W., Bullmore, E.T., & Zeki, S. (1996). A direct demonstration of functional specialization within motion-related visual and auditory cortex of the human brain. *Current Biology*, *6*(8), 1015-1019.

Huys, R., Canal-Bruland, R., Hagemann, N., Beek, P.J., Smeeton, N.J., & Williams, A.M. (2009). Global information pickup underpins anticipation of tennis shot direction. *Journal of Motor Behavior*, *41*(2), 158-171.

Huys, R., Smeeton, N.J., Hodges, N.J., Beek, P.J., & Williams, A.M. (2008). On the dynamic information underlying visual anticipation skill. *Perception & Psychophysics*, *70*(7), 1217-1234.

Hwang, S., Agada, P., Kiemel, T., & Jeka, J.J. (2014). Dynamic reweighting of three modalities for sensor fusion. *PLoS One*, *9*(1), e88132.

Ida, H., Fukuhara, K., & Ishii, M. (2012). Recognition of tennis serve performed by a digital player: comparison among polygon, shadow, and stick-figure models. *PLoS One*, *7*(3), e33879.

Ida, H., Fukuhara, K., Kusubori, S., & Ishii, M. (2011). A study of kinematic cues and anticipatory performance in tennis using computational manipulation and computer graphics. *Behavior Research Methods*, *43*(3), 781-790.

Ida, H., Fukuhara, K., Sawada, M., & Ishii, M. (2011). Quantitative relation between server motion and receiver anticipation in tennis: implications of responses to computer-simulated motions. *Perception*, *40*(10), 1221-1236.

Jeka, J., Allison, L., Saffer, M., Zhang, Y., Carver, S., & Kiemel, T. (2006). Sensory reweighting with translational visual stimuli in young and elderly adults: the role of state-dependent noise. *Experimental Brain Research*, *174*(3), 517-527.

Jeka, J., Oie, K.S., & Kiemel, T. (2000). Multisensory information for human postural control: integrating touch and vision. *Experimental Brain Research*, *134*(1), 107-125.

Johansson, G. (1973). Visual perception of biological motion and a model for its analysis. *Perception & Psychophysics*, *14*, 201-211.

Kandel, E.R., Schwartz, J.H., Jessell, T.M., Siegelbaum, S.A., & Hudspeth, A.J. (2012). *Principles of neural science* (Vol. 5). New York, NY, USA: McGraw-Hill.

Kelly, J.W., Loomis, J.M., & Beall, A.C. (2005). The importance of perceived relative motion in the control of posture. *Experimental Brain Research*, *161*(3), 285-292.

Kemeny, A., & Panerai, F. (2003). Evaluating perception in driving simulation experiments. *Trends in Cognitive Sciences*, *7*(1), 31-37.

Kihara, K., Kawahara, J., & Takeda, Y. (2010). Usability of liquid crystal displays for research in the temporal characteristics of perception and attention. *Behavior Research Methods*, *42*(4), 1105-1113.

Kozlowski, L., & Cutting, J. (1977). Recognizing the sex of a walker from a dynamic point-light display. *Perception & Psychophysics*, *21*(6), 575-580.

Krupinski, E.A., Johnson, J., Roehrig, H., Nafziger, J., Fan, J., & Lubin, J. (2004). Use of a human visual system model to predict observer performance with CRT vs LCD display of images. *Journal of Digital Imaging*, *17*(4), 258-263.

Lagroix, H.E., Yanko, M.R., & Spalek, T.M. (2012). LCDs are better: psychophysical and photometric estimates of the temporal characteristics of CRT and LCD monitors. *Attention, Perception, & Psychophysics*, *74*(5), 1033-1041.

Lanier, J. (2001). Virtually there. *Scientific American*, *284*(4), 66-75.

Le Runigo, C., Benguigui, N., & Bardy, B.G. (2005). Perception-action coupling and expertise in interceptive actions. *Human Movement Science*, *24*(3), 429-445.

Lee, D.N. (1976). A theory of visual control of braking based on information about time-to-collision. *Perception*, *5*(4), 437-459.

Lee, D.N., & Lishman, J.R. (1975). Visual proprioceptive control of stance. *Journal of Human Movement Studies*, *1*(2), 87-95.

Lee, H.Y., Cherng, R.J., & Lin, C.H. (2004). Development of a virtual reality environment for somatosensory and perceptual stimulation in the balance assessment of children. *Computers in Biology and Medicine*, *34*(8), 719-733.

Lishman, J.R., & Lee, D.N. (1973). The autonomy of visual kinaesthesis. *Perception*, *2*(3), 287-294.

Livingstone, M., & Hubel, D. (1988). Segregation of form, color, movement, and depth: anatomy, physiology, and perception. *Science*, *240*(4853), 740-749.

Ma, Y., Paterson, H.M., & Pollick, F.E. (2006). A motion capture library for the study of identity, gender, and emotion perception from biological motion. *Behavior Research Methods*, *38*(1), 134-141.

Mahboobin, A., Loughlin, P.J., Redfern, M.S., & Sparto, P.J. (2005). Sensory re-weighting in human postural control during moving-scene perturbations. *Experimental Brain Research*, *167*(2), 260-267.

Marken, R.S. (2001). Controlled variables: psychology as the center fielder views it. *The American Journal of Psychology*, *114*(2), 259-281.

McBeath, M.K., Shaffer, D.M., & Kaiser, M.K. (1995). How baseball outfielders determine where to run to catch fly balls. *Science*, *268*(5210), 569-569.

McDonnell, R., Jörg, S., McHugh, J., Newell, F., & O'Sullivan, C. (2008). Evaluating the emotional content of human motions on real and virtual characters. In: *Proceedings of the 5th Symposium on Applied Perception in Graphics and Visualization* (pp. 67-74). Los Angeles, CA, USA: ACM.

McLeod, P., & Dienes, Z. (1996). Do fielders know where to go to catch the ball or only how to get there? *Journal of Experimental Psychology: Human Perception and Performance*, *22*(3), 531-543.

McLeod, P., Reed, N., & Dienes, Z. (2006). The generalized optic acceleration cancellation theory of catching. *Journal of Experimental Psychology: Human Perception and Performance*, *32*(1), 139-148.

McLeod, P., Reed, N., Gilson, S., & Glennerster, A. (2008). How soccer players head the ball: a test of Optic Acceleration Cancellation theory with virtual reality. *Vision Research*, *48*(13), 1479-1487.

Mellet, E., Laou, L., Petit, L., Zago, L., Mazoyer, B., & Tzourio-Mazoyer, N. (2010). Impact of the virtual reality on the neural representation of an environment. *Human Brain Mapping*, *31*(7), 1065-1075.

Menozzi, M., Lang, F., Näpflin, U., Zeller, C., & Krueger, H. (2001). CRT versus LCD: effects of refresh rate, display technology and background luminance in visual performance. *Displays*, *22*(3), 79-85.

Mentley, D.E. (2002). State of flat-panel display technology and future trends. *Proceedings of the IEEE*, *90*(4), 453-459.

Miles, H.C., Pop, S.R., Watt, S.J., Lawrence, G.P., & John, N.W. (2012). A review of virtual environments for training in ball sports. *Computers & Graphics*, *36*(6), 714-726.

Montagne, G., Buekers, M., de Rugy, A., Camachon, C., & Laurent, M. (2002). Control of human locomotion under various task constraints. *Experimental Brain Research*, *143*(1), 133-136.

Moraes, R., & Patla, A. (2006). Determinants guiding alternate foot placement selection and the behavioral responses are similar when avoiding a real or a virtual obstacle. *Experimental Brain Research*, *171*(4), 497-510.

Newell, K.M. (1991). Motor skill acquisition. *Annual Review of Psychology*, *42*, 213-237.

Nishiike, S., Okazaki, S., Watanabe, H., Akizuki, H., Imai, T., Uno, A., Kitahara, T., Horii, A., Takeda, N., & Inohara, H. (2013). The effect of visual-vestibulosomatosensory conflict induced by virtual reality on postural stability in humans. *The Journal of Medical Investigation*, *60*(3-4), 236-239.

Nyberg, L., Lundin-Olsson, L., Sondell, B., Backman, A., Holmlund, K., Eriksson, S., Stenvall, M., Rosendahl, E., Maxhall, M., & Bucht, G. (2006). Using a virtual reality system to study balance and walking in a virtual outdoor environment: a pilot study. *Cyberpsychology & Behavior*, *9*(4), 388-395.

O'Connor, S.M., & Kuo, A.D. (2009). Direction-dependent control of balance during walking and standing. *Journal of Neurophysiology*, *102*(3), 1411-1419.

Oie, K.S., Kiemel, T., & Jeka, J.J. (2001). Human multisensory fusion of vision and touch: detecting non-linearity with small changes in the sensory environment. *Neuroscience Letters*, *315*(3), 113-116.

Peirce, J.W. (2007). PsychoPy--Psychophysics software in Python. *Journal of Neuroscience Methods*, *162*(1-2), 8-13.

Pelli, D.G. (1997). The VideoToolbox software for visual psychophysics: transforming numbers into movies. *Spatial Vision*, *10*(4), 437-442.

Pelphrey, K.A., Mitchell, T.V., McKeown, M.J., Goldstein, J., Allison, T., & McCarthy, G. (2003). Brain activity evoked by the perception of human walking: controlling for meaningful coherent motion. *The Journal of Neuroscience*, *23*(17), 6819-6825.

Peper, L., Bootsma, R.J., Mestre, D.R., & Bakker, F.C. (1994). Catching balls: how to get the hand to the right place at the right time. *Journal of Experimental Psychology: Human Perception and Performance*, *20*(3), 591-612.

Perani, D., Fazio, F., Borghese, N.A., Tettamanti, M., Ferrari, S., Decety, J., & Gilardi, M.C. (2001). Different brain correlates for watching real and virtual hand actions. *Neuroimage*, *14*(3), 749-758.

Peterka, R.J. (2002). Sensorimotor integration in human postural control. *Journal of Neurophysiology*, *88*(3), 1097-1118.

Peterka, R.J., & Loughlin, P.J. (2004). Dynamic regulation of sensorimotor integration in human postural control. *Journal of Neurophysiology*, *91*(1), 410-423.

Petrini, K., Pollick, F.E., Dahl, S., McAleer, P., McKay, L.S., Rocchesso, D., Waadeland, C.H., Love, S., Avanzini, F., & Puce, A. (2011). Action expertise reduces brain activity for audiovisual matching actions: an fMRI study with expert drummers. *Neuroimage*, *56*(3), 1480-1492.

Plumert, J.M., Kearney, J.K., Cremer, J.F., & Recker, K. (2005). Distance perception in real and virtual environments. *ACM Transactions on Applied Perception*, *2*(3), 216-233.

Pollick, F.E., Fidopiastis, C., & Braden, V. (2001). Recognising the style of spatially exaggerated tennis serves. *Perception*, *30*(3), 323-338.

Pollick, F.E., Hill, H., Calder, A., & Paterson, H. (2003). Recognising facial expression from spatially and temporally modified movements. *Perception*, *32*(7), 813-826.

Pollick, F.E., Paterson, H.M., Bruderlin, A., & Sanford, A.J. (2001). Perceiving affect from arm movement. *Cognition*, *82*(2), B51-61.

Prinz, W. (1997). Perception and action planning. *European Journal of Cognitive Psychology*, *9*(2), 129-154.

Ranganathan, R., & Carlton, L.G. (2007). Perception-action coupling and anticipatory performance in baseball batting. *Journal of Motor Behavior*, *39*(5), 369-380.

Riecke, B.E., Väljamäe, A., & Schulte-Pelkum, J. (2009). Moving sounds enhance the visually-induced self-motion illusion (circular vection) in virtual reality. *ACM Transactions on Applied Perception*, *6*(2), 1-27.

Rose, F.D., Brooks, B.M., & Rizzo, A.A. (2005). Virtual reality in brain damage rehabilitation: review. *Cyberpsychology & Behavior*, *8*(3), 241-262; discussion 263-271.

Runeson, S., & Frykholm, G. (1983). Kinematic specification of dynamics as an informational basis for person-and-action perception: expectation, gender recognition, and deceptive intention. *Journal of Experimental Psychology: General*, *112*(4), 585-615.

Rushton, S.K., Harris, J.M., Lloyd, M.R., & Wann, J.P. (1998). Guidance of locomotion on foot uses perceived target location rather than optic flow. *Current Biology*, *8*(21), 1191-1194.

Rushton, S.K., & Wann, J.P. (1999). Weighted combination of size and disparity: a computational model for timing a ball catch. *Nature Neuroscience*, *2*(2), 186-190.

Sanchez-Vives, M.V., & Slater, M. (2005). From presence to consciousness through virtual reality. *Nature Reviews Neuroscience*, *6*(4), 332-339.

Savelsbergh, G.J., Whiting, H.T., & Bootsma, R.J. (1991). Grasping tau. *Journal of Experimental Psychology: Human Perception and Performance*, *17*(2), 315-322.

Saygin, A.P., Wilson, S.M., Hagler, D.J., Jr., Bates, E., & Sereno, M.I. (2004). Point-light biological motion perception activates human premotor cortex. *The Journal of Neuroscience*, *24*(27), 6181-6188.

Schneider, G.E. (1969). Two visual systems. *Science, 163*(3870), 895-902.

Schutz-Bosbach, S., & Prinz, W. (2007). Perceptual resonance: action-induced modulation of perception. *Trends in Cognitive Sciences, 11*(8), 349-355.

Shim, J., Carlton, L.G., Chow, J.W., & Chae, W.S. (2005). The use of anticipatory visual cues by highly skilled tennis players. *Journal of Motor Behavior, 37*(2), 164-175.

Sifakis, E., Neverov, I., & Fedkiw, R. (2005). Automatic determination of facial muscle activations from sparse motion capture marker data. *ACM Transactions on Graphics, 24*(3), 417-425.

Simpson, G., Johnston, L., & Richardson, M. (2003). An investigation of road crossing in a virtual environment. *Accident Analysis & Prevention, 35*(5), 787-796.

Soechting, J.F., & Berthoz, A. (1979). Dynamic role of vision in the control of posture in man. *Experimental Brain Research, 36*(3), 551-561.

Sparto, P.J., Redfern, M.S., Jasko, J.G., Casselbrant, M.L., Mandel, E.M., & Furman, J.M. (2006). The influence of dynamic visual cues for postural control in children aged 7-12 years. *Experimental Brain Research, 168*(4), 505-516.

Sperry, R.W. (1952). Neurology and the mind-brain problem. *American Scientist, 40*(2), 291-312.

Stoffregen, T.A. (1985). Flow structure versus retinal location in the optical control of stance. *Journal of Experimental Psychology: Human Perception and Performance, 11*(5), 554-565.

Stoffregen, T.A., Schmuckler, M.A., & Gibson, E.J. (1987). Use of central and peripheral optical flow in stance and locomotion in young walkers. *Perception, 16*(1), 113-119.

Tarr, M.J., & Warren, W.H. (2002). Virtual reality in behavioral neuroscience and beyond. *Nature Neuroscience, 5 Suppl*, 1089-1092.

Todorov, E., Shadmehr, R., & Bizzi, E. (1997). Augmented feedback presented in a virtual environment accelerates learning of a difficult motor task. *Journal of Motor Behavior, 29*(2), 147-158.

Tresilian, J.R. (2005). Hitting a moving target: perception and action in the timing of rapid interceptions. *Perception & Psychophysics, 67*(1), 129-149.

Troje, N.F. (2002). Decomposing biological motion: a framework for analysis and synthesis of human gait patterns. *Journal of Vision, 2*(5), 371-387.

Ungerleider, L.G. (1982). Two cortical visual systems. *Analysis of Visual Behavior*, 549-586.

Vaina, L.M., Solomon, J., Chowdhury, S., Sinha, P., & Belliveau, J.W. (2001). Functional neuroanatomy of biological motion perception in humans. *Proceedings of the National Academy of Sciences, 98*(20), 11656-11661.

van Asten, W.N., Gielen, C.C., & Denier van der Gon, J.J. (1988). Postural adjustments induced by simulated motion of differently structured environments. *Experimental Brain Research, 73*(2), 371-383.

van der Kamp, J., Savelsbergh, G., & Smeets, J. (1997). Multiple information sources in interceptive timing. *Human Movement Science, 16*(6), 787-821.

van Loon, E.M., Khashawi, F., & Underwood, G. (2010). Visual strategies used for time-to-arrival judgments in driving. *Perception, 39*(9), 1216-1229.

Vanrie, J., & Verfaillie, K. (2004). Perception of biological motion: a stimulus set of human point-light actions. *Behavior Research Methods, Instruments, & Computers, 36*(4), 625-629.

Vetter, T., & Troje, N.F. (1997). Separation of texture and shape in images of faces for image coding and synthesis. *Journal of the Optical Society of America A*, *14*(9), 2152-2161.

Vignais, N., Bideau, B., Craig, C., Brault, S., Multon, F., Delamarche, P., & Kulpa, R. (2009). Does the level of graphical detail of a virtual handball thrower influence a goalkeeper's motor response? *Journal of Sports Science & Medicine*, *8*(4), 501.

Wann, J.P., Rushton, S., & Mon-Williams, M. (1995). Natural problems for stereoscopic depth perception in virtual environments. *Vision Research*, *35*(19), 2731-2736.

Wann, J.P., Swapp, D., & Rushton, S.K. (2000). Heading perception and the allocation of attention. *Vision Research*, *40*(18), 2533-2543.

Warren, W.H., Jr., Kay, B.A., Zosh, W.D., Duchon, A.P., & Sahuc, S. (2001). Optic flow is used to control human walking. *Nature Neuroscience*, *4*(2), 213-216.

Warren, W.H., Kay, B.A., & Yilmaz, E.H. (1996). Visual control of posture during walking: functional specificity. *Journal of Experimental Psychology: Human Perception and Performance*, *22*(4), 818-838.

Watson, G., Brault, S., Kulpa, R., Bideau, B., Butterfield, J., & Craig, C. (2011). Judging the 'passability' of dynamic gaps in a virtual rugby environment. *Human Movement Science*, *30*(5), 942-956.

Williams, A.M., Huys, R., Cañal-Bruland, R., & Hagemann, N. (2009). The dynamical information underpinning anticipation skill. *Human Movement Science*, *28*(3), 362-370.

Witmer, B.G., & Singer, M.J. (1998). Measuring presence in virtual environments: a presence questionnaire. *Presence*, *7*(3), 225-240.

Woollacott, M., & Shumway-Cook, A. (2002). Attention and the control of posture and gait: a review of an emerging area of research. *Gait Posture*, *16*(1), 1-14.

Wright, M.J., Bishop, D.T., Jackson, R.C., & Abernethy, B. (2011). Cortical fMRI activation to opponents' body kinematics in sport-related anticipation: expert-novice differences with normal and point-light video. *Neuroscience Letters*, *500*(3), 216-221.

Yoonessi, A., & Yoonessi, A. (2011). A glance at psychophysics software programs. *Basic and Clinical Neuroscience*, *2*(3), 73-75.

Zaal, F.T., & Michaels, C.F. (2003). The information for catching fly balls: judging and intercepting virtual balls in a CAVE. *Journal of Experimental Psychology: Human Perception and Performance*, *29*(3), 537-555.

Zago, M., Bosco, G., Maffei, V., Iosa, M., Ivanenko, Y.P., & Lacquaniti, F. (2004). Internal models of target motion: expected dynamics overrides measured kinematics in timing manual interceptions. *Journal of Neurophysiology*, *91*(4), 1620-1634.

In: Advances in Visual Perception Research
Editor: Thomas Heinen

ISBN: 978-1-63482-455-2
© 2015 Nova Science Publishers, Inc.

Chapter 13

Effects of Using Two Different Augmented Feedback Devices on the Learning Process of Modeled Movements

***Konstantinos Velentzas*[1,*]*, Christoph Schütz*[2] *and Thomas Schack*[1,2]**

[1]Bielefeld University, Faculty of Psychology and Sport, Germany
[2]Center of Excellence - Cognitive Interaction Technology (CITEC), Bielefeld University, Germany

Abstract

New technologies allow learners to receive performance relevant information (visual, auditory) simultaneously to a task execution. Extended or augmented feedback seems to increase motivation, support cognition and accelerate rehabilitation. In the field of motor control and learning, Schmidt and Young (1991) indicate that more experimental studies should be conducted in order to clarify and extend the effects of augmented feedback. The main effort of the present study is to investigate the effects of using two different augmented feedback devices on performing a movement reproduction task. 45 Students participated in this study. Group one (n = 15) received performance (posture) related information via open head mounted display whereas group two (n = 15) used a closed head mounted display. The third group (n = 15) practiced without any performance feedback. Both feedback groups enhanced their execution similarity to the given model from pre to post test. The results are in line with the findings of other studies and show that augmented feedback using new technological devices can be also beneficial in sport and exercise science where modeled movements should be replicated.

Keywords: movement reproduction, head-mounted display, model, sport

* ...eld University, Faculty of Psychology and Sport, Universitaetsstr. 25, 33615 Bielefeld, Germany. Email: ...s.velentzas@uni-bielefeld.de

Introduction

In motor learning contexts, demonstrations are often used as a means of conveying information to learners about how to perform a skill (Magill, 2007). This approach is often conceptualized as *observational learning* (McCullagh & Weiss, 2001). It is based on Bandura's social learning theory (Bandura, 1977) and it is widely applied in field of motor control and motor learning (Dowrick, 1999). According to Bandura (1986), the received visual information during observational learning supports learners' attentional focus, the recall and the behavioral adaptation process by a future reproduction of the observed task, as well as the motivation of the learners.

In the early seventies new computer technologies (i.e., software, hardware) were used in order to manipulate, and analyze human behaviors and to control learning effects in "real life" resembling environments. This technological application is being declared as virtual reality. Virtual reality users immerse completely into an artificial world, whereas the user is not able to perceive any information from the real world (Heim, 1993). The person-environment interaction — implying verbal information, overlay of body (or body parts) movements, as well as manipulation of virtual objects — into a virtual reality environment contains only a part of the in reality comprehended information while the sensorimotor feedback is moderately missed resulting in a so called *out of body experience* (e.g., Levy, 1998). Recent technologies developed in topics such as robotics, telemanipulation and military, extended the utilization of virtual reality by enriching the reality with computer generated information which is designated as augmented reality or augmented feedback (Milgram, Takemura, Utsumi, & Kishino, 1994). On the one hand, augmented feedback supported training has similarities to traditional learning methods like those of learning with pictures or video feedback training. On the other hand, it differs clearly concerning the technical components and predominantly the way and the time feedback is provided.

Nowadays, in the field of educational science, augmented information is brought up for discussion as a substantial component which can support and facilitate the movement learning and optimization of movement patterns by supporting cognition (Ronsse et al., 2011), enhancing motivation (Freitas & Campos, 2008; Magill & Anderson 2012), guiding perception (Wulf & Prinz, 2001), eliminating fear (Azuma et al., 2001), and increasing learning experience by supporting apprentices to take control over the learning process (Newell, 1991; Wishart, Lee, & Cunningham, 2002). These effects attribute to the fact that virtual (sensory) information in augmented reality gets integrated in real time into the perception system during the actual movement execution. Augmented feedback is thus on a continuum between reality and virtual reality (Milgram et al., 1994). Particularly, in augmented reality, a specific pool of information is generated, which can be implemented into the learning process (real time feedback; Heidemann et al., 2004). The reality (perceived information) of a participating person gets superimposed with computer-generated virtual information in real time. In other words, techniques marked as augmented reality refer to an online imbedding of movement or environmental relevant information into the reality of the participant.

The most common applied augmented reality technical devices in the field of sport and exercise science are presentation screens, audio signals, and, more recently, head mounted displays, which are used to provide the participant with real time information regarding their own performance similarly to the self observation (Magill & Anderson, 2012; Liebermann et al., 2002). Due to this last specific property, an essential parameter of the technical supplementary system is that it should be exactly calibrated and be able to adapt to the participants' movement (Milgram et al., 1994). Several studies in sport and/or rehabilitation domains are accomplished using special developed devices as the combination of visual and auditory feedback (i.e., Liebermann et al, 2002; Todorov, Shadmehr, & Bizzi, 1997) as well as gaming platforms combined with movement analysis and outcome evaluation (Fery & Ponserre, 2001; Sanchez, 2011). Nevertheless, the existing research findings regarding the effects of augmented reality on learning and performance process are still inconsistent (Shelton & Hadley, 2004). The lack of information is mentioned by Schmidt and Young (1991) as follows: "[...] But despite the inherent interest in kinematic feedback, several factors reviewed here have operated to inhibit its study, the most important of which has been the lack of a suitable laboratory task and paradigm" (Schmidt & Young, 1991, p. 13).

In an earlier experimental setting, Shea and Wulf (1999) used a balance task in order to determine the effects of augmented feedback in combination with the manipulation of the participants' attentional focus orientation (internal versus external focus). Four groups of participants were asked to balance on a stabilometer and keep this in the horizontal position for at least 90 seconds. The platform position was presented on a computer monitor providing the feedback groups with visual feedback about the current position of their own feet (or some marking lines on the stabilometer) during performance. The participants of the no-feedback training condition were instructed only to keep their feet at the same height while the participants of the other group were instructed to keep the marking lines at the same height. The results supported the assumption that the effects of augmented feedback training increase when coupled with an external focus of attention (see also Magill & Anderson 2012; Wulf & Shea, 2004). However, augmented feedback can be seen as advancement in the area of self-observation and motor learning.

However, taking into account that new technologies, such as the head mounted displays – which avouch an increased viewability (Tanaka, Kishino, & Miyamae, 2008) – are not widely used in sport and exercise science, researchers should make an effort to clarify for instance which devices or which format of information is more beneficial (i.e., performance vs. goal oriented) in enhancing performance. The application of head mounted displays is associated with few limitations (Shelton & Hedley, 2004). First, participants wearing closed head mounted displays get visual feedback from an external perspective (camera), but at the same time they lose important visual input from their own perspective. Second, closed head mounted displays are most often binocular, causing a discomfort regarding eyestrain and fatigue (e.g., Azuma et al., 2001). Contradictory, the development of the open (see through) displays permits for instance a visual combination of one's own perspective with these of the coach/judges perspective providing increased visual interaction and convenience. In spite of the aspect just mentioned, the increased flow of information could induce a cognitive overload and thus a decrease in performance (cf., Mayer & Moreno, 2003). Finally, the camera perspective seems to be a crucial factor, which can lead to differential learning effects (see also, Shea, Wright, Wulf, & Whitacre, 2000).

Nevertheless, the rapid development of the technical components (computing, 3D video sequences, simulations and online movement analyses, technical devices, etc.) permit the question of which technical setup is more appropriate in supporting learning and optimizing simple self-paced movement skills, and further to which extend the effects of specific augmented reality training are stable during time (i.e., Lee, 2012)? The main aim of the present study is to compare the effects of two different technical devices (open vs. closed head mounted display) on the execution quality (i.e. replication of a body posture) of a complex throwing movement task.

Method

Participants

Forty-five right-handed undergraduate students (16 females and 29 males) volunteered to participate in this study (M_{age} = 24.5 years, SD_{age} = 2.8). The participants were randomly assigned into three groups. The first group (n = 15) practiced the experimental task receiving simultaneous augmented feedback by an open head-mounted display (*OHMD*). The second group (n = 15) participated wearing a closed head-mounted display (*CHMD*). The third group (n = 15) was treated as a control group (*CG*). Participants of the control group practiced without any extended feedback information. Prior to the investigation, all participants were informed about the purpose of the study and provided written informed consent in accordance with the ethical guidelines of the local university, which are in line with the APA (6th ed.) guidelines and the declaration of Helsinki (2008).

Motor Task

The experimental task was a controlled underhand throw with the non-dominant hand, on to a circular target of 50 cm diameter dyed on the wall. The middle of the target was marked by a red dot of 5 cm diameter. The participants were instructed to throw a hacky sack as close as possible to the target's middle, reproducing at the same time a clearly defined movement pattern (Figure 1). Additionally, participants were asked to execute the goal-movement only by moving their arm avoiding other body-parts' displacement.

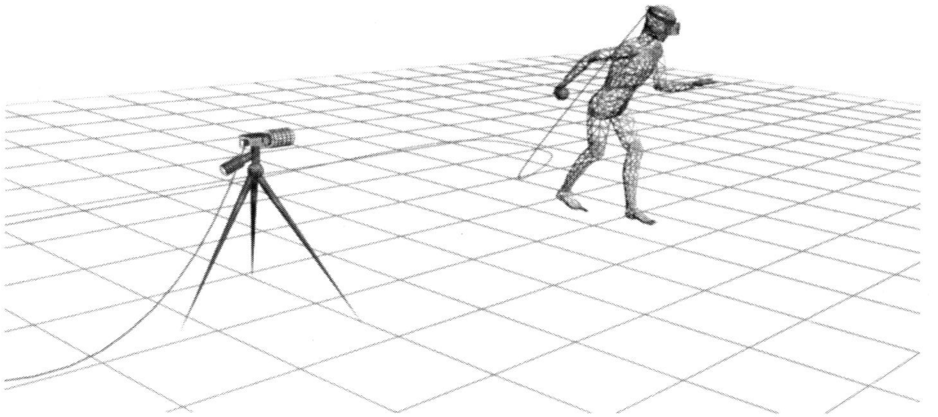

Figure 1. Artificial demonstration of the experimental setting.

The experimental task was appropriate for the study's proposal, due to the fact that it is easy to execute, its spatial properties are restricted (two-dimensional non-dynamic movement), and the participants' movement quality can be videotaped, simultaneously evaluated, and feeded back to the participant.

Apparatus

For the present study and in order to analyze performance simultaneously to task execution (augmented feedback), reflective markers were placed over the left wrist, elbow, shoulder, and hip, of the participants. In addition, three high-speed infrared Nexus (*VICON®*) cameras were utilized. The markers were tracked from the VICON movement analysis system at 140 Hz. An additional camera (Basler® A602-fc operating also at 140 Hz) was used to feedback participants' movements through the head mounted display. Two different head mounted displays were applied to provide participants with augmented feedback. For the CHMD group a Cyberman closed head mounted display (Auvisio®; up to 640 × 480 pixel) was applied (Figure 2a). For the OHMD group a see-through Military-micro head mounted display (Liteye®; true color VGA, up to 800 × 600 pixel) was used (Figure 2b).

Both systems were modified in order to receive the digital information via wireless signal. In order to fulfill this last requirement, specific computer software was developed, which integrated the information of the Vicon system and the video data of the external perspective. The target area was videotaped by a digital camera HDR-CX520 (Sony®, 50 Hz). Finally, two freestyle hacky sacks were used as objects, which should be thrown towards the target area.

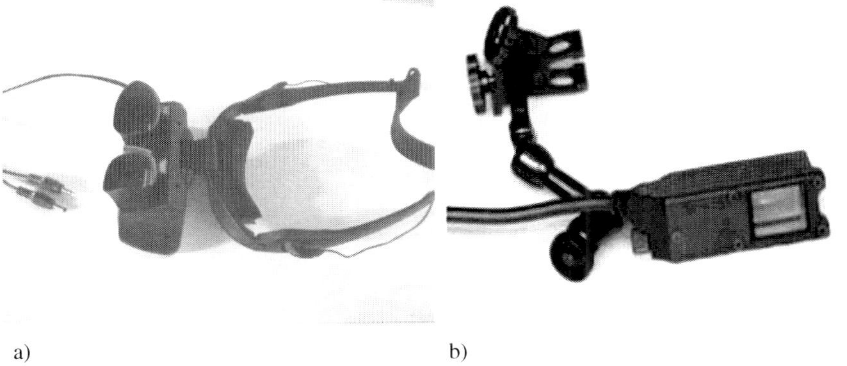

a) b)

Figure 2. Illustration of the used technical devices a) Closed head mounted display. b) Open head mounted display.

Procedure

For the present study a three (condition) × two (measure) design was used. Following five practice throws, participants of each group were asked to perform six blocks of ten throws each in the respective treatment condition. Although, nine joint body angles of the arm (wrist, elbow and shoulder) for the front swing (beginning), between, and release posture were defined as a set of constraints needed for a successful skill mastering, which should be replicated. At the same time these data served as a reference to control movement replication and to feedback kinematical invariance (actual and attended movement) in real time. The desired movement posture was individualized for each participant accordingly to participants' body scheme.

Prior to each block the movement requirements were presented (start, between, and final posture) to the participants as row of headers. The participants were asked to position themselves behind a marking line (5 × 15 cm) located 240 cm away from the target. The feet / body posture (cf., Figure 1) was determined in order to warranty a stable and comfortable position and at the same time to reduce further degrees of freedom for the given movement. The participants were instructed to avoid body displacement and to accomplish the task by moving only their non-dominant arm. The participants of both experimental groups received augmented visual information about their own movement from a lateral perspective (90°) during movement execution (Basler camera located at 260cm from the participation area) including an overlay of the target movement. The pre and post measurement were performed without head mounted display or any knowledge of performance (i.e. Ranganathan & Newell, 2009).

Results

The main goal of the present study was to examine the effects of using two different augmented reality systems in the learning process of a complex movement. Due to the fact that we were interested in performance changes within groups, no baseline correction were performed but only *t*-tests were calculated for paired dependent samples regarding the average angle differences between the actual and the anticipated goal movement. The analysis showed that both experimental groups significantly increased performance from pre to post test whereas the control group showed no significant performance changes concerning the movement execution.

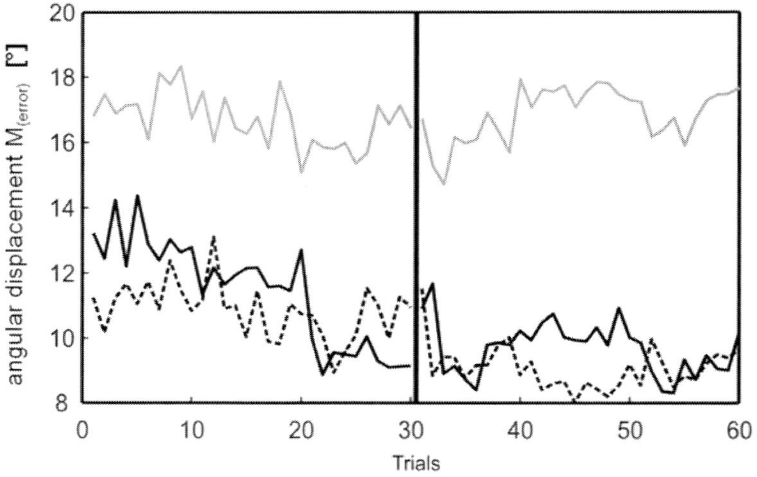

Figure 3. Graphical presentation of the measured differences between actual and aimed task execution.

More precisely, we performed separated t-Tests between pre and post test scores, elucidating that the posture of the OHMD group (—) participate significantly better from pre to post test ($t = 2.29$, $p = .031$). The same result was found for the CHMD group (--), $t = 2.34$, $p = .023$. There were no significant performance changes for the participants of the control group (—), $t = .91$, $p > .05$; Figure 3).

Discussion

The main aim of this study was to assess the effects of using two different feedback devices (open vs. closed head mounted display) in the learning process of a complex movement under the light of the augmented feedback and self-observation. The effects of augmented feedback were investigated through several studies, which demonstrated that its application may facilitate learning to a greater degree as compared to traditional learning (Caljouw, van der Kamp, & Savelsbergh, 2004; Yuen, Yaoyuneyong, & Johnson, 2011). Extended visual information increases a sense of familiarity between actual and goal movements, supports feelings of confidence, motivation and control and helps overcome performance errors.

For the present investigation, 45 students were randomly assigned into three groups. One of the groups received simultaneously to the task execution performance related feedback through an open head mounted display, whereas a closed mounted display was applied to the second experimental group. The third group (control group) practiced without any performance-related feedback. The results of the study yield that augmented feedback training is significantly more effective compared to traditional training when the main aim of the intervention is the qualitative replication of an observed movement. More specifically, both experimental groups performed significantly more similar on the demanded task after the involvement of augmented feedback. Regarding the control group no performance changes were found after the traditional training session.

Our results support the existing findings from the educational field and at the same time offer a new perspective for sport science. The mastery of complex movement skills is always related to expenditure of time and hard training sessions. New technologies can be used in order to accelerate learning processes and/or optimizing skill performance. Furthermore, it can be suggested that augmented feedback can also be applied as implementation for modeling or imagery training (i.e. by using overlays or eliminating disturbing environmental information). Nevertheless, it has to be illustrated that the application of such devices and their combination with traditional physical training should be scrutinized as well as that the hardware and software has to be developed in spite of an individualized utilization.

Some limitations of the study concerning the design have to be discussed. At first the closed head mounted display and the missed visual information about the result do not permit the verification of the training effect on the throw accuracy (movement outcome). Second, the missed manipulation check does not allow an interpretation of the results in conjunction with an optimization of the visual strategies or of the movement coordinative pattern. Nonetheless the results are encouraging for scientists and practitioners who should make some effort to specify the function of augmented feedback in motor control and learning and at the same time to make it more suitable to everyday training.

Acknowledgment

The project was financed by the German Federal Institute for Sport Science (BISp).

References

Azuma, R.T., Baillot, Y., Behringer, R., Feiner, S., Julier, S., & MacIntyre, B. (2001). Recent advances in augmented reality. *Computer Graphics and Applications*, *21*, 34–47.

Bandura, A. (1977). Self-efficacy: Toward a unifying theory of behavioral change. *Psychological Review*, *84*, 191–215.

Bandura, A. (1986). *Social foundations of thought and action: A social cognitive theory.* Englewood Cliffs, NJ: Prentice Hall.

Caljouw, S.R., van der Kamp, J., & Savelsbergh, G.J.P. (2004). Catching optical information for the regulation of timing. *Experimental Brain Research, 155*, 427–438.

Dowrick, P. W. (1999). A review of self modeling and related interventions. *Applied & Preventive Psychology*, *8*, 23–39.

Fery, Y. A., & Ponserre, S. (2001). Enhancing the control of force in putting by video game training. *Ergonomics*, *44*, 1025–1037.

Freitas, R., & Campos, P. (2008). SMART: a System of augmented reality for teaching 2nd grade students. *Proceedings of the 22nd British Computer Society Conference on Human Computer Interaction*, 27–30. Liverpool, UK.

Heidemann, G., Bax, I., Bekel, H., Bauckhage, C., Wachsmuth, S., Fink, G., Pinz, A., Ritter, H. & Sagerer, G. (2004). Multimodal interaction in an augmented real Multimodal interaction in an augmented reality scenario. In R. Sharma, T. Darrell, M.P. Harper, G. Lazzari & M. Turk (Eds.), *6th International Conference on Multimodal Interfaces* (Proceedings of ICMI State College PA, 53–60). USA: ACM.

Heim, M. (1993). *The Metaphysics of Virtual Reality*. New York: Oxford University Press.

Lee, K. (2012). Augmented reality in education and training. *Technological Trends*, *2*, 13–21.

Levy, P. (1998). *Becoming virtual: Reality in the digital age*, New York: Plenum Trade.

Liebermann, D.G.,Katz, L.,Hughes, M. D.,Bartlett,R.M., McClements,J., & Franks, I.M. (2002). Advances in the application of information technology to sport performance. *Journal of Sports Sciences*, *10*, 755–769.

Magill, R.A. (2007). *Motor learning and control: Concepts and applications* (8th ed.). New York: McGraw-Hill.

Magill, R. A., & Anderson, D. I. (2012). The roles and uses of augmented feedback in motor skill acquisition. In N. Hodges & A. M. Williams (Eds.), *Skill Acquisition in Sport: Research, Theory and Practice*, 3–21, London: Routledge.

Mayer, R. E., & Moreno, R. (2003). Nine ways to reduce cognitive load in multimedia learning. *Educational Psychologist*, *38*, 43–52.

McCullagh, P., & Weiss, M.R. (2001). Modeling: Considerations for motor skill performance and psychological responses. In R.N. Singer, H.A. Hausenblas, & C.M. Janelle (Eds.), *Handbook of sport psychology* (2nd ed.), 205–238. New York: Wiley.

Milgram, P., Takemura, H., Utsumi, A., & Kishino, F. (1994). Augmented reality: a class of displays on the reality- virtuality continuum. *Telemanipulator and Telepresence Technologies*. Boston: MA.

Newell, K. M. (1991). Motor skill acquisition. *Annual Review of Psychology*, *42*, 213-237.

Ranganathan, R., & Newell, K. M. (2009). Influence of augmented feedback on coordination strategies. *Journal of Motor Behavior*, *4*, 317–330.

Ronsse, R., Puttemans, V., Coxon, J. P., Goble, D. J., Wagemans, J., Wenderoth, N., & Swinnen, S. P. (2011). Motor learning with augmented feedback: modality-dependent behavioral and neural consequences. *Cerebral Cortex*, *21*, 1283–1294.

Sanchez, C. A. (2011). Enhancing visuospatial performance through video game training to increase learning in visuospatial science domains. *Psychonomic Bulletin & Review*, *19*, 58–65.

Schaik, P. V., Blake, J., Pernet, F., Spears, I., & Fencott, C. (2008). Virtual Augmented Exercise Gaming for Older Adults. *Cyber Psychology & Behavior*, *11*, 103–106.

Schmidt, R. A., & Young, D. E. (1991). Methodology for motor learning: a paradigm for kinematic feedback. *Journal of Motor Behavior*, *23*, 13–24.

Shea, C. H., & Wulf, G. (1999). Enhancing motor learning through external-focus instructions and feedback. *Human Movement Science*, *18*, 553–571.

Shea, C. H., Wright, D. L., Wulf, G., & Whitacre, C. (2000). Physical and observational practice afford unique learning opportunities. *Journal of Motor Behavior*,*32*, 27–36.

Shelton, B. E., & Hedley, N. R. (2004). Exploring a cognitive basis for learning spatial relationships with augmented reality. *Technology, Instruction, Cognition and Learning*, *4*, 323–357.

Tanaka, K., Kishino, Y., Miyamae, M., Terada, T., Nishio, S. (2008). An information layout method for an optical see-through head mounted display focusing on the viewability. In: *Proceedings of the Seventh IEEE International Symposium on Mixed and Augmented Reality*, 15–18 September, 2008, Cambridge, UK, 139–142.

Todorov, E., Shadmehr, R., & Bizzi, E. (1997). Augmented feedback presented in a virtual environment accelerates learning of a difficult motor task. *Journal of Motor Behavior*, *29*, 147–158.

Yuen, S., Yaoyuneyong, G., & Johnson, E. (2011). Augmented reality: An overview and five directions for AR in education. *Journal of Educational Technology Development and Exchange*, *4*, 119–140.

Wishart, L. R., Lee, T. D., Cunningham, S. J., & Murdoch, J. E. (2002). Age-related differences and the role of augmented visual feedback in learning a bimanual coordination pattern. *Acta Psychologica*, *110*, 247–263.

Wulf, G., & Prinz, W. (2001). Directing attention to movement effects enhances learning: A review. *Psychonomic Bulletin & Review*, *8*, 648–660.

Wulf, G., & Shea, C.H. (2004). Understanding the role of augmented feedback: The good, the bad, and the ugly. In A.M. Williams, & N.J. Hodges (Eds.). *Skill acquisition in sport: Research, theory and practice*, 121–144. N.Y.: Routledge.

In: Advances in Visual Perception Research
Editor: Thomas Heinen

ISBN: 978-1-63482-455-2
© 2015 Nova Science Publishers, Inc.

Chapter 14

Why Encode Limb and Body Displacements in the Velocity Domain? Neurophysiological and Behavioral Evidence

*Luc Tremblay** *and John de Grosbois*
University of Toronto, Canada

Abstract

Performing voluntary actions often requires using more than one sensory modality. However, different modalities provide information in different domains. For example, vision primarily gathers information in the positional domain while the inner ear primarily encodes information in the acceleration domain. This chapter presents neurophysiological and behavioral evidence for the use of visual and vestibular information in the velocity domain during perceptual and sensorimotor activities. Specifically, for activities of daily living requiring the use of visual and vestibular information, it is argued that the central nervous system preferentially converts sensory cues into the velocity domain prior to implementing the multisensory combination and integration processes relevant to perception and action.

Keywords: speed; perception; action; vision; vestibular

* Centre for Motor Control, Faculty of Kinesiology and Physical Education, University of Toronto, 55 Harbord St., Toronto, ON, M5S 2W6, Canada. Email: luc.tremblay@ utoronto.ca.

Introduction

Reaching for a cup of coffee involves much more than planning a spatial trajectory or a final position. Once visual information about the target to be attained has been encoded, the central nervous system must often compute sensorimotor transformations involving modalities other than vision. However, different modalities gather information in different domains (i.e., position, velocity, acceleration). The core idea in the following sections is that sensorimotor transformations may be optimally computed in the velocity domain.

When reaching to a target object with the upper-limb, the central nervous system must consider the spatial arrangements between the eye, head, trunk and limb (see Crawford, Medendorp, & Marotta, 2004; Flanders, Helms Tillery, & Soechting, 1992; Henriques, Klier, Smith, Lowy, & Crawford, 1998). The position of the target on the retina must be contrasted with input from the muscle spindles of oculomotor muscles to encode the eye orientation relative to the head. In turn, muscle spindles of neck muscles provide information about the head orientation relative to the trunk. In addition, because visual information is not sufficient by itself to determine absolute head location is space (see Blouin, Labrousse, Simoneau, Vercher, & Gauthier, 1998; Cohen, 1961; Vaitl, Mittelstaedt, Saborowski, Stark, & Baisch, 2002), vestibular information is also used to successfully reach for targets in our environment (see Figure 1).

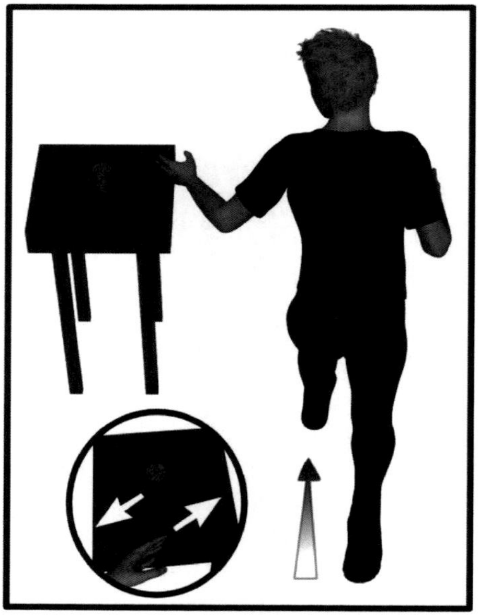

Figure 1. A depiction of a situation where visual and vestibular information must be contrasted to disentangle motion of the target in space vs. motion of the head relative to the target. Resolving such ambiguity is necessary to successfully reach for an object in the depicted dynamic condition. Inset: the relative visual motion of the hand and the target. This original figure was inspired by Gomi (2008) Figure 1.

Thus, being able to reach to a target presented on the retina requires contrasting visual and vestibular information to disentangle motion of the target in space vs. motion of the head relative to the target (e.g., Bresciani, Blouin, Popov, Bourdin, Sarlegna, Vercher, & Gauthier,

2002). As a result, one constraint facing the central nervous system is to perform multisensory comparisons from modalities that provide information in different domains (i.e., position vs. velocity[1] vs. acceleration).

The retina provides information in the positional domain. Retinal cells primarily respond to the presence of light on specific locations of the retina (e.g., Meister & Tessier-Lavigne, 2013). As a result, visual information is fundamentally in the positional domain. To provide a contrast, the vestibular system provides information in the acceleration domain. The hair cells of the semi-circular canals and the otoliths respond to changes in linear and angular head accelerations (e.g., Goldberg, Walker, & Hudspeth, 2013). Interestingly, there is neurophysiological and behavioral evidence supporting the idea that visual and vestibular information are processed in the velocity domain to perform voluntary sensorimotor behaviors. Further, such processing of multisensory information in the velocity domain extends to perceptual processes.

Visuomotor Processing and the Velocity Domain

Neurophysiological Evidence of Visuomotor Processes

Bullock, Cisek, and Grossberg (1998) forwarded a cortical model primarily designed to explain the use of proprioceptive information when dealing with obstacles or perturbations during voluntary arm movements. Recognizing the imperative of visuomotor transformations when performing voluntary actions, they proposed that a visual input is used to generate a difference vector (see also Buneo & Andersen, 2006; Prablanc, Echallier, Jeannerod, & Komilis, 1979; Vindras & Viviani, 1998). For example, according to Bullock et al. (1998), positional information about a target location, which is obtained via visual information, is used to compute a difference vector (i.e., in Brodmann's area 5). The next processing step in that model is to use the difference vector to compute a desired velocity vector (e.g., in Brodmann's area 4). Such desired velocity vector is the sole source of signals that are transmitted to the dynamic gamma motor neurons. That is, visual information from the spatial / position domain must be transformed into the velocity domain before being used to initiate a voluntary arm movement. Such a view has been corroborated by other neurophysiological evidence.

Ashe and Georgopoulos (1994) performed multiple linear regression analyses between cell discharge activity and four characteristics of reaching movements: target direction, hand position, hand velocity, and hand acceleration. The cells analyzed were from the primary motor cortex (i.e., Brodmann's area 4) and Brodmann's area 5 from monkeys. While the target direction was most strongly associated with activity in these cortical areas (i.e., Brodmann's area 5: see also Buneo, Jarvis, Batista, & Anderson, 2002), the second most important characteristic was hand velocity. Specifically, for 55 and 57% of the cells in Brodmann's areas 4 and 5, the first ranked movement parameter was target direction,

[1] The term velocity will be employed throughout this chapter while the term speed will be avoided. This is primarily for brevity purposes but also because of the association of neurophysiological processes with vector information processing (e.g., vector-integration-to-endpoint model: see Bullock, Cisek, & Grossberg, 1998; Bullock & Grossberg, 1988).

respectively. In contrast, for 27 and 25% of the cells of the same areas, the first ranked movement parameter was hand velocity. Finally, for the same areas, hand position was the first ranked parameter for only 17 and 18% of the cells. This led Ashe and Georgopoulos to conclude the existence of a "strong relation of both areas to target direction and movement velocity, less to position, and even less to acceleration" (p. 599). Referring to the thesis of the current chapter, it is also important to note that direction is not solely associated with the positional domain as the velocity domain can include both a direction and a magnitude (cf. speed). Nevertheless, the evidence brought forward by Ashe and Georgopoulos is in line with the model from Bullock et al. (1998: see also Cisek, Grossberg, & Bullock, 1998). As well, more recent neurophysiological evidence provided direct support for the importance of the velocity domain for the control of neuromotor behaviors.

Churchland, Santhanam, and Shenoy (2006) provided compelling evidence for the importance of the velocity domain in neuromotor processing through the manipulation of limb velocity of voluntary reaching movements. Monkeys were taught to perform a three-stage trial type. First, the hand has to be stabilized on a start position for 400-500 ms. Second, a target appeared and was "jittered" to instruct the monkey to wait before initiating the reach. During that period, the target and a central cue were either green or red, instructing the monkey whether the reaching movement had to be slow or fast, respectively. Third and last, the target became stable and the central cue disappeared, which was the cue to initiate the reaching movement. The training period allowed the monkey to associate a peak limb velocity criterion with a successful trial and a reward. The velocity criteria were set according to the reaching distances (i.e., 3 to 12 cm). The main analyses of their study were related to neural activity recordings from cells in the primary motor and dorsal premotor cortices (i.e., Brodmann's areas 4 and 6, respectively). The novel finding of that study was that activity in the measured cortical areas during the movement preparation period was strongly associated with the velocity of the to-be-performed reaches and not necessarily associated with spatial characteristics (e.g., distance, direction). Such results further support the importance of the velocity domain for the preparation of voluntary movements.

Overall, both neurophysiological theoretical modeling and empirical evidence have supported the concept that limb velocity represents a core movement preparation component. Albeit limited to specific areas of the monkey brain, a theoretical model and neurophysiological evidence provide a clear rationale for converting visual signals into the velocity domain prior to sending commands to the motor neurons. Corroborating evidence can be extracted from neuro-behavioral investigations performed with humans.

Behavioral Evidence of Visuomotor Processes

The seminal work of Woodworth (1899) provided evidence that humans perform upper-limb movements in distinct phases. Based on sensory information available prior to movement initiation, the first phase of the trajectory (i.e., ballistic or initial impulse) propels the limb towards the target. Then, based on sensory information gathered during the ballistic phase, the second phase of the trajectory (i.e., current control) implements amendments to bring the limb onto the target. Of particular relevance to this chapter are the kinematic criteria employed to segregate the ballistic and current control phases of a movement.

Meyer, Abrams, Kornblum, Wright, and Smith (1988) employed a series of kinematic criteria to segregate the primary submovement (i.e., ballistic phase) and secondary submovements (i.e., current control phase). The velocity of a wrist rotation movement was employed to identify the start of the primary submovement. Then, the end of the primary submovement could be identified with a zero crossing in the velocity profile or a re-acceleration (i.e., with or without a zero acceleration crossing). As a result, the first increase in velocity was deemed to be the start of the primary submovement. Subsequently, a zero crossing in the velocity profile or a subsequent increase in velocity after reaching peak limb velocity was deemed to represent secondary submovements. Increases in velocity were thus deemed as central components for the parsing of iterative trajectory submovements, even if the idea of iterative trajectory amendments has been subsequently challenged.

Elliott, Carson, Goodman, and Chua (1991) asked participants to make reaching movements of the upper limb with a stylus. The experimental conditions included reaches made with and without vision under instructions to emphasize accuracy or speed. Participants exhibited more discrete trajectory amendments for movements performed with the instructions to be accurate than with the instructions to go fast. However, there were no reliable differences in the number of submovements for reaches made with than without vision. Instead, it was the time between peak limb velocity and movement end that reliably differed between the trials with and without vision. Elliott et al. (1991) suggested that voluntary movements may be comprised of many overlapping trajectory amendments that are not necessarily detectable via increases in limb velocity but still yield longer times between peak limb velocity and movement end. Overall, these behavioral studies indicate that information about the phases of a limb movement can be reliably parsed using the velocity profile of a movement (see also Chua & Elliott, 1993; Elliott, Hansen, Grierson, Lyons, Bennett, & Hayes, 2010; Jeannerod, 1988). Therefore, despite arguments regarding the sequencing of online trajectory amendments between Meyer et al. (1988) and Elliott et al. (1991), both lines of investigations emphasize the importance of limb velocity in extracting information about online control mechanisms.

Notably, the above lines of research employed vision withdrawal manipulations that took place immediately after the velocity of the limb or the effector departed from zero. If sensorimotor processes are performed in the velocity domain, manipulating vision before the limb velocity significantly departs from zero (0) could in fact minimize the chances of detecting sensorimotor processes that depend on limb velocity. In contrast, manipulating vision at different limb velocity criteria rather than time or position could prove a useful method to assess sensorimotor mechanisms.

Using vision manipulations as a function of limb velocity during upper-limb reaching movements, Tremblay, Hansen, Kennedy, and Cheng (2013) supported the idea that some portions of the trajectory do not significantly contribute to the control of movement endpoint (e.g., Carlton, 1992). Vision was manipulated via liquid-crystal goggles on the basis of the real-time limb velocity (i.e., goggles changed state within 10 ms of the limb meeting a velocity criterion). In the first experiment, vision could be made available or not during the entire movement (i.e., Vision or No-Vision), or available above or below a limb velocity criterion of 0.8 m/s (i.e., VHigh or VLow) (see Figure 2). The endpoint precision or variable error (i.e., standard deviation of endpoint distribution) contrasts were as follows: Vision ~ VHigh < No-Vision ~ VLow. That is, seeing when the limb travels at velocities above 0.8 m/s yields comparable endpoint precision than seeing throughout the movement. In contrast, seeing when the limb travels at velocities below 0.8 m/s did not yield any better endpoint precision than not seeing throughout the movement. Further, endpoint precision was significantly better when seeing the limb travelling above than below 0.8 m/s. In the second experiment of Tremblay et al. (2013), real-time limb velocity criteria ranging from 0.8 to 1.2 m/s were employed.

The endpoint variability results yielded support for the idea that amendments to the initial impulse (i.e., impulse regulation processes: see Elliott et al., 2010) are made when the limb travels between 0.8 and 0.9 m/s, while amendments based on contrasts between limb and target positions (i.e., limb-target regulation processes: see Elliott et al., 2010) are made when the limb travels above 1.0 m/s. Considering that commands sent to motor neurons presumably require transformations of the visual signals into the velocity domain (Bullock et al., 1998; Cisek et al., 1998), it is possible that information in the velocity domain is relevant for both the planning (e.g., Churchland et al., 2006) and the online control of upper-limb movements (re.: results of Tremblay et al., 2013). Nevertheless, these results provided further evidence for the importance of the velocity domain when assessing sensorimotor functions. Be it more, such importance of real-time limb velocity for sensorimotor processes extends to perceptual processes.

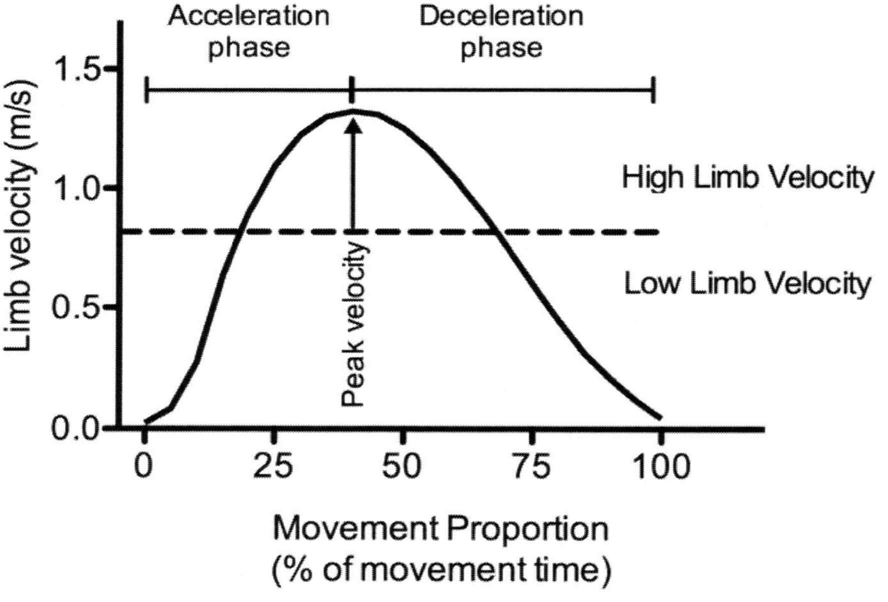

Figure 2. A depiction of the vision at high (VHigh) and low (VLow) limb velocity conditions from Tremblay et al. (2013). The above plot depicts a smoothed average velocity profile over proportions of movement time, peak velocity as well as the acceleration and deceleration phases. In the VHigh condition, vision was provided when the limb velocity was above 0.8 m/s, whereas in the VLow condition, vision was provided when the limb velocity was below 0.8 m/s.

Using an audio-visual illusion wherein one or two beeps influence the perception of one or two flashes (see Andersen, Tiippana, & Sams, 2004; Shams, Kamitani, & Shimojo, 2000; Shams, Kamitani, & Shimojo, 2002), Tremblay and Nguyen (2010) showed that the relative contribution of visual and auditory information to the perception of visual events is modulated as a function of real-time limb velocity. Typically, the presentation of a single beep with two flashes yields the perception of a single flash (i.e., fusion illusion: see Andersen et al., 2004). By presenting one or two beeps with one or two flashes at various times relative to movement onset (0-250 ms), Tremblay and Nguyen (2010) showed that the strength of the fusion illusion was weaker when the stimuli were presented at the times corresponding to the higher limb velocities (see Figure 3). Specifically, higher limb velocities at the stimulus midpoint were associated with a decreased likelihood of being influenced (i.e., fooled) by the number of beeps when judging the number of flashes. In an unpublished experiment, these results were replicated and expanded, showing that: 1) the fusion illusion was strongest in a control condition wherein no movements were required (i.e., at rest); and 2) the control condition and presentation conditions associated with the lowest limb velocities yielded comparable fusion illusion strengths.

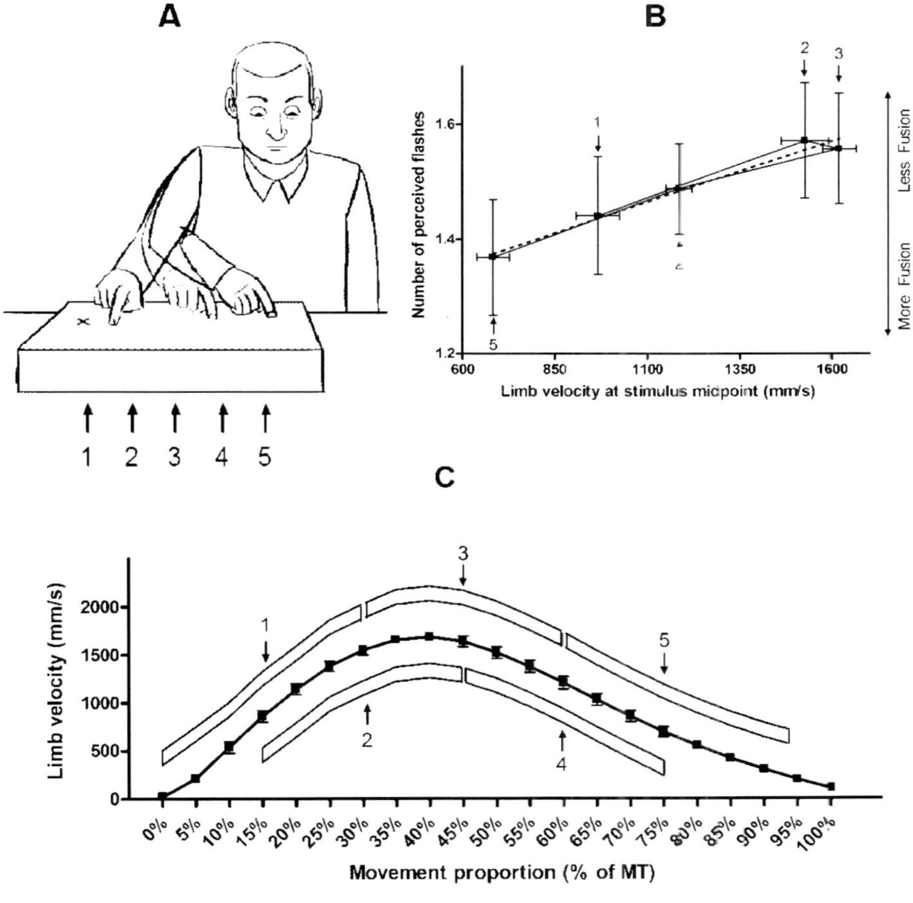

Figure 3. Experimental Task, Limb Velocity vs. the Fusion Illusion, and Average Velocity Profile. Reproduced from Tremblay and Nguyen (2010), licensed under CC By 3.0. (doi:10.1371/journal.pone.0008952.g002). Panel A: Depiction of the experimental task. Panel B: Mean number of perceived flashes for the 2 flashes and 1 beep condition (i.e., fusion illusion stimulus) at the different stimulus midpoints. Panel C: Average limb velocity profile with depiction of stimuli presentation (white boxes) and stimuli midpoints (arrows). The stimulus onset conditions are numbered as follows: 1 = 0 ms, 2 = 50 ms, 3 = 100 ms, 4 = 150 ms, and 5 = 200 ms relative to movement onset.

Altogether, there is a decreased susceptibility to be influenced by an audio-visual illusion at the high velocity stages of a movement. These results further support the above-mentioned proposal that processing sensory information in the velocity domain is important before (e.g., Churchland et al., 2006) and during a movement (e.g., Tremblay et al., 2013).

The importance of information in the velocity domain for the control of a voluntary upper-limb movement clearly extends to the perception of visual events. While the behavioral research cited above needs further replications and investigations, it emphasizes the importance of the velocity domain for central nervous system processing because it allows for the evaluation of multisensory contributions to optimal perceptual estimates (e.g., Ernst & Bülthoff, 2004). Interestingly, the vestibular system offers parallels to the above-mentioned contributions of the visual system.

Vestibulomotor Processing and the Velocity Domain

Neurophysiological Evidence of Vestibulomotor Processing

Ventre-Dominey (2014) provided a review of the neural pathways involved in the processing of vestibular information. Two main pathways were emphasized in that review. One pathway includes the temporal cortex, which processes visual and vestibular information to encode the velocity of self-motion. This first pathway is deemed to be most relevant for the encoding and processing of head accelerations into the velocity domain, to implement vestibulo-ocular control processes. The need to convert the head acceleration into the velocity domain is justified considering that vestibular inputs must ultimately be employed to send commands to static (i.e., alpha) or dynamic (i.e., gamma) motor neurons, which implies position or velocity commands, respectively. The second pathway highlighted by Ventre-Dominey projects through the parietal cortex and contributes to the "storage" of velocity information. Such pathway is deemed to be involved in extrapersonal and self-referential space encoding. Because the head acceleration (i.e., vestibular) signals are ultimately encoded to identify body position relative to objects and/ or in space, the conversion of head accelerations into the velocity domain is mathematically necessary before being able to encode position. Altogether, the model forwarded by Ventre-Dominey presents neurophysiological arguments as to how information from the vestibular system, which encodes head accelerations, must be converted into the velocity domain information in order to be used for eye movement control and body position encoding in space.

Behavioral Evidence of Vestibulomotor Processing

The suggestion made by Ventre-Dominey (2014) is substantiated by the behavioral literature. For example, Pulaski, Zee, and Robinson (1981) tested the vestibulo-ocular reflex response at various angular velocities of the head. The participants exhibited strong relationships between the head and the eye velocity, up to an individual velocity limit. On average, the head angular velocity was strongly related to the eye angular velocity, until approximately 350 degrees per second. This relationship between head and eye velocity represents further empirical evidence of the vestibular pathway involving the temporal cortex (Ventre-Dominey, 2014).

In terms of the vestibular pathway involving the parietal cortex and contributing to the perception of the body in space (Ventre-Dominey, 2014), support for the "storage" of velocity information was reported by Tremblay, Kennedy, Paleressompoulle, Borel, Mouchnino, and Blouin (2013). Participants were passively rotated and asked to reproduce the perceived rotation with a manipulandum (see Figure 4). Symmetric and asymmetric angular acceleration profiles were employed (i.e., shape of acceleration phase being the same / symmetric or different / asymmetric than shape of deceleration phase). One main finding was that the gains between the perceived and actual body rotations were significantly greater before than after the maximum angular velocity of the body (see Figure 4).

It is likely that these greater gains observed before than after peak velocity of the body rotation were due to velocity storage mechanisms. As highlighted by Ventre-Dominey (2014: see also Raphan, Matsuo, & Cohen, 1979), the central nervous system can accumulate velocity information by integrating acceleration signals over time. Because natural head acceleration profiles tend to be symmetric, the acceleration phase is highly predictive of the deceleration phase. It is thus efficient for the central nervous system to prioritize the use of acceleration information over time through velocity storage mechanisms to encode body rotation information. Indeed, the angular velocity of the body was more associated with the perceptual judgments of body rotation than the angular acceleration, providing further empirical support for the notion that vestibular signals need to be encoded in the velocity domain in order to be used for encoding body position in space.

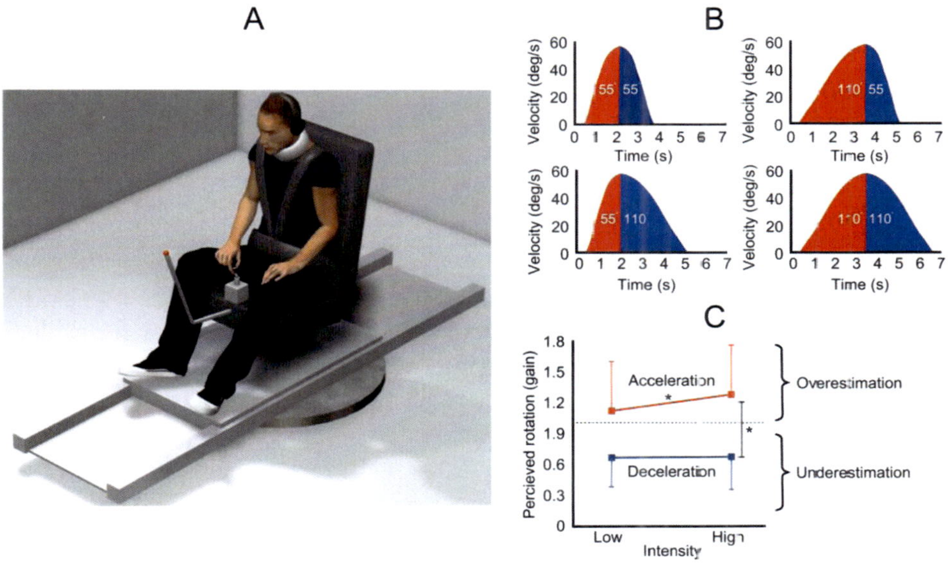

Figure 4. Amalgamation and adaptation of figures originally published in Tremblay et al. (2013b). Biases in the perception of self-motion during whole-body acceleration and deceleration. *Frontiers in Integrative Neuroscience,* 7(90), 1–10. Panel A: Depiction of the experimental setup. Panel B: Chair angular velocity profiles. Panel C: Gains between the perceived and actual body rotations during the acceleration and deceleration phases.

Moreover, the segregation of different phases of vestibular information encoding prior to and after peak velocity is analogous to the phases of online visuomotor regulation (e.g., Elliot et al., 1991). Together, the above lines of evidence prompt the need for the central nervous system to make multisensory contrasts when performing some activities of daily living.

Multisensory Combination, Integration and Conclusion

Information from the visual and vestibular systems must be compared to make optimal multisensory judgments. One model that helps predict how sensory signals are integrated to optimize perceptual and motor performance is the Maximum Likelihood Estimator (MLE) model (see Ernst & Banks, 2002; Fetsch, DeAngelis, & Angelaki, 2010; Knill & Saunders, 2003; Ghahramani, Wolpert, & Jordan, 1997). Mathematically, this model was presented as:

$$\text{Estimate} = \sum_i (w_i \times \hat{S}_i) \quad \text{with } w_i = \frac{1/\sigma_i^2}{\sum_j (1/\sigma_j^2)} \qquad \text{(Eq. 1)}$$

where $\hat{S}_i$ represents the estimate of a particular modality, and w_i represents the weight associated with it. This weight, (i.e., w_i), is computed as the proportional inverse variance of the estimate relative the total (i.e., the linear sum) of the inverse variances associated with all (i.e., *j*) contributing estimates (see Equation 1). If the estimates are combined in accordance to the MLE, then the variance of the combined estimate is lower than the variance of individual estimates alone (see Equation 2).

$$\sigma_{AB}^2 = \frac{\sigma_A^2 \times \sigma_B^2}{\sigma_A^2 + \sigma_B^2} \qquad \text{(Eq. 2)}$$

To support this model, Ernst and Banks (2002) manipulated visual and haptic signals to ascertain the contribution of both modalities to the perceived dimension of a graspable object. The relative contribution of visual and haptic information was significantly altered based on the amount of noise present in the visual signal, which was introduced via depths displacements of dots. More importantly, in order "to be integrated, the sensory estimates must be in the same units" (Ernst & Bülthoff, 2004, p. 163). Although estimates of a target location or an object size should intuitively be performed in the positional domain, encoding position and acceleration information when our body moves into space could be optimally integrated by transforming the visual and vestibular information into the velocity domain.

It is important to note that the thesis of this chapter does not challenge the idea that position, direction, distance, and other spatial characteristics can also be crucial domains of multisensory integration for the preparation and execution of voluntary movements (e.g., Ashe & Georgopoulos, 1994; Messier & Kalaska, 2000; van Beers, Wolpert, & Haggard,

2002). As such, the proposal that multisensory integration may be performed in the velocity domain might be limited to situations when the body is subject to accelerations and when vestibular signals are crucial to making a perceptual estimate or performing a goal-directed movement. That is, multisensory integration processes performed in the velocity domain would likely yield optimal performance if the encoding of head position (i.e., via vestibular inputs) is processed relative to other relevant information (e.g., step or door handle height) that requires afferent inputs in the position domain (e.g., via visual inputs). Such an approach would surely yield better performance than integrating the vestibular acceleration signals twice or, even worse, differentiating the visual position signals twice.

The use of whole body movements presents methodological challenges (e.g., motion capture), which could explain the relatively common use of transient and non-moving stimuli in scientific investigations. However, stable stimuli requiring minimal motor responses may fail to elicit all multisensory combination and integration capacities of the brain. For example, if a stimulus is not moving, there may be no need to process vestibular information and disentangle stimulus motion from self-motion. As a result, neurophysiological and behavioral studies employing stable stimuli without body or arm movements may be investigating a rather limited proportion of the brain's capabilities. Indeed, many activities of daily living require head rotations/ displacements in addition to limb movements, which would thus prompt visual-vestibular comparisons that may be optimally performed in the velocity domain.

Overall, it is suggested that the optimal integration of visual and vestibular information is made in the velocity domain, at least when making upper-limb reaching movements that includes head motion. It is acknowledged that such a view does not negate the existence of multisensory contrasts performed in other domains (i.e., position and acceleration) as well as other mechanisms influencing basic motor functions (e.g., grasping a tennis ball vs. a light bulb: see Marteniuk, MacKenzie, Jeannerod, Athenes & Dugas, 1987; see also Buckingham, Cant, & Goodale, 2009). Simply, the importance of the velocity domain for perceptual and sensorimotor functions is clearly supported by neurophysiological and behavioral evidence.

Acknowledgments

This research was supported by the Natural Sciences and Engineering Research Council of Canada (NSERC) as well as the Canada Foundation for Innovation (CFI) and the Ontario Research Fund (ORF).

References

Andersen, T.S., Tiippana, K., & Sams, M. (2004). Factors influencing audiovisual fission and fusion illusions. *Brain Research*, *21*(3), 301–308.

Ashe, J., & Georgopoulos, A.P. (1994). Movement parameters and neural activity in motor cortex and area 5. *Cerebral Cortex*, *4*(6), 590–600.

Blouin, J., Labrousse, L., Simoneau, M., Vercher, J., & Gauthier, G.M. (1998). Updating visual space during passive and voluntary head-in-space movements. *Experimental Brain Research*, *122*, 93–100.

Buckingham, G., Cant, J.S., & Goodale, M.A. (2009). Living in a material world: how visual cues to material properties affect the way that we lift objects and perceive their weight. *Journal of Neurophysiology*, *102*(6), 3111–3118.

Bullock, D., Cisek, P., & Grossberg, S. (1998). Cortical networks for control of voluntary arm movements under variable force conditions. *Cerebral Cortex*, *81*(1), 48–62.

Bullock, D., & Grossberg, S. (1988). Neural dynamics of planned arm movements: Emergent invariants and speed-accuracy properties during trajectory formation. *Psychological Review*, *95*(1), 49–90.

Bresciani, J.P., Blouin, J., Popov, K., Bourdin, C., Sarlegna, F., Vercher, J.L., & Gauthier, G.M. (2002). Galvanic vestibular stimulation in humans produces online arm movement deviations when reaching towards memorized visual targets. *Neuroscience Letters*, *318*(1), 34–38.

Buneo, C.A., & Andersen, R.A. (2006). The posterior parietal cortex: Sensorimotor interface for the planning and online control of visually guided movements. *Neuropsychologia*, *44*(13), 2594–2606.

Buneo, C.A, Jarvis, M.R., Batista, A.P., & Andersen, R.A. (2002). Direct visuomotor transformations for reaching. *Nature*, *416*(6881), 632–636.

Carlton, L. (1992). Visual processing time and the control of movement. In L. Proteau, & D. Elliott (Eds.), *Advances in Psychology: Vision and Motor Control* (pp. 3–32). Amsterdam: North-Holland.

Chua, R., & Elliott, D. (1993). Visual regulation of manual aiming. *Human Movement Science*, *12*(4), 365–401.

Churchland, M.M., Santhanam, G., & Shenoy, K.V. (2006). Preparatory activity in premotor and motor cortex reflects the speed of the upcoming reach. *Journal of Neurophysiology*, *96*(6), 3130–3146.

Cisek, P., Grossberg, S., & Bullock, D. (1998). A cortico-spinal model of reaching and proprioception under multiple task constraints. *Journal of Cognitive Neuroscience*, *10*(4), 425–444.

Cohen, L. A. (1961). Role of eye and neck proprioceptive mechanisms in body orientation and motor coordination. *Journal of Neurophysiology*, *24*, 1–11.

Crawford, J.D., Medendorp, W.P., & Marotta, J.J. (2004). Spatial transformations for eye-hand coordination. *Journal of Neurophysiology*, *92*(1), 10–19.

Elliott, D., Carson, R., Goodman, D., & Chua, R. (1991). Discrete vs. continuous visual control of manual aiming. *Human Movement Science*, *10*, 393–418.

Elliott, D., Hansen, S., Grierson, L.E.M., Lyons, J., Bennett, S.J., & Hayes, S.J. (2010). Goal-directed aiming: two components but multiple processes. *Psychological Bulletin*, *136*(6), 1023–1044.

Ernst, M.O., & Banks, M.S. (2002). Humans integrate visual and haptic information in a statistically optimal fashion. *Nature*, *415*(24), 429–433.

Ernst, M.O., & Bülthoff, H.H. (2004). Merging the senses into a robust percept. *Trends in Cognitive Sciences*, *8*(4), 162–169.

Fetsch, C.R., DeAngelis, G.C., & Angelaki, D.E. (2010). Visual-vestibular cue integration for heading perception: Applications of optimal cue integration theory. *The European Journal of Neuroscience*, *31*(10), 1721–1729.

Flanders, M., Helms Tillery, S.I., & Soechting, J.F. (1992). Early stages in a sensorimotor transformation. *Behavioral and Brain Sciences*, *15*, 309–362.

Ghahramani, Z., Wolpert, D.M., & Jordan, I. (1997). Computational models of sensorimotor integration. In P. Morasso, & V. Sanguineti (Eds.), *Advances in psychology: Self organization, computational maps, and motor control* (pp. 117–147). Amsterdam: North-Holland.

Goldberg, M.E., Walker, M.F., & Hudspeth, A.J. (2013). The vestibular system. In E.R. Kandel, J.H. Schwartz, T.M. Jessel, S.A. Siegelbaum, & A.J. Hudspeth (Eds.) *Principles of Neural Science* (pp. 917-934), New York: McGraw-Hill.

Gomi, H. (2008). Implicit online corrections of reaching movements. *Current Opinion in Neurobiology*, *18*(6), 558–564.

Henriques, D.Y.P., Klier, E.M., Smith, M.A., Lowy, D., & Crawford, J.D. (1998). Gaze-Centered Remapping of Remembered Visual Space in an Open-Loop Pointing Task. *The Journal of Neuroscience*, *18*(4), 1583–1594.

Jeannerod, M. (1988). *The neural and behavioural organization of goal-directed movements.* Oxford: Oxford University Press.

Knill, D.C., & Saunders, J.A. (2003). Do humans optimally integrate stereo and texture information for judgments of surface slant? *Vision Research*, *43*(24), 2539–2558.

Marteniuk, R.G., MacKenzie, C.L., Jeannerod, M., Athenes, S., & Dugas, C. (1987). Constraints on Human Arm Movement Trajectories. *Canadian Journal of Psychology*, *41*(3), 365–378.

Messier, J., & Kalaska, J.F. (2000). Covariation of primate dorsal premotor cell activity with direction and amplitude during a memorized-delay reaching task. *Journal of Neurophysiology*, *84*, 152–165.

Meister, M., & Tessier-Lavigne, M. (2013). Low-level visual processing: The retina. In E.R. Kandel, J.H. Schwartz, T.M. Jessel, S.A. Siegelbaum, & A.J. Hudspeth (Eds.) *Principles of Neural Science* (pp. 577-601), New York: McGraw-Hill.

Meyer, D.E., Abrams, R.A., Kornblum, S., Wright, C.E., & Smith, J.E. (1988). Optimality in human motor performance: Ideal control of rapid aimed movements. *Psychological Review*, *95*(3), 340–370.

Prablanc, C., Echallier, J.E., Jeannerod, M., & Komilis, E. (1979). Optimal response of eye and hand motor systems in pointing at a visual target: II Static and dynamic visual cues in the control of hand movement. *Biological Cybernetics*, *35*, 183–187.

Pulaski, P.D., Zee, D.S., & Robinson, D.A. (1981). The behavior of the vestibulo-ocular reflex at high velocities of head rotation. *Brain Research*, *222*, 159–165.

Raphan, T., Matsuo, V., & Cohen, B. (1979). Brain Velocity Storage in the Vestibulo-Ocular Reflex Arc. *Experimental Brain Research*, *248*, 229–248.

Shams, L., Kamitani, Y., & Shimojo, S. (2000). What you see is what you hear. *Nature*, *408*, 788–788.

Shams, L., Kamitani, Y., & Shimojo, S. (2002). Visual illusion induced by sound. *Cognitive Brain Research*, *14*(1), 147–152.

Tremblay, L., Hansen, S., Kennedy, A., & Cheng, D.T. (2013). The utility of vision during action: multiple visuomotor processes? *Journal of Motor Behavior*, *45*(2), 91–99.

Tremblay, L., Kennedy, A., Paleressompoulle, D., Borel, L., Mouchnino, L., & Blouin, J. (2013). Biases in the perception of self-motion during whole-body acceleration and deceleration. *Frontiers in Integrative Neuroscience*, *7*(90), 1–10.

Tremblay, L., & Nguyen, T. (2010). Real-time decreased sensitivity to an audio-visual illusion during goal-directed reaching. *PLoS ONE*, *5*(1), 1–4.

Vaitl, D., Mittelstaedt, H., Saborowski, R., Stark, R., & Baisch, F. (2002). Shifts in blood volume alter the perception of posture: further evidence for somatic graviception. *International Journal of Psychophysiology*, *44*(1), 1–11.

Van Beers, R.J., Wolpert, D.M., & Haggard, P. (2002). When feeling is more important than seeing in sensorimotor adaptation. *Current Biology*, *12*(10), 834–837.

Ventre-Dominey, J. (2014). Vestibular function in the temporal and parietal cortex: distinct velocity and inertial processing pathways. *Frontiers in Integrative Neuroscience*, *8*(53), 1–13.

Vindras, P., & Viviani, P. (1998). Frames of reference and control parameters in visuomanual pointing. *Journal of Experimental Psychology. Human Perception and Performance*, *24*(2), 569-591.

Woodworth, R.S. (1899). The accuracy of voluntary movement. *Psychological Review*, *3*(2), 1–114.

In: Advances in Visual Perception Research
Editor: Thomas Heinen

ISBN: 978-1-63482-455-2
© 2015 Nova Science Publishers, Inc.

Chapter 15

Sensorimotor Integration: A Special Emphasis on Visual Inputs for Goal-Directed Movements

Jan M. Hondzinski*[*] *and Chelsea M. Soebbing
Louisiana State University, Baton Rouge, LA, US

Abstract

Performances of many activities of daily living rely on the proper integration of different sensory and motor systems. In neurologically healthy people the CNS integrates sensory cues into task commands to control performances. Use of visual inputs from central and peripheral visual fields can facilitate the online control of movement and form spatial memories about a target goal, the environment, or both. Thus after people execute a motor program or a set of commands to produce the movement, they can attempt to match hand movement to the spatial perceptions of remembered target locations to complete the goal with a certain amount of accuracy. Orientation of gaze, environmental illumination, and access to visual inputs about the movement can influence this goal-directed precision. A special phenomenon of reaching to remembered target locations along the earth-fixed vertical in illuminated and dark environments exists such that upright individuals will end reaches in the dark either lower than reaches to remembered target locations in an illuminated environment or lower than remembered target locations. Experimental outcomes revealed that error differences between performances in dark and illuminated environments observed for upright individuals were also observed individuals lying supine. These findings show that the phenomenon of reaching lower in the dark is not limited to upright individuals or based on an egocentric movement direction along the longitudinal body axis.

Keywords: allocentric cues; Earth-fixed vertical; endpoint errors; kinematics; body orientations

---

[*] Corresponding author: Jan M. Hondzinski. School of Kinesiology, Louisiana State University, 112 Huey P. Long Fieldhouse, Baton Rouge, LA 70803. E-mail: jhondz1@lsu.edu.

Sensorimotor Integration

Sensorimotor integration is imperative for the proper motor control needed to produce coordinated movements. Healthy people commonly rely on multiple sensory systems to perform what may appear as the simplest of tasks. The seemingly effortless and basic task of reaching toward an object, for example, requires control over multiple muscles to coordinate arm, head, and eye movements. In this case proprioceptive sensations used for arm, head, and eye position combine with visual cues for target location to assist with task performance. To perform a task well the central nervous system (CNS) must integrate available sensations, ignore distracting inputs, and account for task requirements such as accuracy and speed. Understanding the sensorimotor control of such ordinary activities is significant, as it offers insight to the resiliency of the nervous system to determine whether and how the CNS can compensate for temporary or permanent deficits to complete various tasks. Such understanding can lead researchers and clinicians to devise the proper treatment for those with neural impairment.

Many studies on hand-eye coordination for discrete goal-directed arm movements in the seated individual exist independently from studies on standing posture control. Yet several discrete, whole body, goal-directed movements commonly performed during daily activities allow for functional independence. Upper limb goal-directed movements utilize inputs from and actions of the eyes, head, and upper limb(s), while posture control to remain upright involves inputs from and actions of additional body segments depending on whether the person is seated or standing. Reaching from a standing position involves simultaneous control of the reaching goal and maintenance of posture (Berret, Bonnetblanc, Papaxanthis, and Pozzo, 2009; Pozzo, Stapley, and Papaxanthis, 2002). Combining these actions is not simply additive, as moving the upper limbs influences body posture (Bouisset and Zattara, 1981, 1987; Cordo and Nashner, 1982; Friedli, Hallett, and Simon, 1984; Gantchev and Dimitrova, 1996; Hodges and Richardson, 1997) and altering body posture can influence movements of the upper limbs (Pozzo et al., 2002). Sensorimotor links for these goal-directed actions become obvious considering that sensory reductions in vision (Hondzinski and Cui, 2006; Hondzinski and Kwon, 2009; Soechting and Flanders, 1989b) or the upper limbs (Prablanc, Pelisson, and Goodale, 1986) can alter focal control used for reaching, while reductions in visual input (Collins and De Luca, 1995), somatosensations of the lower limb (Clement, Gurfinkel, Lestienne, Lipshits, and Popov, 1984; Gaveau and Papaxanthis, 2011; Jeka, Oie, and Kiemel, 2000; Teasdale and Simoneau, 2001), and vestibular inputs (Black and Nashner, 1984; Foley, 1978) can alter posture stability. In fact reductions in lower limb sensations can also influence upper limb reaching accuracy in a goal-directed task involving a step to suggest people possessing normal visual acuity and somatosensations in the upper limb cannot completely compensate for the lower limb sensory deficits (Hondzinski, Li, and Welsch, 2010).

Whether the performance occurs from a seated or standing body orientation, control of discrete, goal-directed movements involves a complex integration of sensory and motor systems. Although various sensory systems contribute to performances of these volitional tasks, the emphasis of this chapter is on the use of visual contributions for controlling endpoint accuracy.

Visuomotor Integration

Most people use visual inputs to perform basic tasks of grooming, eating, and transport. Visual inputs used to perceive object locations can match movements to objects (Bridgeman and Stark, 1991), however movements do not always match visual perceptions influenced by illusions (Bridgeman, Kirch, and Sperling, 1981), as context information affects cognitive judgments, not movement (Coello and Iwanow, 2006) Endpoint errors often exist when spatial perceptions of object locations are memorized. Thus having participants point or reach to remembered locations of visual targets offers great insight to how spatial perceptions are used for controlling movement. Comparing performances of movements to remembered target locations with movements to veridical target locations or a control condition allows for insight to such control. In the control conditions updates of precise location of the target can match the intended outcome of the pointing device, such as a fingertip or handheld pen tip, through online visual inputs. When the spatial location of the target is remembered, participants must rely on a preprogrammed movement plan or try to match the pointing device to the memorized target location to complete the goal. The following text provides background information on spatial memory and the use of different visual fields for reaches to remembered target locations, which aids in the understanding of experimental methodologies and outcomes for visuomotor integration use in goal-directed reaches.

Spatial Memory

Tasks involving reaching or pointing to remembered target locations utilize the concept of spatial memory or visual working memory. Briefly stated, working memory, which is described in detail in most psychology or motor learning textbooks, involves the encoding and interim storage of recently introduced information to be retrieved and used to initiate and possibly complete a cognitive or motor task (Magill, 2004, p. 169). When using spatial memory for goal-directed movements, the task-relevant information for location of the target is memorized for a short period prior to making a motor response toward the remembered location (Pierrot-Deseilligny, Muri, Rivaud-Pechoux, Gaymard, and Ploner, 2002). Clearly, anything that diminishes or augments remembering the target location can influence the motor response toward the remembered target, including endpoint precision. Goal-directed reaches to remembered target locations feature a spatial memory component, making it one item of particular interest that influences the motor response.

Spatial memory decay persists as a well-known influence on remembered target locations, influencing subsequent endpoint accuracy. Not only does the decay of spatial memory begin immediately following removal of visual inputs (Heath, Westwood, and Binsted, 2004; Keele and Posner, 1968; Westwood, Heath, and Roy, 2001), electrophysiological evidence reveals that the visual perception decay begins within hundreds of milliseconds (ms) (Cruikshank, Caplan, and Singhal, 2012) and continues with increasing time; at least up to 3 seconds (s) (Cruikshank, Caplan, and Singhal, 2014). Some researchers have used the error bias saturation rate of 2 s (Elliott and Madalena, 1987) to indicate the completion of spatial memory decay (Glover, 2004). Introducing a longer delay from either 500 ms to 2 s (Westwood, Heath, and Roy, 2003) or from 2 s to 5 s (Heath and Binsted, 2007) can result in greater variable errors when moving in darkness, revealing continued spatial memory instability as time passes. Variable errors which remain similar between 2 s and 5 s delay conditions when the reaching cursor and start position remain visible throughout the trial, emphasize that visual cues related to the actual movement can decrease the variability of the final reaching positions (Heath and Westwood, 2003) and limit spatial memory decay.

Visual Fields

People use various parts of their visual field when performing daily tasks. Although the roles of central and peripheral vision are not completely segregated, humans use different viewing fields to perform different tasks. The central visual field represents the area of highest visual clarity (Sivak and MacKenzie, 1992; Figure 1) thus people who lose central vision have difficulties performing many tasks, such as reading, which rely on the ability to detect physical characteristics of objects (Legge, Rubin, Pelli, and Schleske, 1985; Sekuler and Blake, 1994).The peripheral visual field allows people to detect certain spatial characteristics of the environment such as relative movement between object and observer, explaining why mobility is compromised in people with reduced peripheral vision (Black et al., 1997). Distinguishing central and peripheral vision and their corresponding viewing fields can vary in the literature, emphasizing the fact that no strict cutoff between the two exists.

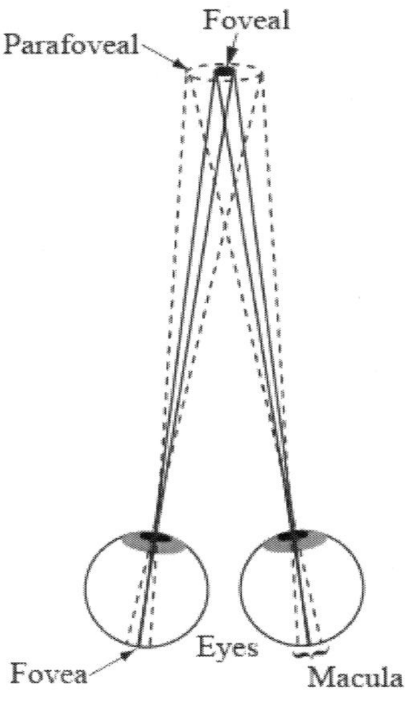

Figure 1. Central visual field.

Central vision, defined here as vision using the central viewing field, closely corresponds to the direction of gaze (Sivak and MacKenzie, 1992). Gaze direction relies on the orientation of the eyes within the environment, thus the orientation of light reflecting off objects and onto the macula, which is located on the central portion of the retina. The macula covers approximately ± 6° (Fawzi, Lee, Acton, Laine, and Smith, 2011) to ± 8° (Hood et al., 2014) of the visual field. Its bullseye arrangement contains the fovea—the centermost region covering less than ± 2° degrees of the retina, the parafovea—the next concentric ring approximating ± 5° of the retina, and the perifovea—the last concentric ring (Harb et al., 2012). Figure 1 depicts the foveal and parafoveal regions or the central 10° of central visual field, which has been used to define central vision (Provis, Dubis, Maddess, and Carroll, 2013) and to indicate central scotoma or central vision loss (Kwon et al., 2012).

Peripheral vision represents vision using the peripheral visual field, which corresponds to the viewing field outside the center of gaze direction. The peripheral visual field of the retina has a low density of cones and is dominated by rods. The highest density of rods ranges from 10°-21° eccentricity from the fovea depending on direction (Curcio, Sloan, Kalina, and Hendrickson, 1990; Jonas, Schneider, and Naumann, 1992). Clarity of the visual image decreases more rapidly in the periphery, which extends up to 130° of the visual arc vertically and 200° of the visual arc horizontally, due to photoreceptor reduction (Harrington, 1964).

Attention differs for location of object presentation in various parts of the visual field (Ando, Kida, and Oda, 2002; Ando, Kokubu, Kida, and Oda, 2002), thus contributes to responses to the given input. Studies on the abilities of people to detect and react to objects in the central and peripheral visual fields offer insight to such temporal responses (Ando, Kida, and Oda, 2001; Ando, Kida, et al., 2002; Ando, Kida, and Oda, 2004; Niechwiej-Szwedo, McIlroy, Green, and Verrier, 2005). Figure 2 shows how participants' reaction times to produce quick horizontal head movements in response to eccentrically presented visual stimuli differ. The distribution of retina cell densities best explains the alterations in reaction times that vary with stimulus presentation at different eccentricities (Payne, 1966; Rains, 1963). Alterations in cell density lead to varied transmission speeds across neural pathways and correspond to changes in reaction time (Poggel and Strasburger, 2004). This explanation illuminates why the shortest responses exist for 10°-20° target presentation eccentricities (Payne, 1966; Rains, 1963), while longer responses can exist at a 4° eccentricity yet most often exist for large eccentricities (Figure 2).

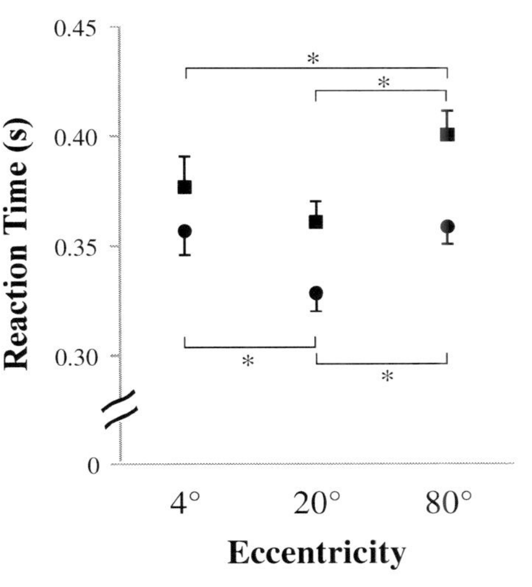

Figure 2. Mean values of reaction time for quick horizontal head rotations toward right or left shoulders in the same direction (circles) and the opposite direction (squares) of visual stimuli presented at 4°, 20°, and 80° peripheral eccentricities are presented. Asterisks indicate significant differences between corresponding data points. Error bars represent 1 standard error (Kwon and Hondzinski, 2010).

Although neural anatomy can be used to dictate central vision based on the retinal distribution of the cone and rod photoreceptors, divergent projections from photoreceptors pass through the underlying cells, the primary visual pathway, and beyond, suggesting links between central and peripheral field projections (e.g. Hadjikhani and Tootell, 2000).Regardless of this overlap, strategies of visuomotor control used exclusively for responses to stimuli projected only on the central retina may not generalize to responses for peripheral target presentation, while responses to stimuli projected only on the peripheral retina may not generalize to responses for central target presentation. Moreover, spatial responses to visual stimuli presented across different retinal eccentricities vary from the temporal responses and correspond directly to accuracy used for goal-directed movements.

Goal-Directed Precision

Gaze Direction Influences

People can look directly at the target of interest, while reaching toward its spatial location or look one direction while reaching toward a target in their peripheral visual field. Reaching toward an object in the peripheral visual field is less than desirable when precision is of interest, because the signals for the direction of gaze, as indicated indirectly by head orientation (Daghestani, Anderson, and Flanders, 2000; Flanders, Daghestani, and Berthoz, 1999; Hondzinski, 2004) or directly through records of eye and head integrations (Admiraal, Keijsers, and Gielen, 2003; Henriques and Crawford, 2000, 2002; Henriques, Klier, Smith, Lowy, and Crawford, 1998; Hondzinski and Cui, 2006; Hondzinski and Kwon, 2009), influence hand movement for goal-directed tasks.

Not only has gaze direction been considered a common coordinate axis for hand placement in space (Admiraal et al., 2003; Admiraal, Keijsers, and Gielen, 2004; Carrozzo, Stratta, McIntyre, and Lacquaniti, 2002; McIntyre, Stratta, and Lacquaniti, 1997), it has been considered a neural input for hand placement during manual tracking tasks (Soechting, Engel, and Flanders, 2001) and for placement of the hand and other body segments during performances of goal-directed tasks involving movement of the whole body (Hondzinski and Cui, 2006; Hondzinski and Kwon, 2009).

With supporting links between gaze direction and hand placement, orienting a person's gaze away from the object of interest presents a new source of potential error for manual control. Participants allowed to saccade the eyes toward a remembered target location in the peripheral visual field will look and point short of the remembered location, thus moving less distance than required to reach the point of interest (Bock and Eckmiller, 1986; Enright, 1995; Prablanc, Echallier, Komilis, and Jeannerod, 1979).These results contribute to the evidence for a common neural network for the gaze and limb control (Admiraal et al., 2004; Engel, Anderson, Gomez, and Soechting, 2004; Engel, Anderson, and Soechting, 2000; Engel and Soechting, 2003; Soechting et al., 2001).Such a network would have to incorporate the eccentrically remembered target location in cases for which the gaze remains directed eccentrically during movement performance. In the past errors in retinal eccentricity have been used to explain the increase in final azimuth endpoint errors for eccentrically directed gaze along a horizontal plane (Bock, 1986; Henriques and Crawford, 2000, 2002; Henriques et al., 1998). Recently researchers blame poor approximations in hand position for the gaze-dependent reach errors, which are limited to the horizontal direction (Dessing, Oostwoud Wijdenes, Peper, and Beek, 2009). Seated individuals often make final endpoint errors more eccentric than remembered target locations, thus overshooting laterally remembered targets (Beurze, Van Pelt, and Medendorp, 2006; Bock, 1986; Dessing et al., 2009; Henriques and Crawford, 2000, 2002; Henriques et al., 1998; McGuire and Sabes, 2009; Pouget, Ducom, Torri, and Bavelier, 2002). In these cases people end reaches left of the veridical target location when looking right and end reaches right of the veridical target location when looking left. Examples of undershooting target locations do exist and have been blamed on perceptual compressions of visual space (Heath and Binsted, 2007; Sheth and Shimojo, 2001) and a poor spatial encoding of eye position (Prablanc et al., 1979) or target amplitude (Bock and Eckmiller, 1986) that degrades with eccentric head orientations (Roll, Bard, and Paillard, 1986). Researchers explain the lateral overshooting for a seated person seems most robust when gaze is diverted primarily with only eye movements in a dark environment (Hondzinski and Kwon, 2009), hand movements are in the radial direction (Bock, 1986), and body movements are restricted, as instances of reaching less eccentric than remembered target locations also exist for unrestricted body movements (Hondzinski, 2004; Hondzinski and Cui, 2006; Hondzinski and Kwon, 2009).

Support for a common neural network for the gaze and limb control has its limitations. One limitation results from the evidence that separate mechanisms control movement direction and amplitude (Bock and Arnold, 1993; Favilla, Gordon, Hening, and Ghez, 1990; Hening, Favilla, and Ghez, 1988; Hondzinski and Cui, 2006; McIntyre, Stratta, and Lacquaniti, 1998; Soechting and Flanders, 1989a, 1989b). Strong links between gaze and limb control are based primarily on azimuth error comparisons of gaze direction and limb position. Movements orthogonal to the direction of the gaze can offer greater perceptible alterations in vision compared to those that occur in depth. For instance, when viewing an object, it is much easier to estimate that it has moved 5 cm right, left, down, or up orthogonal to the line-of-sight rather than 5 cm closer or further away along gaze direction. The spread in endpoint errors along the gaze vector (Admiraal et al., 2003, 2004; Carrozzo et al., 2002; McIntyre et al., 1997, 1998) emphasize this point. Other limitations of the common neural network for gaze and limb control result from changes in illumination and the availability of environmental spatial cues.

Illumination and Spatial Cues

Performing a goal-directed movement in complete darkness introduces specific challenges to participants that do not exist when performing goal-directed movements in dimly lit or illuminated environments. Spatial memory decay appears less stable over time in darkness, as indicated by greater variability in movement errors in dark compared to full vision conditions (Elliott and Hansen, 2010; Heath and Binsted, 2007; Hondzinski and Cui, 2006; Hondzinski and Kwon, 2009; Westwood et al., 2003). People also cannot fixate targets well in the dark. Not only does an upshift in fixation occur with a dark background illumination compared to a light background illumination (Barash, Melikyan, Sivakov, and Tauber, 1998) but an unconscious radial drift in binocular gaze position (the crossing of left and right gaze vectors) away from the participants also exists in dark environments (Admiraal et al., 2003, 2004). The upshift in fixation and drift in gaze do not explain why some participants undershot remembered radial target locations in darkness (Coello and Iwanow, 2006; Darling and Miller, 1993; McIntyre et al., 1997, 1998; Soechting and Flanders, 1989b), why small fixation errors do not correlate well with small endpoint errors in a dark environment (Henriques, Medendorp, Gielen, and Crawford, 2003), or why participants' reaching errors in the vertical direction do not always match gaze direction (Admiraal et al., 2004; Henriques and Crawford, 2000; Henriques et al., 1998; Hondzinski and Cui, 2006). Apparently the common neural network for gaze and limb control represents more of an approximation without visual inputs.

People who reach toward a remembered target location in the dark will generally complete the task with more error bias and/or greater error variability in their movement than reaches performed toward a veridical target location or remembered target location in an illuminated environment (Heath and Westwood, 2003; Heath et al., 2004; Hondzinski and Cui, 2006; Hondzinski and Kwon, 2009; Westwood et al., 2001). Providing visual updates of the movement itself can enhance movement precision even when targets are remembered (Admiraal et al., 2003, 2004; Heath, 2005; Heath and Westwood, 2003; Prablanc et al., 1986). Adding visual cues about environment can also improve movement accuracy (Admiraal et al., 2003, 2004; Hondzinski and Cui, 2006; Hondzinski and Kwon, 2009), however, error improvements will depend on specific requirements of the task, which seem to accompany more challenging conditions (Desmurget, Pelisson, Rossetti, and Prablanc, 1998). For example, participants who reach to remembered target locations with an illuminated fingertip and illuminated points to define the otherwise dark environment decreased endpoint error bias and variability compared to reaches performed with only an illuminated fingertip or in complete darkness (Admiraal et al., 2003, 2004). In contrast only decreases in azimuth error variability were observed for participants who reached to remembered target locations in an illuminated room compared to complete darkness (Hondzinski and Cui, 2006; Hondzinski and Kwon, 2009). Although similar task requirements existed among studies, background luminance did differ to potentially challenge the participants to a greater extent and offer an explanation for differences in error bias observed between conditions (Admiraal et al., 2003, 2004).

Controlling amplitude of goal-directed reaches can vary by direction. Examples of undershooting (Elliott and Hansen, 2010; Heath, 2005), overshooting (Adamovich, Berkinblit, Fookson, and Poizner, 1998; Berkinblit, Fookson, Smetanin, Adamovich, and Poizner, 1995; Coello and Iwanow, 2006) and over- and undershooting (McIntyre et al., 1997, 1998; Westwood et al., 2003) remembered target locations in the main direction (usually radial direction) of movement exist. When overshooting and undershooting are reported, people often overshoot near locations and undershoot far locations (Admiraal et al., 2003; Brown, Knauft, and Rosenbaum, 1948; Darling and Miller, 1993; Heath and Binsted, 2007; Soechting and Flanders, 1989a, 1989b). Researchers blame the error accruing sensorimotor transformations for the inaccurate endpoints, which exist when reaching to remembered target locations (Soechting and Flanders, 1989a, 1989b).

Although smaller lateral and vertical reaching errors often exist when compared to radial errors, possibly because of the good approximation of a common input for gaze and limb control, there is a systematic vertical error that occurs in darkness such that people have a tendency to reach below remembered target locations or below reaches to remembered target locations when the background is illuminated. Information on this tendency to "reach lower in the dark" will be presented in the next section in an introduction to a research study on this topic.

Spatial Cues and Precision along the Earth-Fixed Vertical: A Research Study

Introduction

Goal-directed upper extremity movements, such as reaching or pointing tasks, are commonly utilized to complete activities of daily living. The seemingly effortless coordination of the eyes, head, and upper limbs, as well as the lower limbs when a person reaches while standing upright, masks the detailed sensorimotor transformations required by the CNS to complete the task accurately. When reaching to a visually defined target quickly and accurately, participants utilize visual guidance to modify the movement (Chua and Elliott, 1993; Elliott and Hansen, 2010). Reaches to remembered target locations often result in different endpoint errors when compared to reaching to veridical target locations (Darling and Miller, 1993; Heath and Westwood, 2003; Heath et al., 2004; Hondzinski and Cui, 2006; Hondzinski and Kwon, 2009; Westwood et al., 2001). Use of visual inputs for online control of hand position during movements can improve endpoint accuracy for reaching to remembered target locations (Admiraal et al., 2003, 2004; Heath, 2005; Heath and Westwood, 2003; Prablanc et al., 1986; Sarlegna and Blouin, 2010). In fact, imperceptibly misleading visual inputs of online reaching control can decrease movement accuracy (Sarlegna et al., 2004) and emphasize the subtle differences that can influence CNS control for movement precision.

Endpoint errors, the primary measure of endpoint precision, can differ in size depending on the spatial dimension. In three dimensional space large overshooting and/or undershooting error bias and greater variability often occur after people reach to remembered target locations along the radial or anterior/posterior directions (Adamovich et al., 1998; Admiraal et al., 2003; Berkinblit et al., 1995; Darling and Miller, 1993; Heath and Binsted, 2007; Heath et al., 2004; McIntyre et al., 1997, 1998; Soechting and Flanders, 1989b; Westwood et al., 2001, 2003). Errors along orthogonal directions also occur and are often, yet not always (Adamovich et al., 1998; Berkinblit et al., 1995), smaller.

Endpoint errors can occur whether the reach to a remembered target location is performed in an environment with or without the availability of allocentric cues (Admiraal et al., 2003, 2004; Hondzinski and Cui, 2006; Hondzinski and Kwon, 2009; Soechting and Flanders, 1989b). With the greater variability in spatial memory decay (Heath and Binsted, 2007), an upshift in fixation (Barash et al., 1998), and an unconscious radial drift in binocular gaze away from the observer (Admiraal et al., 2003, 2004) in dark environments, it is easy to predict why reaches to remembered target locations in an illuminated environment commonly produce smaller error bias and/or variability in movement than reaches to remembered target locations in darkness (Heath and Westwood, 2003; Heath et al., 2004; Hondzinski and Cui, 2006; Hondzinski and Kwon, 2009; Westwood et al., 2001). However, a less intuitive and less predictive phenomenon exists for the vertical dimension of upright individuals reaching to remembered target locations in illuminated and dark environments.A systematic offset appears in a dark environment, in which upright participants frequently reach below either the remembered target location or a control reference. This phenomenon of reaching lower in darkness has occurred while sitting (Adamovich et al., 1998; Berkinblit et al., 1995; Brown et al., 1948; Crawford, Henriques, and Vilis, 2000; Henriques and Crawford, 2000; Henriques et al., 1998), standing (Admiraal et al., 2003; Smetanin and Popov, 1997; Soechting and Flanders, 1989b; Wnuczko and Kennedy, 2011), or stepping forward (Admiraal et al., 2004; Flanders et al., 1999; Hondzinski and Cui, 2006). In these experiments starting upper limb positions ranged from a straight arm with hand down by the thigh (Wnuczko and Kennedy, 2011) to a bent arm with hand at eye level (Adamovich et al., 1998) and although several targets required an upward movement component of the hand (Wnuczko and Kennedy, 2011), downward movement components also existed (Adamovich et al., 1998; Berkinblit et al., 1995; Flanders et al., 1999; Hondzinski and Cui, 2006). Methodological differences correspond to use of different muscles as well as extension and flexion of the joints, eliminating these differences as possible explanatory factors for lower reaches in darkness.

The reference point for lower reaches and type of remember target location have varied across studies. Since the systematic error reference can vary by the location of remembered targets (Hondzinski and Cui, 2006; Soechting and Flanders, 1989b), the term dark phenomenon does not always signify reaches relative to veridical target locations. Lower reaches relative to the actual remembered target location, to the endpoints for remembered reaches in illuminated environments, to the endpoints for remembered reaches with an illuminated pointer, or to a combination of these exist. Emphasis in this study will be on visually remembered target locations placed in the surrounding environment, rather than targeted body locations using proprioceptive cues or kinesthetically remembered target locations, to offer greater insight to this particular phenomenon of visuomotor integration.

Currently, no clear explanation for the dark phenomenon exists. Methods in previous studies allow some insight to potential contributing factors, predominantly from an exclusionary perspective. Although sensorimotor transformations have been used to explain general endpoint imprecision for under- and overshooting remembered target locations (Soechting and Flanders, 1989a, 1989b), only a few researchers have tried to explain the dark phenomenon, specifically.The few studies used to investigate the phenomenon directly offer some illuminating insights to guide future experiments.

People may use different egocentric reference points for pointing in illuminated and dark environments. Figure 3 shows two final endpoints of arm movement to illustrate the eyes or the shoulder as an egocentric reference point. Blindfolded participants directed the shoulder-finger line of their straight arm toward target locations on the floor, suggesting the use of the shoulder as a reference point for pointing direction in darkness (Wnuczko and Kennedy, 2011). The same participants aligned the fingertip with eyes directed to the floor target locations in an illuminated environment, suggesting use of the eyes as a reference point for pointing direction in normal room lighting. Note that directing the shoulder-finger line towards the target places the endpoint of the fingertip lower than that its endpoint if it were aligned with the gaze direction (Figure 3), that occurs with the dark phenomenon, yet pointing accuracy to remembered target location is maintained. These results do not explain the lower reaches that occur in darkness when participants actually reach to place the fingertip on a remembered target location (Adamovich et al., 1998; Admiraal et al., 2003, 2004; Berkinblit et al., 1995; Flanders et al., 1999; Hondzinski and Cui, 2006; Soechting and Flanders, 1989b), rather than just pointing toward the remembered target. It seems unlikely that participants would use one strategy for pointing toward a remembered target location and one for reaching to its location. Future studies could determine if using the shoulder as a reference point in the dark still exists for conditions when reaching using multi-joint arm movements, from different body orientations, and in dark environments without the use of blindfolds.

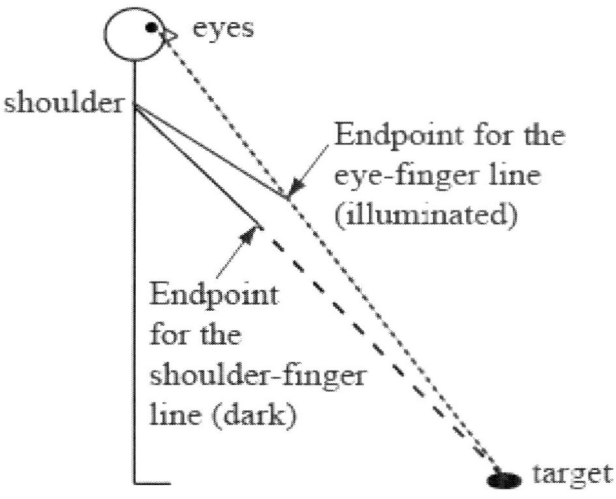

Figure 3. Representations of an eye-centered and shoulder-centered egocentric frame of reference. Arms of the stick figure represent final reach position to the given target in illuminated and dark environments. The shoulder-finger line (dashed line) and eye-finger line (dotted line) are directed toward the center of the target illustrating the difference in fingertip locations for each condition.

Gravitational influences on vertically directed arm trajectory control (Gentili, Cahouet, and Papaxanthis, 2007; Papaxanthis, Pozzo, and Schieppati, 2003) may also exist for endpoint control in the dark. Errors associated with the dark phenomenon align with the earth-fixed vertical in the direction of the gravitational vector for upright individuals, making gravitational influences a good candidate as a potential explanatory factor. Evidence for gravitational influences on endpoint control in darkness ensues from studies involving one- and two-dimensional reaches. People made shorter upward movement excursions for long distances and longer downward movement excursions for short and long distances when asked to manually estimate remembered target-to-target distances on a vertical slide in the dark (Brown et al., 1948).

Authors used these outcomes as evidence for gravitation influences for one-dimensional distance estimations. Performances in which reaching to remembered target locations with eyes closed resulted in significantly greater negative, thus more egocentrically inferior, errors for standing than those for the supine or prone body orientations (Smetanin and Popov, 1997). In that study remembered targets located on flat surfaces parallel to the frontal plane of each participant allowed for two-dimensional egocentric error calculations along the superior/inferior and medial/lateral directions. Analyses of errors along the earth-fixed vertical were not determined for all body orientations. Instead authors compared the greater superior bias while lying down to the greater inferior/downward bias while upright and used it as evidence for gravitational influences on reach accuracy. These data indicate that restrictive lower reaches in the dark observed in upright individuals are not egocentric. Asking participants to point to a remembered target location rather than estimate target-to-target distance in an unencumbered space, which eliminates surface restrictions on movement and tactile feedback, and evaluating errors along the earth-fixed vertical would expand upon previous work by offering insights to the potential of gravitational influences over vertical endpoint control in three dimensional (3D) space.

Clearly, further exploration is warranted to make conclusions about gravitational influences and/or use of a shoulder reference point on endpoint accuracy in the dark, especially when tactile feedback of the reaching goal is not provided. The purpose of the following experiment was to take the first step towards better understanding the dark phenomenon in 3D space.

Methods

Seven females and three males participated in the experiment. Ages ranged between 19 and 22 years with an average mass of 67.72 ± 11.3 kg, height of 168.42 ± 8.5 cm, and dominant arm length of 67.69 ± 4.4 cm. Participants were right-handed, had no known neurological or musculoskeletal problems to influence task performance, and uncorrected or corrected visual acuity better than 20/30. Although visual acuity for one participant was worse than the accepted normal acuity of 20/20, participants had no difficulty viewing targets and were within the accepted acuity of 20/40 for commercial driving in the United States (Owsley and McGwin, 1999). Each participant read and signed informed consent prior to participating in the experimental procedures approved by the University's Institutional Review Board.

Reflective markers were placed on each shoulder and the elbow, wrist, and tip of a handheld pen of the dominant arm. Marker movements were monitored at 60 Hz during task performance using a four-camera passive-marker digital video system (Qualysis Medial AB, SE).

Figure 4 shows the experimental setup. Three targets (1.5 cm diameter fishing anchors) were presented individually to participants at shoulder level and 30 cm superior (shoulder+30) and inferior (shoulder-30) to shoulder level along the body's mid-sagittal plane. Participants stood UPRIGHT or laid SUPINE on a padded table with the feet a self-selected comfortable distance apart and the dominant arm bent at the elbow to approximately 90°. Target distance was one half the dominant arm length (range 30.5 cm - 38.1 cm) for the UPRIGHT body orientation. In the SUPINE body orientation, the distance between the platform underneath the participant and the targets were 5 cm greater than one half the arm length added to the foot length of each participant to account for the slightly forward body position that occurs during upright stance. Order of body orientation was randomized so that half the participants began UPRIGHT while the other half began SUPINE.

Participants were asked to reach and place the tip of a handheld pen just in front of the REAL target or remembered target location, thus receiving no tactile feedback of endpoint locations. A trial would proceed as follows. Prior to movement, a participant would anchor their gaze on a presented target for approximately 2 s. After a "ready", pause (~1 s), "go" signal, participants were instructed to make a single reaching movement to an actual target (REAL) or remembered target location at a comfortable pace and hold that position for 1-2 s until given a "relax" signal. They were instructed to look at the REAL target or its remembered location throughout the trial. Movements in remembered target trials occurred in normal room lighting (LIGHT) or complete darkness (DARK). Targets were removed from sight manually for LIGHT and DARK remembered target trials. Participants were unaware of when the DARK trials would occur as the "ready" signal cued not only target removal by an investigator but also lights-out so the participants did not observe target removal or their movement in this condition.

Participants performed about 5 practice trials to acquaint themselves with the protocol before performing 54 reaching movements (6 trials for REAL, LIGHT, and DARK visual conditions at shoulder, shoulder+30, and shoulder-30 target levels for SUPINE and UPRIGHT body orientations). Trial order was organized in 3 groups. Two trials for each visual condition for each target level were randomized within a group. Data were collected in 2-minute intervals with at least 1 minute of rest between intervals. Trials were repeated when participants did not follow directions (i.e. made obvious movement corrections, moved before the "go" signal, or touched the target in REAL trials). Extra trials were randomly presented and performed in cases when all planned and repeated trials were completed and time was left in the 2 minute data collection interval and used to replace substandard trials obtained during collection (i.e., those in which markers were blocked or obvious extra movement occurred that were not observed during data collection).

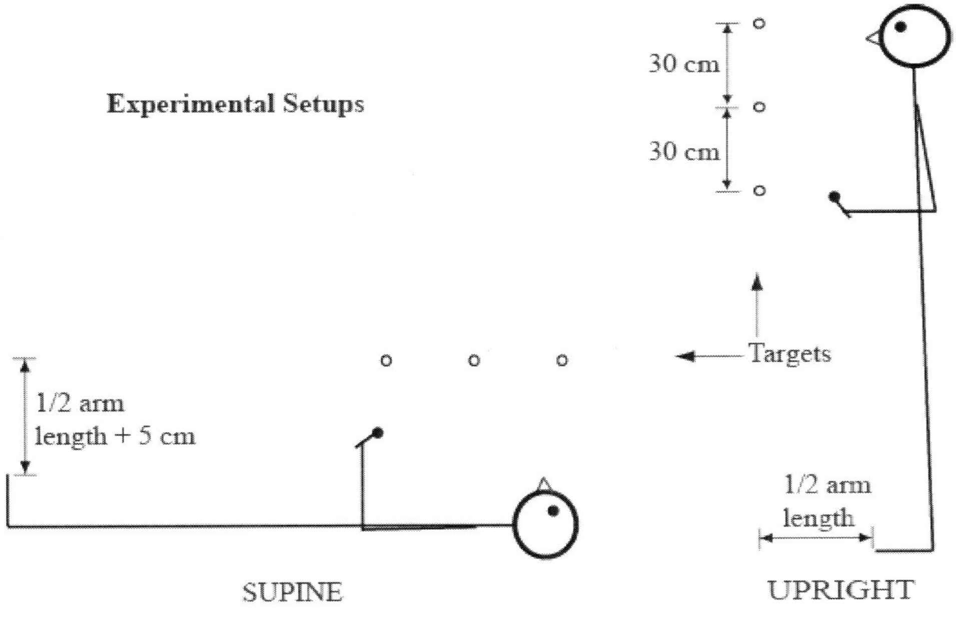

Figure 4. The experimental setups for SUPINE and URIGHT body orientations are shown. Stick figures approximate starting position prior to reaches. The padded table is not shown for the supine orientation.

A 2nd order lowpass Butterworth filter with a 6 Hz cutoff frequency was used to filter position data of each marker. The pen tip position data were differentiated with respect to time to obtain movement velocity. Plots of trial velocity data with a line representing 5% of peak pen tip velocity allowed for manual identification of the frames at movement onset and end similar to previous work (Gaveau and Papaxanthis, 2011). Start and endpoint values correspond to average of five frames of data just prior to movement onset and after movement end, respectively. The primary variable of interest was linked to endpoint accuracy. Endpoint errors corresponded to errors along the gravitational or external z-axis, of the pen tip marker. Each trial error for LIGHT and DARK visual conditions was calculated relative to the mean values of REAL trials for a given target, visual condition, body orientation, and participant. Note that endpoint error for a remembered trial equaled the final trial z-value minus the final mean REAL z-value. Positive errors represented final endpoints that were more superior than the average location of REAL endpoints in the UPRIGHT body orientation and more anterior than the average REAL endpoints in the SUPINE body orientation. Errors in the x- and y-directions were also determined using similar methods and used to describe final endpoint precision. Secondary variables were determined to offer insight to reaching movements. Displacement (DISPL) was calculated as the 3D distance between pen tip marker at movement start and end. Movement time (MT) was determined as the number of frames between movement start and end divided by the data collection frequency of 60 Hz. Peak velocity (PV) was determined as the maximum tangential velocity during movement of a given trial.

Average values and standard deviations of each variable for each person, visual condition (VIS = DARK, LIGHT), and body orientation (ORIENT = SUPINE, UPRIGHT) were calculated. Data were analyzed using a 2 x 2 repeated measures ANOVA test to determine whether each variable differed according to VIS, ORIENT, or a VIS x ORIENT interaction. Tukey's HSD test was used when appropriate. Significance level was set at $\alpha = 0.05$. Partial eta squared was used to report effect size (ES). Correlations of endpoint errors and displacement with PV and MT for trials across and within participants were determined using Pearson's R to offer potential insight to movement control strategies for goal-directed movements.

Results

Figure 5 shows the final reaching position of the arm and pen tip assemblies for one participant after reaching to remembered target locations. Only pen tip data are shown for reaching to REAL target locations. Note that regardless of body orientation final reaches to remembered target locations could end above or below final reaches to REAL target locations and final pen tip locations for DARK trials often ended more inferior than final pen tip locations for LIGHT trials. Analyses for endpoint errors across all participants support these latter observations.

The main effect of VIS on endpoint error ($F(1,9) = 44.91$, $p < 0.0001$; ES = 0.83) revealed that participants had more positive mean endpoint errors in LIGHT than in DARK conditions (Figure 6A). Interestingly, error bias was smallest for the DARK condition (i.e., means close to 0) to suggest that overall participants were more accurate when reaching in the DARK than in the LIGHT. Although some participants produced greater scatter in their endpoint errors when reaching to certain remembered target locations in the dark (see shoulder and shoulder-30 target levels for UPRIGHT conditions, Figure 5), analyses on variable errors across participants did not reveal significant outcomes ($p > 0.05$).

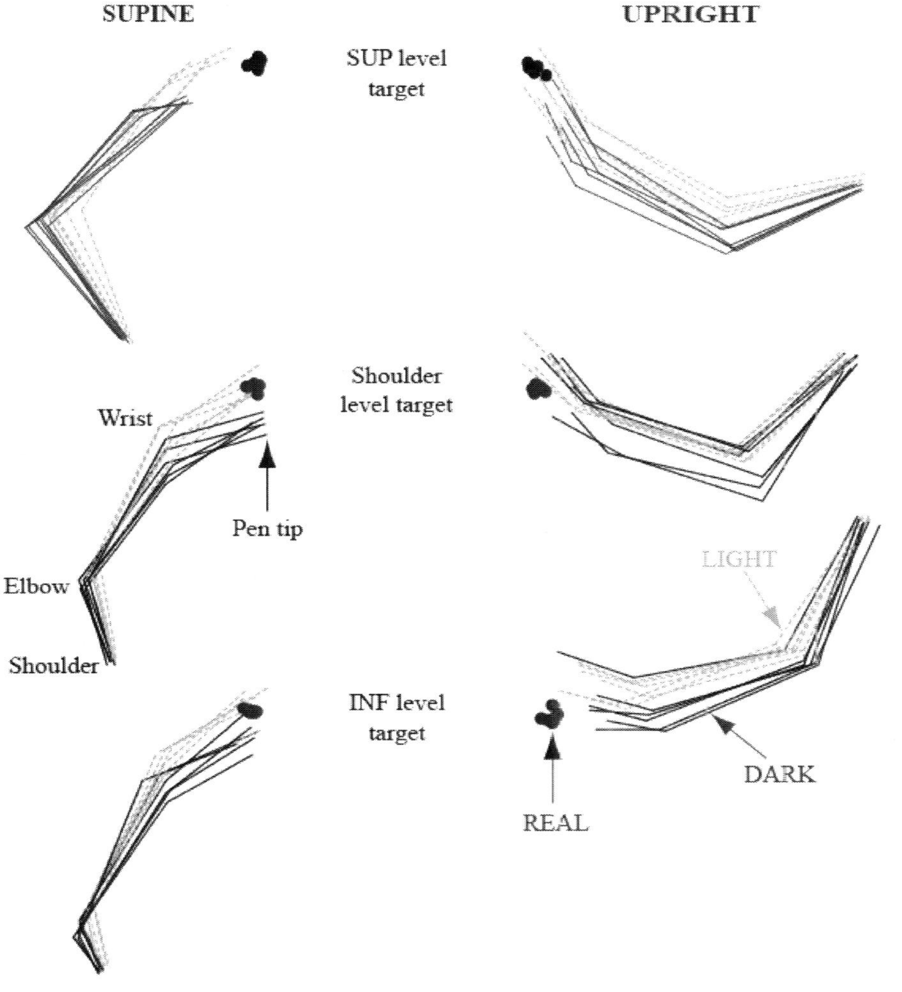

Figure 5. Plots represent final reach locations for all trials from one right handed participant. Filled black circles represent final pen tip locations for REAL trials. Final arm stick figures of the shoulder, elbow, wrist, and pen tip are shown for LIGHT (dashed gray lines) and DARK (solid black lines) visual conditions after reaching. Plots for the SUPINE body orientation are plotted from an inferior view (left panels), while plots for the UPRIGHT body orientation are plotted from a medial view (right panels) for each target level.

Errors for directions orthogonal to the earth fixed vertical were also determined to offer insight to final endpoint locations in 3D for each body orientation. Figure 7 shows the mean endpoint errors in each direction for each visual condition for all subjects. Data are plotted relative to mean reaches to REAL target locations and show that in addition to reaching higher (more anterior for SUPINE and more superior for UPRIGHT), participants also ended reaches about 1 cm to the left regardless of body orientations. They also reached about 2 cm more inferior when SUPINE and 0.6 cm more anterior in the LIGHT and 0.3 cm more posterior in the DARK when UPRIGHT. Plots show that the largest standard deviations were along the direction of target placement (posterior-anterior for SUPINE and superior-inferior for UPRIGHT).

Main effects of VIS were also observed for DISPL ($F(1,9) = 38.99$, $p < 0.001$; ES = 0.76), MT ($F(1,9) = 9.53$, $p < 0.05$; ES = 0.51), as well as variability of DISPL ($F(1,9) = 8.79$, $p < 0.05$; ES = 0.49) and PV ($F(1,9) = 6.50$, $p < 0.05$; ES = 0.42). On average participants produced greater excursions (Figure 5B), yet took a less time (Figure 5C) to produce their reaches in the LIGHT when compared to the DARK condition. Variability of DISPL and PV were also greater for reaches produced in the LIGHT relative to the DARK (data not shown).

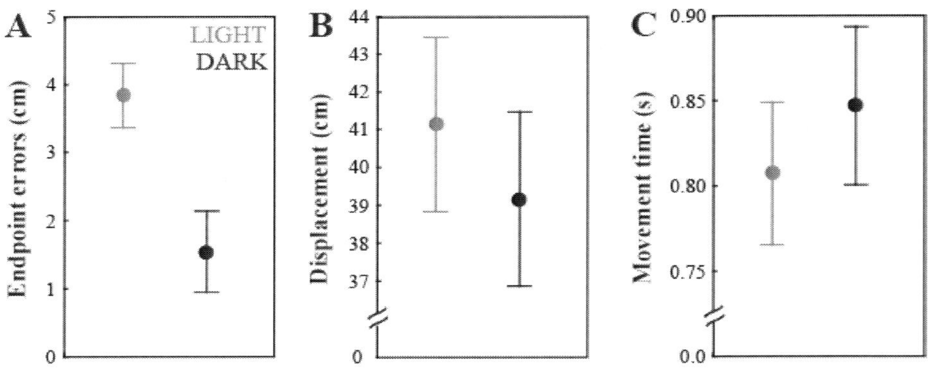

Figure 6. Plots represent the main effect of VIS on endpoint errors (A), displacement (B), and Movement time (C). Mean values ± 1 standard error are shown for LIGHT (gray) and DARK (black) visual conditions.

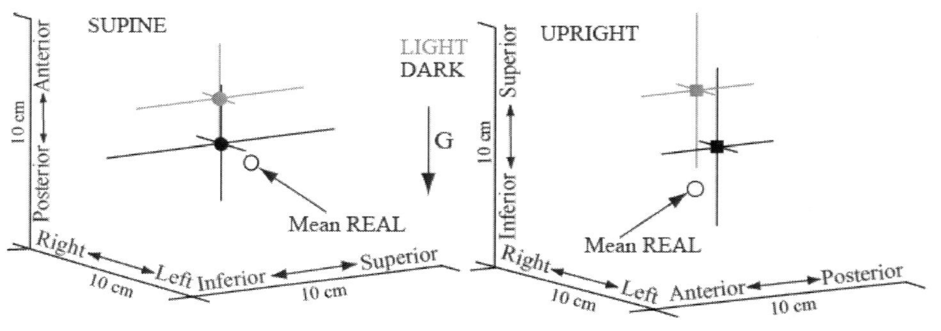

Figure 7. Plots represent final endpoint errors in each dimension in LIGHT (gray) and DARK (black) conditions for SUPRINE (left) and UPRIGHT (right) body orientations. Filled symbols represent systematic errors and line segments represent ±1 standard deviation for each dimension. Open circles represent mean locations of final reaches in the REAL condition.

Analyses revealed main effects of ORIENT on MT ($F(1,9) = 7.12$, $p < 0.05$; ES = 0.44), PV ($F(1,9) = 5.14$, $p < 0.05$; ES = 0.36), and the variability of DISPL ($F(1,9) = 12.06$, $p < 0.01$; ES = 0.57) and PV ($F(1,9) = 19.46$, $p < 0.005$; ES = 0.68). Mean MT was longer in SUPINE (0.86 s) than UPRIGHT (0.79 s) body orientations and corresponded to greater PV in UPRIGHT (115.8 cm/s) than SUPINE (97.2 cm/s) body orientations. Greater variability in DISPL and PV was also observed for SUPINE than UPRIGHT body orientations (data not shown). Analyses indicated no significant interaction effects for the given variables.

Correlations between each planned variable pair for LIGHT trials and DARK trials yielded several significant associations across participants (Table 1). For most target levels significant correlations between error and DISPL, DISPL and PV, and DISPL and MT across participants were observed. Within subject comparisons indicated that the positive association for error and DISPL across subjects was only true for half the participants when reaching to the shoulder level target in the LIGHT. In this case participants produced more positive errors for greater movement excursions. Positive correlations for DISPL and PV were most consistent for across and within subject analyses and reveal that participants moved at faster peak speeds for greater movement excursions. The significant negative correlations between DISPL and MT across subjects indicate that the participants who produced greater movement excursions did so in a shorter duration. The remaining significant across subject correlations were not consistent across targets, within visual conditions, or within participants.

Discussion

This experiment was designed to explore the dark phenomenon of reaching lower along a vertical axis in darkness compared to an illuminated environment. The experiment offered the first step to better understand the phenomenon for 3D reaching movements. No tactile feedback was provided to participants in the current study who were asked to reach to remembered 3D target locations from upright and supine body orientations in illuminated and dark environments.

Table 1. Correlation Results

Visual Condition	Target Level	Error DISPL	Error PV	Error MT	DISPL PV	DISPL MT
LIGHT	Shoulder+30	0.27$^{(0)}$	ns	0.29$^{(2)}$	**0.79$^{(8)}$**	-0.31$^{(2)}$
	Shoulder	**0.33$^{(5)}$**	ns	ns	**0.88$^{(6)}$**	-0.33$^{(0)}$
	Shoulder-30	ns	ns	ns	**0.85$^{(8)}$**	-0.29$^{(2)}$
DARK	Shoulder+30	0.39$^{(0)}$	0.32$^{(1)}$	ns	**0.82$^{(8)}$**	-0.34$^{(2)}$
	Shoulder	0.44$^{(3)}$	0.23$^{(3)}$	ns	**0.84$^{(8)}$**	-0.34$^{(0)}$
	Shoulder-30	0.27$^{(4)}$	ns	ns	**0.81$^{(7)}$**	-0.29$^{(2)}$

r-values are provided in cases where significant correlations ($p < 0.05$) were observed for the given comparisons across participants. The number in parentheses indicates the number of individual participants with corresponding significant correlations. Bold text indicates significant correlations for at least half the participants.

Note: DISPL=displacement; PV=peak velocity; MT=movement time; ns=not significant.

Reaching from a supine body orientation is less practiced than reaches performed while upright. Reaches associated with lying supine took longer to perform, achieved smaller peak velocities, and resulted in greater variability in displacement and peak velocity than those made while upright. These outcomes resemble those of performance of a simple novel task in which people complete the task slower during initial practice (Gottlieb, Corcos, Jaric, and Agarwal, 1988). The less practiced task of reaching while supine produced differences from the more practiced task of reaching while upright, yet effects of visual condition on the different variables did not differ by body orientation.

Participants reaching in complete darkness vertically undershot, thus ended lower than, endpoints in an illuminated environment. The present results correspond with the dark phenomenon outcomes that exists for upright participants (Adamovich et al., 1998; Admiraal et al., 2003, 2004; Berkinblit et al., 1995; Crawford et al., 2000; Flanders et al., 1999; Henriques and Crawford, 2000; Henriques et al., 1998; Hondzinski and Cui, 2006; Smetanin and Popov, 1997; Soechting and Flanders, 1989b; Wnuczko and Kennedy, 2011) and expand upon previous outcomes for participants reaching in one (Brown et al., 1948) and two (Smetanin and Popov, 1997) dimensions. The vertical undershooting in the present work did not correspond to vertical undershooting of visually remembered target locations (Adamovich et al., 1998; Berkinblit et al., 1995; Crawford et al., 2000; Henriques and Crawford, 2000; Henriques et al., 1998) or kinesthetically remembered target locations (Adamovich et al., 1998; Adamovich, Berkinblit, Fookson, and Poizner, 1999). On average participants reaching in the dark vertically overshot, thus reached slightly higher than, remembered target location along the vertical axis (Figure 6A). Interestingly, participants ended reaches higher still in the LIGHT condition, vertically overshooting remembered target locations twice as far as in the DARK. Higher reaches in an illuminated environment usually occur for reaches to lower level remembered target locations for participants who step forward while reaching (Flanders et al., 1999; Hondzinski and Cui, 2006). Undoubtedly the use of allocentric inputs for online control of goal-directed movements do not have to improve endpoint accuracy bias for reaching to remembered target locations along the vertical as observed elsewhere (Berkinblit et al., 1995; Hondzinski and Cui, 2006).

Ordinarily displacements closely match endpoint errors. The differences in vertical error bias parallel 3D movement excursions as indicated by mean displacement outcomes. The smaller displacements in the DARK relative to the LIGHT conditions indicate shorter movement excursions in darkness and correspond to shorter upward movement excursions in the dark when estimating relatively long distances on a vertical slide (Brown et al., 1948). Significant positive across subject correlations between 3D displacements and endpoint errors for most target levels in LIGHT and DARK conditions indicate an overall tendency for errors to increase with longer movement excursions for each target level and visual condition. However, this trend was not consistent within subjects and can be explained by the greater displacement variability between visual conditions that was not observed for vertical endpoint variability. Two explanations for differences between displacement variability and endpoint variability include: (1) having participants approximate their starting hand position may have increased start position variability and could explain greater variability in displacement and not endpoint errors and (2) comparing 3D displacements to one-dimensional errors could also account for these differences. Follow-up testing using repeated measures ANOVAs to determine VIS and ORIENT effects on vertical displacements and start position z-values revealed no significant effects on the variability of vertical displacements or start position z-values ($P > 0.05$). Thus starting hand position was not to blame for difference between variability in 3D displacement and endpoint errors. Therefore, the greater variability in 3D displacement resulted from displacement alterations along dimensions orthogonal to vertical.

The larger movement excursions and greater vertical overshooting of remembered target locations observed in the LIGHT condition took less time to complete than the shorter movement excursions identified in the DARK (Figures 5B and 5C). Although the temptation to use the speed-accuracy trade-off to explain the greater accuracy in the DARK condition exists, correlations results across and within subjects show few significant associations of endpoint errors with PV and MT to support this statement. These data support previous results that show movements with longer durations do not always increase endpoint accuracy in illuminated environments (Hondzinski et al., 2010). However, the longer movement excursions associated with shorter movement durations and faster peak speeds (Table 1) suggest temporal influences on movement amplitudes (Fitts, 1954).

Gravitational influences on control of vertically directed arm trajectories with similar movement endpoints have been identified (Gentili et al., 2007), thus cannot be extrapolated to endpoint precision control.

Data from the present study expand upon results which indicated potential gravitational influences on endpoint accuracy for restricted movements which limit errors to less than three dimensions (Brown et al., 1948; Smetanin and Popov, 1997). Ending below the remembered reach location in an illuminated environment happened to fall along the gravitational vector to emphasize that the phenomenon of reaching lower in the dark occurs along the external earth-fixed axis and not the longitudinal body axis, making the directional pull of gravity a potential explanation for the lower endpoint error in the dark. However, the current results also revealed that participants frequently produce shorter movement excursions in darkness, confounding outcomes. Although the gravitational pull could have caused the shorter movement excursions for slow movements (Fisk, Lackner, and DiZio, 1993), the smaller movement excursions in the dark, which have been observed in other dimensions (Admiraal et al., 2003; Brown et al., 1948; Darling and Miller, 1993; Elliott and Hansen, 2010; Heath, 2005; Heath and Binsted, 2007; Soechting and Flanders, 1989b) may result from other influences, which are still unclear. Whether the CNS utilizes gravitational cues for endpoint precision to help explain differences in dark and illuminated environments remains to be tested, as potential influences of the gravitational pull and shorter movement excursions were not isolated in the current study.

Although the current data provide some evidence that gravitational influences may explain the dark phenomenon for 3D reaching movements, resolving this issue requires further examination. Future studies should include different body orientations and different starting hand positions. Asking inverted (upside down) participants to point to remembered target locations in DARK and LIGHT environments and having them start with the hand down by the side or up by the head allows for separation of gravitational influences and endpoint excursions. Endpoints in darkness terminating below those in an illuminated environment in all body orientations and arm start positions would offer support for gravitational influences on movement precision differences between visual conditions. This would correspond to more inferior errors when pointing while upright and more superior errors when pointing while inverted.

Errors which correspond to shorter movement amplitudes regardless of body orientation or starting hand position would eliminate gravitational influences as an explanation for the dark phenomenon. Data from our laboratory provide evidence for shorter movement excursions that in some case are definitely not influenced by pull the gravity (Soebbing, 2014). However, causes for shorter movement excursions warrant further investigation.

References

Adamovich, S. V., Berkinblit, M. B., Fookson, O., and Poizner, H. (1998). Pointing in 3D space to remembered targets. I. Kinesthetic versus visual target presentation. *Journal of Neurophysiology,* 79(6), 2833-2846.

Adamovich, S. V., Berkinblit, M. B., Fookson, O., and Poizner, H. (1999). Pointing in 3D space to remembered targets. II. Effects of movement speed toward kinesthetically defined targets. *Experimental Brain Research,* 125(2), 200-210.

Admiraal, M. A., Keijsers, N. L. and Gielen, C. C. (2003). Interaction between gaze and pointing toward remembered visual targets *Journal of Neurophysiology,* 90(4), 2136-2148.

Admiraal, M. A., Keijsers, N. L. and Gielen, C. C. (2004). Gaze affects pointing toward remembered visual targets after a self-initiated step. *Journal of Neurophysiology,* 92(4), 2380-2393.

Ando, S., Kida, N. and Oda, S. (2001). Central and peripheral visual reaction time of soccer players and nonathletes. *Perceptual and Motor Skills,* 92(3 Pt 1), 786-794. doi: 10.2466/pms.2001.92.3.786.

Ando, S., Kida, N. and Oda, S. (2002). Practice effects on reaction time for peripheral and central visual fields. *Perceptual and Motor Skills,* 95(3 Pt 1), 747-751.

Ando, S., Kida, N. and Oda, S. (2004). Retention of practice effects on simple reaction time for peripheral and central visual fields. *Perceptual and Motor Skills,* 98(3 Pt 1), 897-900.

Ando, S., Kokubu, M., Kida, N., and Oda, S. (2002). Attention can be oriented to intermediate locations within the large area of the visual field. *Perceptual and Motor Skills,* 95(3 Pt 1), 806-812. doi: 10.2466/pms.2002.95.3.806.

Armer, M. C., Nilaweera, W. U., Rivers, T. J., Dasgupta, N. M., and Beloozerova, I. N. (2013). Effect of light on the activity of motor cortex neurons during locomotion. *Behavioural Brain Research,* 250, 238-250. doi: 10.1016/j.bbr.2013.05.004.

Barash, S., Melikyan, A., Sivakov, A., and Tauber, M. (1998). Shift of visual fixation dependent on background illumination. *Journal of Neurophysiology,* 79(5), 2766-2781.

Berkinblit, M. B., Fookson, O. I., Smetanin, B., Adamovich, S. V., and Poizner, H. (1995). The interaction of visual and proprioceptive inputs in pointing to actual and remembered targets. *Experimental Brain Research,* 107(2), 326-330.

Berret, B., Bonnetblanc, F., Papaxanthis, C., and Pozzo, T. (2009). Modular control of pointing beyond arm's length. *Journal of Neuroscience,* 29(1), 191-205. doi: 10.1523/JNEUROSCI.3426-08.2009.

Beurze, S. M., Van Pelt, S. and Medendorp, W. P. (2006). Behavioral reference frames for planning human reaching movements. *Journal of Neurophysiology,* 96(1), 352-362. doi: 10.1152/jn.01362.2005.

Black, A., Lovie-Kitchin, J. E., Woods, R. L., Arnold, N., Byrnes, J., and Murrish, J. (1997). Mobility performance with retinitis pigmentosa. *Clinical and Experimental Optometry,* 80(1), 1-12.

Black, F. O. and Nashner, L. M. (1984). Postural disturbance in patients with benign paroxysmal positional nystagmus. *Annals of Otology, Rhinology, and Laryngology,* 93(6 Pt 1), 595-599.

Bock, O. (1986). Contribution of retinal versus extraretinal signals towards visual localization in goal-directed movements. *Experimental Brain Research,* 64(3), 476-482.

Bock, O. and Arnold, K. (1993). Error accumulation and error correction in sequential pointing movements. *Experimental Brain Research,* 95(1), 111-117.

Bock, O. and Eckmiller, R. (1986). Goal-directed arm movements in absence of visual guidance: evidence for amplitude rather than position control. *Experimental Brain Research,* 62(3), 451-458.

Bouisset, S. and Zattara, M. (1981). A sequence of postural movements precedes voluntary movement. *Neuroscience Letters,* 22(3), 263-270.

Bouisset, S. and Zattara, M. (1987). A sequence of postural adjustments precedes voluntary movement. *Neuroscience Letters,* 22, 263-270.

Bridgeman, B., Kirch, M. and Sperling, A. (1981). Segregation of cognitive and motor aspects of visual function using induced motion. *Perception & Psychophysics,* 29(4), 336-342.

Bridgeman, B. and Stark, L. (1991). Ocular proprioception and efference copy in registering visual direction. *Vision Research,* 31(11), 1903-1913.

Brown, J. S., Knauft, E. B. and Rosenbaum, G. (1948). The accuracy of positioning reactions as a function of their direction and extent. *American Journal of Psychology,* 61(2), 167-182.

Carrozzo, M., Stratta, F., McIntyre, J., and Lacquaniti, F. (2002). Cognitive allocentric representations of visual space shape pointing errors. *Experimental Brain Research,* 147 (4), 426-436.

Chua, R. and Elliott, D. (1993). Visual regulation of manual aiming. *Human Movement Science,* 12, 365-401.

Clement, G., Gurfinkel, V. S., Lestienne, F., Lipshits, M. I., and Popov, K. E. (1984). Adaptation of postural control to weightlessness. *Experimental Brain Research,* 57(1), 61-72.

Coello, Y. and Iwanow, O. (2006). Effect of structuring the workspace on cognitive and sensorimotor distance estimation: no dissociation between perception and action. *Perception & Psychophysics,* 68(2), 278-289.

Collins, J. J. and De Luca, C. J. (1995). The effects of visual input on open-loop and closed-loop postural control mechanisms. *Experimental Brain Research,* 103(1), 151-163.

Cordo, P. J. and Nashner, L. M. (1982). Properties of postural adjustments associated with rapid arm movements. *Journal of Neurophysiology,* 47(2), 287-302.

Crawford, J. D., Henriques, D. Y. and Vilis, T. (2000). Curvature of visual space under vertical eye rotation: implications for spatial vision and visuomotor control. *The Journal of Neuroscience,* 20(6), 2360-2368.

Cruikshank, L. C., Caplan, J. B. and Singhal, A. (2012). Human electrophysiological reflections of the recruitment of perceptual processing during actions that engage memory. *Journal of Vision,* 12(6). doi: 10.1167/12.6.29.

Cruikshank, L. C., Caplan, J. B. and Singhal, A. (2014). A perception-based ERP reveals that the magnitude of delay matters for memory-guided reaching. *Experimental Brain Research,* 232(7), 2087-2094. doi: 10.1007/s00221-014-3897-x.

Curcio, C. A., Sloan, K. R., Kalina, R. E., and Hendrickson, A. E. (1990). Human photoreceptor topography. *Journal of Comparative Neurology,* 292(4), 497-523. doi: 10.1002/cne.9029204 02.

Daghestani, L., Anderson, J. H. and Flanders, M. (2000). Coordination of a step with a reach. *Journal of Vestibular Research: Equilibrium & Orientation,* 10(2), 59-73.

Darling, W. G. and Miller, G. F. (1993). Transformations between visual and kinesthetic coordinate systems in reaches to remembered object locations and orientations. *Experimental Brain Research,* 93(3), 534-547.

Desmurget, M., Pelisson, D., Rossetti, Y., and Prablanc, C. (1998). From eye to hand: planning goal-directed movements. *Neuroscience & Biobehavioral Reviews,* 22(6), 761-788.

Dessing, J. C., Oostwoud Wijdenes, L., Peper, C. E., and Beek, P. J. (2009). Visuomotor transformation for interception: catching while fixating. *Experimental Brain Research,* 196(4), 511-527. doi: 10.1007/s00221-009-1882-6.

Elliott, D. and Hansen, S. (2010). Visual regulation of manual aiming: a comparison of methods. *Behavior Research Methods,* 42(4), 1087-1095. doi: 10.3758/BRM.42.4.1087.

Elliott, D. and Madalena, J. (1987). The influence of premovement visual information on manual aiming. *The Quarterly Journal of Experimental Psychololgy A,* 39(3), 541-559.

Engel, K. C., Anderson, J. H., Gomez, C. M., and Soechting, J. F. (2004). Deficits in ocular and manual tracking due to episodic ataxia type 2. *Movement Disorders,* 19(7), 778-787.

Engel, K. C., Anderson, J. H. and Soechting, J. F. (2000). Similarity in the response of smooth pursuit and manual tracking to a change in the direction of target motion. *Journal of Neurophysiology* 84(3), 1149-1156.

Engel, K. C. and Soechting, J. F. (2003). Interactions between ocular motor and manual responses during two-dimensional tracking. *Progress in Brain Research,* 142, 141-153.

Enright, J. T. (1995). The non-visual impact of eye orientation on eye-hand coordination. *Vision Research,* 35(11), 1611-1618.

Favilla, M., Gordon, J., Hening, W., and Ghez, G. (1990). Trajectory control in targeted force impulses. VII. Independent setting of amplitude and direction in response preparation. *Experimental Brain Research,* 79, 530-538.

Fawzi, A. A., Lee, N., Acton, J. H., Laine, A. F., and Smith, R. T. (2011). Recovery of macular pigment spectrum in vivo using hyperspectral image analysis. *Journal of Biomedical Optics,* 16(10), 106008. doi: 10.1117/1.3640813.

Fisk, J., Lackner, J. R. and DiZio, P. (1993). Gravitoinertial force level influences arm movement control. *Journal of Neurophysiology,* 69(2), 504-511.

Fitts, P. M. (1954). The information capacity of the human motor control system in controlling the amplitude of movements. *Journal of Experimental Psychology,* 47, 381-391.

Flanders, M., Daghestani, L. and Berthoz, A. (1999). Reaching beyond reach. *Experimental Brain Research,* 126(1), 19-30.

Foley, J. (1978). Vestibulogenic imbalance. *British Medical Journal,* 1(6122), 1244-1246.

Friedli, W. G., Hallett, M. and Simon, S. R. (1984). Postural adjustments associated with rapid voluntary arm movements 1. Electromyographic data. *Journal of Neurology, Neurosurgery, and Psychiatry,* 47(6), 611-622.

Gantchev, G. N. and Dimitrova, D. M. (1996). Anticipatory postural adjustments associated with arm movements during balancing on unstable support surface. *International Journal of Psychophysiology,* 22(1-2), 117-122.

Gaveau, J. and Papaxanthis, C. (2011). The temporal structure of vertical arm movements. *PLoS One,* 6(7), e22045. doi: 10.1371/journal.pone.0022045.

Gentili, R., Cahouet, V. and Papaxanthis, C. (2007). Motor planning of arm movements is direction-dependent in the gravity field. *Neuroscience,* 145(1), 20-32. doi: 10.1016/j.neuroscience.2006.11.035.

Glover, S. (2004). Separate visual representations in the planning and control of action. *Behavioral and Brain Sciences,* 27(1), 3-24; discussion 24-78.

Gottlieb, G. L., Corcos, D. M., Jaric, S., and Agarwal, G. C. (1988). Practice improves even the simplest movements. *Experimental Brain Research,* 73(2), 436-440.

Hadjikhani, N. and Tootell, R. B. (2000). Projection of rods and cones within human visual cortex. *Human Brain Mapping,* 9(1), 55-63.

Harb, E., Hyman, L., Fazzari, M., Gwiazda, J., Marsh-Tootle, W., and Group, C. S. (2012). Factors associated with macular thickness in the COMET myopic cohort. *Optometry and Vision Science,* 89(5), 620-631. doi: 10.1097/OPX.0b013e318251293a.

Harrington, D. O. (1964). *The visual field.* St. Louis, MO: The C. V. Mosby Company.

Heath, M. (2005). Role of limb and target vision in the online control of memory-guided reaches. *Motor Control,* 9(3), 281-311.

Heath, M. and Binsted, G. (2007). Visuomotor memory for target location in near and far reaching spaces. *Journal of Motor Behavior,* 39(3), 169-177. doi: 10.3200/JMBR.39.3.169-178.

Heath, M. and Westwood, D. A. (2003). Can a visual representation support the online control of memory-dependent reaching? Evident from a variable spatial mapping paradigm. *Motor Control,* 7(4), 346-361.

Heath, M., Westwood, D. A. and Binsted, G. (2004). The control of memory-guided reaching movements in peripersonal space. *Motor Control,* 8(1), 76-106.

Hening, W., Favilla, M. and Ghez, C. (1988). Trajectory control in targeted force impulses V. Gradual specification of response amplitude. *Experimental Brain Research,* 71, 116-128.

Henriques, D. Y. and Crawford, J. D. (2000). Direction-dependent distortions of retinocentric space in the visuomotor transformation for pointing. *Experimental Brain Research,* 132(2), 179-194.

Henriques, D. Y. and Crawford, J. D. (2002). Role of eye, head, and shoulder geometry in the planning of accurate arm movements. *Journal of Neurophysiology,* 87(4), 1677-1685.

Henriques, D. Y., Klier, E. M., Smith, M. A., Lowy, D., and Crawford, J. D. (1998). Gaze-centered remapping of remembered visual space in an open-loop pointing task. *The Journal of Neuroscience,* 18(4), 1583-1594.

Henriques, D. Y., Medendorp, W. P., Gielen, C. C., and Crawford, J. D. (2003). Geometric computations underlying eye-hand coordination: orientations of the two eyes and the head. *Experimental Brain Research,* 152(1), 70-78. doi: 10.1007/s00221-003-1523-4.

Hodges, P. W. and Richardson, C. A. (1997). Feedforward contraction of transversus abdominis is not influenced by the direction of arm movement. *Experimental Brain Research,* 114(2), 362-370.

Hondzinski, J. M. (2004). Comparing human reaches across three viewing conditions in a step and reach task. *Neuroscience Letters,* 357(1), 25-28.

Hondzinski, J. M. and Cui, Y. (2006). Allocentric cues do not always improve whole body reaching performance. *Experimental Brain Research,* 174(1), 60-73. doi: 10.1007/s00221-006-0421-y.

Hondzinski, J. M. and Kwon, T. (2009). Pointing control using a moving base of support. *Experimental Brain Research,* 197(1), 81-90. doi: 10.1007/s00221-009-1893-3.

Hondzinski, J. M., Li, L. and Welsch, M. (2010). Age-related and sensory declines offer insight to whole body control during a goal-directed movement. *Motor Control,* 14, 176-194.

Hood, D. C., Nguyen, M., Ehrlich, A. C., Raza, A. S., Sliesoraityte, I., De Moraes, C. G., ... Schiefer, U. (2014). A test of a model of glaucomatous damage of the macula with high-density perimetry: Implications for the locations of visual field test points. *Translational Vision Science and Technology,* 3(3), 5. doi: 10.1167/tvst.3.3.5.

Jeka, J., Oie, K. S. and Kiemel, T. (2000). Multisensory information for human postural control: integrating touch and vision. *Experimental Brain Research,* 134(1), 107-125.

Jonas, J. B., Schneider, U. and Naumann, G. O. (1992). Count and density of human retinal photoreceptors. *Graefes Archive for Clinical and Experimental Ophthalmology,* 230(6), 505-510.

Keele, S. W. and Posner, M. I. (1968). Processing of visual feedback in rapid movements. *Journal of Experimental Psychology,* 77(1), 155-158.

Kwon, M., Ramachandra, C., Satgunam, P., Mel, B. W., Peli, E., and Tjan, B. S. (2012). Contour enhancement benefits older adults with simulated central field loss. *Optometry and Vision Science,* 89(9), 1374-1384. doi: 10.1097/OPX.0b013e3182678e52.

Kwon, T. Y. and Hondzinski, J. M. (2010). *The influence of target eccentricity on ipsilateral and contralateral responses.* Paper presented at the 40th Society for Neuroscience Annual Meeting, San Diego.

Legge, G. E., Rubin, G. S., Pelli, D. G., and Schleske, M. M. (1985). Psychophysics of reading--II. Low vision. *Vision Research,* 25(2), 253-265.

Magill, R. A. (2004). *Motor learning: Concepts and applications* (6th ed.). Boston: McGraw Hill.

McGuire, L. M. and Sabes, P. N. (2009). Sensory transformations and the use of multiple reference frames for reach planning. *Nature Neuroscience,* 12(8), 1056-1061. doi: 10.1038/nn. 2357.

McIntyre, J., Stratta, F. and Lacquaniti, F. (1997). Viewer-centered frame of reference for pointing to memorized targets in three-dimensional space. *Journal of Neurophysiology,* 78(3), 1601-1618.

McIntyre, J., Stratta, F. and Lacquaniti, F. (1998). Short-term memory for reaching to visual targets: psychophysical evidence for body-centered reference frames. *The Journal of Neuroscience,* 18 (20), 8423-8435.

Naito, E. and Ehrsson, H. H. (2001). Kinesthetic illusion of wrist movement activates motor-related areas. *Neuroreport,* 12(17), 3805-3809.

Niechwiej-Szwedo, E., McIlroy, W. E., Green, R., and Verrier, M. C. (2005). The effect of directional compatibility on the response latencies of ocular and manual movements. *Experimental Brain Research,* 162(2), 220-229. doi: 10.1007/s00221-004-2146-0.

Owsley, C. and McGwin, G., Jr. (1999). Vision impairment and driving. *Survey of Ophthalmology,* 43(6), 535-550.

Papaxanthis, C., Pozzo, T. and Schieppati, M. (2003). Trajectories of arm pointing movements on the sagittal plane vary with both direction and speed. *Experimental Brain Research,* 148(4), 498-503. doi: 10.1007/s00221-002-1327-y.

Payne, W. H. (1966). Reaction time as a function of retinal location. *Vision Research,* 6(12), 729-732.

Pierrot-Deseilligny, C., Muri, R. M., Rivaud-Pechoux, S., Gaymard, B., and Ploner, C. J. (2002). Cortical control of spatial memory in humans: the visuooculomotor model. *Annals of Neurology,* 52(1), 10-19. doi: 10.1002/ana.10273.

Poggel, D. A. and Strasburger, H. (2004). Visual perception in space and time--mapping the visual field of temporal resolution. *Acta Neurobiologiae Experimentalis*, 64(3), 427-437.

Pouget, A., Ducom, J. C., Torri, J., and Bavelier, D. (2002). Multisensory spatial representations in eye-centered coordinates for reaching. *Cognition,* 83(1), B1-11.

Pozzo, T., Stapley, P. J. and Papaxanthis, C. (2002). Coordination between equilibrium and hand trajectories during whole body pointing movements. *Experimental Brain Research,* 144(3), 343-350.

Prablanc, C., Echallier, J. F., Komilis, E., and Jeannerod, M. (1979). Optimal response of eye and hand motor systems in pointing at a visual target. I. Spatio-temporal characteristics of eye and hand movements and their relationships when varying the amount of visual information. *Biological Cybernetics,* 35(2), 113-124.

Prablanc, C., Pelisson, D. and Goodale, M. A. (1986). Visual control of reaching movements without vision of the limb. I. Role of retinal feedback of target position in guiding the hand. *Experimental Brain Research,* 62(2), 293-302.

Proske, U. (2006). Kinesthesia: the role of muscle receptors. *Muscle & Nerve,* 34(5), 545-558. doi: 10.1002/mus.20627.

Provis, J. M., Dubis, A. M., Maddess, T., and Carroll, J. (2013). Adaptation of the central retina for high acuity vision: cones, the fovea and the avascular zone. *Progress in Retinal and Eye Research,* 35, 63-81. doi: 10.1016/j.preteyeres.2013.01.005.

Rains, J. D. (1963). Signal luminance and position effects in human reaction time. *Vision Research,* 61, 239-251.

Roll, R., Bard, C. and Paillard, J. (1986). Head orienting contributes to the directional accuracy of aiming at distant targets. *Human Movement Science,* 5(4), 359-371.

Sarlegna, F., Blouin, J., Vercher, J. L., Bresciani, J. P., Bourdin, C., and Gauthier, G. M. (2004). Online control of the direction of rapid reaching movements. *Experimental Brain Research,* 157(4), 468-471. doi: 10.1007/s00221-004-1860-y.

Sarlegna, F. R. and Blouin, J. (2010). Visual guidance of arm reaching: online adjustments of movement direction are impaired by amplitude control. *Journal of Vision,* 10(5), 24. doi: 10.1167/ 10.5.24.

Sekuler, R. and Blake, R. (Eds.). (1994). *Perception.* New York, NY: McGraw-Hill.

Sheth, B. R. and Shimojo, S. (2001). Compression of space in visual memory. *Vision Research,* 41 (3), 329-341.

Sivak, B. and MacKenzie, C. L. (1992). The contributions of peripheral vision and central vision to prehension. In: L. Proteau and D. Elliott (Eds.), *Vision and motor control* (pp. 233-259). Amsterdam, The Netherlands: North-Holland.

Smetanin, B. N. and Popov, K. E. (1997). Effect of body orientation with respect to gravity on directional accuracy of human pointing movements. *European Journal of Neuroscience,* 9(1), 7-11.

Soechting, J. F., Engel, K. C. and Flanders, M. (2001). The Duncker illusion and eye-hand coordination. *Journal of Neurophysiology,* 85(2), 843-854.

Soechting, J. F. and Flanders, M. (1989a). Errors in pointing are due to approximations in sensorimotor transformations. *Journal of Neurophysiology,* 62(2), 595-608.

Soechting, J. F. and Flanders, M. (1989b). Sensorimotor representations for pointing to targets in three-dimensional space. *Journal of Neurophysiology,* 62(2), 582-594.

Soebbing, C. M. (2014). *Can gravitational influences explain endpoint precision between visual conditions?* (Master of Science Master's), Louisiana State University. (etd-01172014-202130).

Teasdale, N. and Simoneau, M. (2001). Attentional demands for postural control: the effects of aging and sensory reintegration. *Gait & Posture,* 14(3), 203-210.

Westwood, D. A., Heath, M. and Roy, E. A. (2001). The accuracy of reaching movements in brief delay conditions. *Canadian Journal of Experimental Psychology,* 55(4), 304-310.

Westwood, D. A., Heath, M. and Roy, E. A. (2003). No evidence for accurate visuomotor memory: systematic and variable error in memory-guided reaching. *Journal of Motor Behavior,* 35 (2), 127-133. doi: 10.1080/00222890309602128.

Wnuczko, M. and Kennedy, J. M. (2011). Pivots for pointing: visually-monitored pointing has higher arm elevations than pointing blindfolded. *Journal of Experimental Psychology. Human Perception and Performance,* 37(5), 1485-1491. doi: 10.1037/a0024232.

Index

D

F

G

H

I

J

K

L

M

Q

R

S

T

U

V

W